Handbook of Clinical Toxicology

Handbook of Clinical Toxicology

Edited by Mary Durrant

hayle
medical

New York

Hayle Medical,
750 Third Avenue, 9th Floor,
New York, NY 10017, USA

Visit us on the World Wide Web at:
www.haylemedical.com

ISBN: 978-1-63241-540-0

Cataloging-in-Publication Data

Handbook of clinical toxicology / edited by Mary Durrant.
    p. cm.
Includes bibliographical references and index.
ISBN 978-1-63241-540-0
1. Clinical toxicology. 2. Toxicology. 3. Clinical medicine. I. Durrant, Mary.
RA1218.5 .H34 2019
615.9--dc23

Table of Contents

Preface

Over the recent decade, advancements and applications have progressed exponentially. This has led to the increased interest in this field and projects are being conducted to enhance knowledge. The main objective of this book is to present some of the critical challenges and provide insights into possible solutions. This book will answer the varied questions that arise in the field and also provide an increased scope for furthering studies.

Toxicology is the discipline that is concerned with the study of adverse reactions of chemical substances on living organisms. The three principal areas of toxicology are medical, clinical and computational toxicology. Clinical toxicology is concerned with the treatment of patients, who have been exposed to toxic substances. It is closely associated with medical toxicology. It is focused on diagnosis and prevention of poisoning and harmful effects caused by toxicants and biological agents. The assessment and treatment of drug overdoses, substance abuse, chemical exposures and industrial accidents are under this domain. This book aims to shed light on some of the unexplored aspects of clinical toxicology and the recent researches in this field. It provides significant information of this discipline to help develop a good understanding of clinical toxicology and related fields. With state-of-the-art inputs by acclaimed experts of this field, it targets students and professionals.

I hope that this book, with its visionary approach, will be a valuable addition and will promote interest among readers. Each of the authors has provided their extraordinary competence in their specific fields by providing different perspectives as they come from diverse nations and regions. I thank them for their contributions.

Editor

A Double-Blind, Placebo-Controlled, Parallel Study Evaluating the Safety of *Bacillus coagulans* MTCC 5856 in Healthy Individuals

Muhammed Majeed[1,2]**, Kalyanam Nagabhushanam**[2]**, Sankaran Natarajan**[1]**, Arumugam Sivakumar**[1]**, Anurag Pande**[2]**, Shaheen Majeed**[2,3] **and Furqan Ali**[1*]

[1]*Sami Labs Limited, 19/1 & 19/2, First Main, Second Phase, Peenya Industrial Area, Bangalore-560 058, Karnataka, India*

[2]*Sabinsa Corporation, 20 Lake Drive, East Windsor, NJ 08520*

[3]*Sabinsa Corporation, 750 Innovation Circle, Payson, UT 84651, USA*

*Corresponding author: Furqan Ali, Sami Labs Limited, 19/1, 19/2, First Main, Second Phase, Peenya Industrial Area, Bangalore-560 058, Karnataka, India, E-mail: furqan@samilabs.com

Abstract

Objective: LactoSpore® containing probiotic strain *Bacillus coagulans* MTCC 5856 has been marketed as a dietary ingredient for nearly two decades. Clinical data on the safety and tolerance has not been evaluated at a dose of 2×10^9 cfu (spores)/day in healthy individuals. Thus, the primary objective of this study was to investigate the safety and tolerability of *B. coagulans* MTCC 5856 in healthy adults.

Study design: A total of 40 participants were randomized into one of two groups in a double-blind, randomized, placebo-controlled parallel study. One group of participants (n=20) were administered *B. coagulans* MTCC 5856 (600 mg tablet), containing 2×10^9 cfu (spores). The control group (n=20) was administered placebo tablets. Safety and tolerability of *B. coagulans* MTCC 5856 was assessed over 30 days by safety laboratory parameters (blood hematology and clinical chemistry parameters), anthropometric measures (weight, BMI, blood pressure and heart rate), adverse events, Bristol stool score, tolerability questionnaire and bowel habit diary.

Results: All laboratory parameters, anthropometric and vital sign measures remained within normal clinical range during the 30 day supplementation. Similar adverse events (AE's) were reported by participants in both the placebo and the *B. coagulans* MTCC 5856 group. The number of bowel movements and the Bristol stool scores were similar between the placebo group and *B. coagulans* MTCC 5856 group during the 30 days of supplementation. Participants also reported that *B. coagulans* MTCC 5856 tablets were tolerable and easy to swallow.

Conclusions: This study has verified that *B. coagulans* MTCC 5856 at a dose of 2×10^9 cfu (spores)/day was safe and tolerable in healthy participants when supplemented for 30 days.

Keywords: *Bacillus coagulans* MTCC 5856; Gut microbiota; LactoSpore®; Probiotic; Safety; Tolerability

Introduction

Intestinal microbiota plays a crucial role in several metabolic processes such as the regulation of intestinal epithelial proliferation, gut maturation, colonization, and resistance and modulation of the intestinal immune response [1-4]. The intestinal metabolome is composed of different species of beneficial and pathogenic bacteria. Beneficial bacterial species have several crucial functions in the intestine; restraining potentially pathogenic or harmful bacteria, activating immune responses, aiding proper digestion and absorption of food and acting as a barrier against harmful bacteria and toxins [5]. More than 500 species of indigenous bacteria colonize the colon and play a crucial role in human health and disease. In healthy individuals, the gut microbiota act as an important modulator of the immune system and serve as a source of non-inflammatory immune stimulation [6]. Modern lifestyle factors such as a poor diet, frequent travel and food or water contaminants in combination with increasing age may disturb the delicate balance of intestinal bacteria. Furthermore, medications such as broad spectrum antibiotics are commonly prescribed to curb infection which unfortunately kills beneficial bacteria disrupting the balance between the non-pathogenic and pathogenic species [7].

Probiotics are microorganisms that when administered in adequate amount provide health benefit to the host organism [8]. They induce health benefits by altering the intestinal microecology, producing antimicrobial compounds, and stimulating the body's immune response. Preparations of *Bacillus coagulans* has been found to contain a large number of viable lactic acid bacilli that retain their viability during storage prior to consumption as the spores are thermostable, survive in gastric secretions, reach and settle in the intestine producing sufficient lactic acid and other antagonistic substances inhibiting the growth of pathogenic bacteria. In vitro and in vivo studies on oral toxicity attest to the safety of *B. coagulans* [9,10]. *B. coagulans* is a probiotic, well known for its clinical efficacy in several human conditions [9-14]. *B. coagulans* based products are efficacious in adults with post-prandial intestinal discomfort, improving their quality of life. A potential for its application in adults with irritable bowel syndrome (IBS) have shown promising results in this arena [11,12,14]. Researchers have also reported on the relationship between *B. coagulans* and the immune system [15,16]. It is a well-established fact that the health benefits and the safety of a probiotic strain is strain specific, and not the species or genus-specific. This was clearly indicated by the Joint Food and Agriculture Organization of the United Nations/World Health Organization and suggested to provide guidance to consumers or clinicians about the type and extent of safety assessments that have been conducted on the probiotic products [8]. Hence, it is a essential to verify the safety aspects of a probiotic strain.

LactoSpore* is a commercial proprietary probiotic preparation containing live spores of *Bacillus coagulans* MTCC 5856 (bearing internal reference number SBC37-01). It is a shelf stable, GRAS affirmed probiotic preparation which produces the beneficial L (+) form of lactic acid in the intestines and inhibits the growth of pathogenic bacteria [17]. Several preparations of *B. coagulans* in powder, tablet and capsule forms have been reported for the treatment of gastrointestinal disorders, vaginal infections, hypercholesterolemia, lactose intolerance, hepatic coma and as an adjuvant to antibiotic therapy in human clinical trials [17-20]. Spores of *B. coagulans* MTCC 5856 strain has the ability to withstand high temperature and reported to be stable during processing and storage of various functional foods [21]. It also reported that the *B. coagulans* MTCC 5856 did not alter either genetically or phenotypically and was found to be consistent over multiple years of commercial production [22]. Animal study revealed that *B. coagulans* MTCC 5856 elicited anti-diarrhoeal activity and inhibited the gastrointestinal motility in fasted rats [23]. However, clinical data on the safety and tolerability of *B. coagulans* MTCC 5856 has not been adequately established in a double-blinded, placebo-controlled study. Thus, the current double-blinded, placebo–controlled two arm study was aimed to evaluate the safety and tolerability of *B. coagulans* MTCC 5856 at a dose of 2×10^9 cfu (spores)/day in healthy adults over a 30 day supplementation period.

Methods and Materials

Product description

B. coagulans MTCC 5856 tablets (600 mg) contained 2×10^9 cfu (spores) (333.33 mg), microcrystalline cellulose, starch, sodium starch glycolate and magnesium stearate. Placebo tablets contained dibasic calcium phosphate, microcrystalline cellulose, starch, and magnesium stearate, No differences in color, taste, texture or packaging were detectable between the two products. Investigational product tablets were sealed in identically-appearing, high-density polyethylene bottles with desiccant.

Ethics and informed consent

The study was reviewed by the Natural Health Products Directorate (NHPD), Health Canada and a research ethics board. Notice of authorization was granted by the NHPD, Ottawa, Ontario (April 10, 2014) and unconditional approval was granted by the Institutional Review Board (IRB Services, Aurora, ON, Canada). This study was conducted in accordance with the ethical principles that have their origins in the Declaration of Helsinki and its subsequent amendments. Informed consent was obtained from each subject at the screening visit (Visit 1) prior to any study-related activities being performed.

Study design

The study design is depicted in figure 1 and disposition of the study participant shown in figure 2. This randomized double-blind clinical study was conducted at a single site (Suite 1440, One London Place, 255 Queens Ave London, ON, Canada). The first subject was enrolled in June 2014 and the last subject completed the study in August 2014.

The sample size for this study was 40 subjects, with 20 subjects randomized to each of the two study arms in a double-blinded manner at a 1:1 ratio. In order to evaluate the primary objective, study assessments were conducted at baseline and day 30. The study consisted of a 30 day intervention period. Subjects met with the investigational team for screening, the baseline/randomization visit and at the end of the study (day 30).

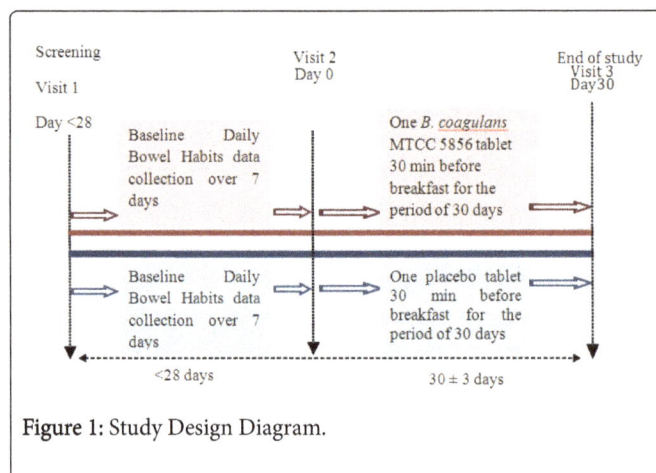

Figure 1: Study Design Diagram.

A description of Visits 1, 2 and 3 with study flow are provided in figure S1. No changes or amendments were made to the approved protocol after the trial commenced and no interim analysis was done during the study period. Independent investigator of the study monitored the progress of all clinical investigations that were conducted and ensured that the protocol is adhered in all aspects. This was a pilot safety study of 40 subjects and therefore the sample size calculation was not carried out. Each participant was assigned a 6-digit randomization code and the investigational products were dispensed by site personnel as per the randomization code list generated by an independent statistician. Double blinding to the investigational products was performed by an independent blinding of the dosing kits and therefore both clinical site staff and participants remained blinded to the treatment received throughout the study duration.

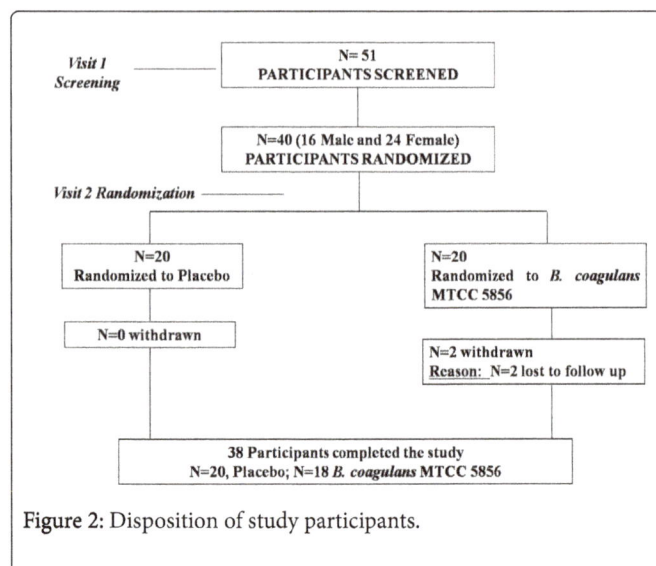

Figure 2: Disposition of study participants.

Selection of study population

A total of 40 healthy adult volunteers (16 males and 24 females) were randomized into two equal groups. All participants met the following eligibility criteria:

Inclusion criteria

1) Male or female ≥ 18 years of age. 2) Females not of child bearing potential, defined as females who had a hysterectomy or oophorectomy, bilateral tubal ligation or were post-menopausal (natural or surgically with >1 year since last menstruation) OR Female subjects of childbearing potential had to agree to use a medically approved method of birth control and have a negative urine pregnancy test result. Acceptable methods of birth control included: a) Hormonal contraceptives including oral contraceptives, hormone birth control patch (Ortho Evra), vaginal contraceptive ring (NuvaRing), injectable contraceptives (Depo-Provera, Lunelle), or hormone implant (Norplant System). b) Intrauterine devices. c) Vasectomy of partner (shown successful as per appropriate follow-up). d) Double barrier method (use of physical barrier by both partners). 3) Healthy as determined by laboratory results and medical history. 4) Normal BMI 18.5-29.9 kg/m^2. 5) Had given voluntary, written, informed consent to participate in the study.

Exclusion criteria

1) Women who were pregnant, breastfeeding, or planning to become pregnant during the course of the trial. 2) Subject had any clinically significant medical condition. 3) Subject required the use of prescribed medications (other than birth control). 4) Use of illicit drugs or history of drug or alcohol abuse within the past 5 years (or had been having more than 2 standard alcoholic drinks per day). 5) Participation in a clinical research trial within 30 days prior to randomization. 6) Clinically significant abnormal laboratory results at screening. 7) Allergy or sensitivity to test product ingredients. 8) Individuals who were cognitively impaired and/or who were unable to give informed consent. (9) Any other condition which in the Investigator's opinion may have adversely affected the subject's ability to complete the study or its measures or which may have posed significant risk to the subject if enrolled in the study.

Interventions

All subjects that met inclusion criteria were randomized into two groups. During the intervention period, one group received *B. coagulans* MTCC 5856 tablets containing 2×10^9 cfu (spores) while the other group received placebo tablets. The intervention period was 30 days in duration. Participants consumed 1 tablet daily 30 minutes before a meal. Participants were instructed to consume the tablet in the morning before breakfast.

Safety Outcomes

Adverse events and laboratory abnormalities

An adverse event (AE) was defined as any untoward medical occurrence in a clinical investigation subject who was administered an investigational product and which did not necessarily have a causal relationship with the treatment [24]. Pre-existing conditions which worsened during the study were to be reported as AEs. During the study, subjects recorded adverse effects in their diary. At each visit the subject was asked "Have you experienced any difficulties or problems since I saw you last?" Any AEs were documented in the study record and were classified according to the description, duration, intensity, frequency, and outcome. The Investigator assessed any AEs and decided causality. Intensity of AEs was graded on a three-point scale (mild, moderate, severe) and reported in detail in the study record.

Serious adverse events

A serious adverse event (SAE) was defined as any AE that resulted in death, a life-threatening adverse event, inpatient hospitalization or prolongation of existing hospitalization, a persistent or significant disability or incapacity and a congenital anomaly/birth defect in the offspring of a subject who received the study treatment. Important medical events that were not immediately life-threatening or resulted in death or hospitalization but may have jeopardized the subject or may have required intervention to prevent one of the outcomes listed above [24].

Laboratory test abnormalities

Laboratory blood tests [complete blood count (CBC), electrolytes, glucose, creatinine, aspartate aminotransferase (AST), alanine transaminase (ALT), gamma-glutamyl aminopeptidase (GGT) and bilirubin] were conducted at screening, baseline/randomization and at the end of study visit (30 days). Laboratory blood tests were analyzed by LifeLabs (London, ON, Canada) by following standardized procedures.

Product tolerability

Participants ranked the *B. coagulans* MTCC 5856 tolerability on a scale of 0 to 10 (0 Representing "not tolerable at all" and 10 Representing "extremely tolerable"). Swallowing difficulty reported by participants by day over 30 days. Patients ranked the ease of swallowing on a scale of 0 to 10 (0 representing "difficult" and 10 representing "not at all difficult"). Participants ranked the performance of the *B. coagulans* MTCC 5856 in terms of ease of swallowing on a scale of 0 to 10 (0 representing "difficult" and 10 representing "not at all difficult"). Similarly, participants ranked the performance of the *B. coagulans* MTCC 5856 in terms of its effect on the stomach such as constipation, diarrhea and cramps on a scale of 0 to 10 (0 Representing "Many Stomach Problems" and 10 Representing "No Stomach Problems").

Daily bowel habits

Participants were asked to maintain a daily bowel habits diary for the 7 days prior to randomization and for the duration of the study (30 days ± 3). Participants recorded the number of bowel movements per day as well as indicating if they experienced a feeling incomplete defecation, straining to start or stop defecation. Participants were provided with the Bristol Stool Scores (BSS) chart to be used to classify their stools [25]. The BSS is a validated score to classify human feces and is a useful tool to measure efficacy of probiotic formulations and their effects on a participants stool consistency. The BSS has 7 score types of classification. A score of 1-2 suggesting constipation, 3 and 4 being the ideal stool form and 5-7 suggesting diarrhea. The information reported by participants in this diary was used to assess if *B. coagulans* MTCC 5856 supplementation caused changes in the bowel habits or consistency during the supplementation.

Data quality assurance

The quality control procedures used in this study included cross-checking all data by research personnel against source document originals. Data entry and verification was executed according to KGK Synergize's Standard Operating Procedures (London, ON, Canada). All raw data and standard operating procedures used in this trial were maintained and archived where appropriate to satisfy regulatory requirements. Frequent monitoring was done during the study. All source documents were reviewed to ensure that all items were completed and that the data provided were accurate and obtained in the manner specified in the protocol.

Data Analysis

Assessment of normality

After the database was locked, but before it was unblinded, the analyzing statistician examined the distribution of all continuous variable endpoints. The Anderson-Darling test of normality was used to determine whether the variable was (1) sufficiently normally distributed to permit its use in parametric statistical tests (i.e. Student's t-test), or (2) sufficiently log-normally distributed to permit the logarithm of that variable to be used in parametric tests, or (3) so intractably non-normal, even with logarithmic transformation as to require non-parametric testing (i.e. Mann-Whitney tests).

Assessment of safety

Summary statistics for continuous variables were computed by treatment and visit as count, mean and standard deviation. Changes from baseline to subsequent time points were summarized the same way. Mean values and mean changes from baseline were compared between products by the unpaired Student t-test, or the non-parametric Mann-Whitney U test. Changes from baseline were tested for within group significance by the paired Student t-test or the Wilcoxon Signed-Ranks test. Summary statistics for discrete variables were tabulated at each time point, for each treatment group and for the combined groups as counts and percentages of group totals. For the assessment of safety laboratory parameters and anthropometric and vital sign measures, the change from baseline was defined as the difference between the value at day 30 and the value at the baseline visit. For the assessment of BSS and average number of bowel movements per day, the baseline was considered to be the average of the 7 day pre-baseline values.

Level of significance and statistical software

Probability (p) values ≤ 0.05 were considered statistically significant. All evaluations were carried out using the software package R 3.03. Data collection during the study and statistical analysis were performed by separate functional groups and a certified, independent statistician respectively.

Results

Forty participants were randomized to either placebo (n=20; 10 males and 10 females) or *B. coagulans* MTCC 5856 (n=20; 6 males and 14 females). The mean age for participants was 33.5 ± 13 years for placebo group and 33.5 ± 14.3 years for *B. coagulans* MTCC 5856 group and demographics were similar between *B. coagulans* MTCC 5856 group and placebo group (Table 1). The average BMI was 24.6 ±

2.7 kg/m^2 for the placebo group and 24.3 ± 3.5 Kg/m^2 for the *B. coagulans* MTCC 5856 group. Two females in the *B. coagulans* MTCC 5856 group withdrew from the study citing personal reasons for opting out of the study.

		Placebo	B. coagulans MTCC 5856	Total	P Value Δ
Gender					
	Female	10	14	24	
	Male	10	6	16	0.333
	Total	20	20	40	
Smokers					
	Ex-Smoker	16	18	34	
	Non-Smoker	1	1	2	
	Smoker	3	1	4	0.797
	Total	20	20	40	
Ethnicity					
	Hispanic	2	3	5	
	Non Hispanic	18	17	35	
	Total	20	20	40	
Races					
	Central American	0	1	1	
	East Asian	1	1	2	
	South Asian	1	1	2	
	South American	0	1	1	
	South East Asian	0	1	1	0.95
	Western European White	18	15	33	
	Total	20	20	40	
Alcohol use					
	None	5	3	8	
	Occasionally	11	9	20	
	Weekly	4	8	12	0.452
	Total	20	20	40	

Table 1: Demographics for all participants randomized into the Study. Δ Independence of treatment assessed by the Fisher's exact test. Probability values ≤ 0.05 are statistically significant.

Treatment compliance

The mean treatment compliance, measured as the number of dosage units taken by participants compared to the number expected to have been taken, was greater than 97% in both groups during the study. One participant had a compliance of 76.7%. Therefore, this participant's data was only used for safety analysis and excluded from tolerability analysis.

Anthropometric and vital signs measures

There were no between group differences at Day 30 in BMI, weight, heart rate, and diastolic blood pressure (DBP) in participants supplemented with *B. coagulans* MTCC 5856 vs those on placebo (Table 2). There was a significant between group difference in systolic blood pressure (SBP) at Day 30 in subjects on placebo vs those on *B. coagulans* MTCC 5856 (p=0.006). This difference reflected an increase in the SBP in the placebo group while those on *B. coagulans* MTCC 5856 showed a decrease. However, the blood pressure in both groups remained within normal and acceptable clinical range at Day 30. Within groups, participants supplemented with *B. coagulans* MTCC 5856, showed no differences in weight, BMI, heart rate and systolic and diastolic blood pressure from baseline to Day 30. However, for participants in the placebo group, all of the anthropometric measures showed no statistically significant difference from baseline to Day 30 except for systolic blood pressure, which increased from baseline to Day 30 (p=0.023) but remained within a normal clinical range.

Parameters		Placebo (N=20)	*B. coagulans* MTCC 5856 (N=18)	P value Δ
Weight (Kg)				
	Baseline (Day 0)	72.2 ± 12.8	68.8 ± 13.6	0.598
	End of Study (Day 30)	71.8 ± 13.5	69.4 ± 14	0.604
	Change From Baseline to Day 30	p = 0.429	p = 0.390	0.968
BMI (kg/m^2)				
	Baseline (Day 0)	24.6 ± 2.7	24.5 ± 3	0.731
	End of Study (Day 30)	24.4 ± 2.9	24.3 ± 3.3	0.869
	Change From Baseline to Day 30	p = 0.381	p = 0.353	0.897
Heart Rate (BPM)				
	Baseline (Day 0)	68.3 ± 7.5	68.9 ± 8.4	0.839
	End of Study (Day 30)	65.9 ± 6.8	69.2 ± 8.6	0.193
	Change From Baseline to Day 30	p = 0.157	p = 0.486	0.159
Systolic Blood Pressure (mmHg)				
	Baseline (Day 0)	100.4 ± 10.3	104.0 ± 9.4	0.253
	End of Study (Day 30)	104.9 ± 10.4	100.0 ± 9.0	0.127
	Change From Baseline to Day 30	p = 0.023	p = 0.100	0.006
Diastolic Blood Pressure (mmHg)				
	Baseline (Day 0)	66.5 ± 7.6	68.4 ± 6.7	0.428
	End of Study (Day 30)	67.4 ± 7.6	69.0 ± 7.9	0.547
	Change From Baseline to Day 30	p = 0.590	p = 0.852	0.796

Table 2: Anthropometrics and Vital Signs for All Participants at Baseline and after 30 Days of Supplementation with *B. coagulans* MTCC 5856 or Placebo BPM, beats per minute; mmHg, millimeter of mercury; kg, kilograms; BMI, body mass index; kg/m^2, kilograms per square meter. Δ Between-group comparisons were made using the unpaired Student's t-test. Within-group comparisons were made using the paired Student's t-test. Probability (p) values ≤0.05 are statistically significant.

Laboratory parameters of safety

There were no differences in the laboratory parameters between participants in the *B. coagulans* MTCC 5856 group and those in the placebo after a 30 day supplementation with *B. coagulans* MTCC 5856 (Table S1). The baseline hemoglobin and hematocrit levels had statistically significant difference between participants supplemented with placebo and those supplemented with *B. coagulans* MTCC 5856 (p=0.017 and p=0.029 respectively). The placebo group consisted of more males (10 males and 10 females) in comparison to the *B. coagulans* MTCC 5856 group (6 males and 10 females). As hemoglobin and hematocrit levels tend to be higher in males compared to females, it is possible that the variation in gender between the two groups may be attributed to this difference. However, these differences did not carry through to Day 30 and values remained similar between groups after the supplementation period. Within groups, participants on placebo showed a decrease in mean corpuscular hemoglobin (p=0.027), and potassium concentration (p=0.017) and an increase in fasting glucose (p=0.015) and eGFR (p=0.022). The *B. coagulans* MTCC 5856 group showed a decrease from baseline in the red blood cell distribution width (RDW) after the 30 day supplementation (p=0.003). However all values remained within normal acceptable laboratory range. No other changes were seen between or within groups after the 30 day supplementation.

Adverse effect

A total of 9 AEs were reported in the placebo group by 8 participants. Six of these AEs were categorized as gastrointestinal with 1 AE (upset stomach) considered by the qualified investigator (QI) as "unlikely related" to the investigational product (IP) and 5 AEs (nausea, upset stomach, bloating, borborygmus, abdominal cramps and stomach ache) considered by the QI to be "possibly" related to the investigational product. One AE was classified as a nervous system disorder; participant in the placebo group reported experiencing headache which was mild in severity and categorized as unlikely related to the IP by the QI. One AE was classified as infections and infestations; participant in the placebo group reported a cold, mild in severity and it was categorized as not related to the IP. Participant 031 in the placebo group accidently consumed gasoline during work which caused upset stomach and loose bowel movements, this AE was categorized as injury, poisoning and procedural complications and the AE classified as not related to IP. All AE's resolved without participants having to discontinue the study products.

In the *B. coagulans* MTCC 5856 group, 10 AEs were reported by 5 participants. Six of these were classified as gastrointestinal with 2 AEs (bloating and diarrhea) considered by the QI as "unlikely" related to the IP and 4 AEs (stomach pain, nausea, upset stomach and bloating) considered by the PI as "possibly" related to the IP. Two nervous system disorders (headache) were experienced by participants in the *B. coagulans* MTCC 5856 group. All nervous system disorder AEs were classified to be unlikely related to the IP. One AE experienced by a participant in the *B. coagulans* MTCC 5856 group was categorized as General Disorder and Administration site conditions. This AE was reported as fever and upset stomach and considered by the PI as unlikely related to the IP. One infection and infestation AEs was reported in the *B. coagulans* MTCC 5856 group (stomach flu) and was considered to be unlikely related to investigational product by the QI. All AEs resolved without participants having to discontinue the study products.

Tolerability

Participants ranked the IP tolerability, performance in term of ease of swallowing, and its effect on the stomach on a scale 0 to 10. The tolerability, swallowing difficulty and effect on the stomach was similar between placebo and *B. coagulans* MTCC 5856. Over the 30 days supplementation period, participants ranked the product to be tolerable with the mean tolerability of 9.02 ± 1.76 for placebo and 9.00 ± 1.96 for *B. coagulans* MTCC 5856 (0 represents "not tolerable at all" and 10 represents "extremely tolerable") (Figure 3). The participants also reported that both the placebo and *B. coagulans* MTCC 5856 were easy to swallow during the 30 days with the mean difficulty of 8.75 ± 1.66 for placebo and 8.82 ± 1.67 for *B. coagulans* MTCC 5856 (0 representing "difficult" and 10 representing "not at all difficult") (Figure 3). Both placebo and *B. coagulans* MTCC 5856 had minimal effect on the stomach such as constipation, diarrhea and cramps over the 30 days of supplementation. The effect of the product on the stomach was reported by participants as a mean of 8.94 ± 1.85 for placebo and a mean of 8.82 ± 2.24 for *B. coagulans* MTCC 5856 (0 representing "Many Stomach Problems" and 10 Representing "No Stomach Problems") over the 30 days of supplementation (Figure 3).

Bowel habits

There were no differences between groups in the daily number of bowel movements in either placebo or *B. coagulans* MTCC 5856 during the 7 days pre-dose period or the 30 day supplementation period (Table 3). The average number of bowel movements showed that there were no between group differences in this parameter for participants receiving either placebo or *B. coagulans* MTCC 5856 the 30 days supplementation (Table 3).

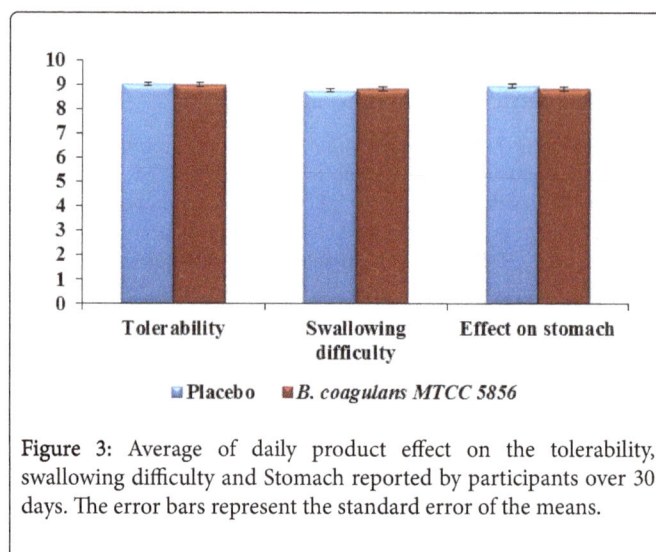

Figure 3: Average of daily product effect on the tolerability, swallowing difficulty and Stomach reported by participants over 30 days. The error bars represent the standard error of the means.

Week of Study	Placebo	*B. coagulans* MTCC 5856	P value Δ
	(N=20)	(N=18)	
Baseline (Day 0)	1.32 ± 0.42	1.19 ± 0.51	0.416
End of Study (Day 30)	1.14 ± 0.45	1.19 ± 0.75	0.842
Change From Day 0 to Day 30	p=0.123	p=0.864	0.509

Table 3: The average number of daily bowel movements of all participants during the 30 Day supplementation with either *B. coagulans* MTCC 5856 or Placebo. Δ Between-group comparisons were made using the unpaired Student's t-test. Within-group comparisons were made using the paired Student's t-test.

During the 30 days of supplementation, there were no between group differences in the number of participants who experienced at least one bowel movement that required straining to start defecation (Table 4) or to stop defecation (Table 5) in the placebo vs *B. coagulans* MTCC 5856 group.

Week of Study	Straining	Placebo	*B. coagulans* MTCC 5856	P value Δ
		(N=20)	(N=18)	
Baseline (Day 0)	No	12	11	1
	Yes	7	9	
End of Study (Day 30)	No	7	14	0.187
	Yes	4	2	

Table 4: Number of participants who experienced at least one bowel movement that required straining to start defecation, during the 30 day supplementation with *B. coagulans* MTCC 5856 or Placebo. Δ Between-group comparisons were made using the Fisher's exact test.

Similarly, there were no differences between subjects who experienced at least one "Feeling of Incomplete Defecation", during the

30 Day supplementation with either *B. coagulans* MTCC 5856 or Placebo (Table 6).

Week of Study	Straining	Placebo (N=20)	*B. coagulans* MTCC 5856 (N=18)	P value Δ
Baseline (Day 0)	No	17	15	0.407
	Yes	2	5	
End of Study (Day 30)	No	11	15	1
	Yes	0	1	

Table 5: Number of participants who experienced at least one bowel movement that required straining to stop defecation, during the 30 Day supplementation with either *B. coagulans* MTCC 5856 or Placebo. Δ Between-group comparisons were made using the Fisher's exact test.

Week of Study	Incomplete Defecation	Placebo (N=20)	*B. coagulans* MTCC 5856 (N=18)	P value Δ
Baseline (Day 0)	No	13	8	0.111
	Yes	6	12	
End of Study (Day 30)	No	11	16	-
	Yes	0	0	

Table 6: Number of subjects who experienced at least one "Feeling of Incomplete Defecation", in a given week, during the 30 Day supplementation with either *B. coagulans* MTCC 5856 or Placebo. Δ Between-group comparisons were made using the Fisher's exact test.

Bristol stool score

The Bristol Stool form scale provides illustrations of the seven stool types, which can be used to help fill out the **stool diary** [25]. It remains in use as a research tool to evaluate the effectiveness of treatments for various conditions of the bowel, as well as a clinical communication aid. Over the 30 day supplementation period, *B. coagulans* MTCC 5856 did not show any adverse effects on the consistency of the faeces of participants. There were no between group differences in the daily BSS for participants in the placebo vs *B. coagulans* MTCC 5856 during the pre-dose week (baseline) (data not shown). The average BSS were not different between the placebo and the *B. coagulans* MTCC 5856 group (Table 7).

Week of Study	Placebo (N=20)	*B. coagulans* MTCC 5856 (N=18)	P value Δ
Baseline (Day 0)	3.76 ± 0.63	3.91 ± 0.86	0.608
End of Study (Day 30)	3.61 ± 0.62	4.40 ± 0.87	0.275
Change from Baseline to Day 30	p=0.336	p=0.021	0.022

Table 7: The average BSS for all participants during the 30 Day supplementation with either *B. coagulans* MTCC 5856 or Placebo. Δ Between-group comparisons were made using the unpaired Student's t-test. Within-group comparisons were made using the paired Student's t-test.

Discussion and Conclusions

Oral administration of *B. coagulans* was found to be safe in several subchronic, chronic and reproductive toxicity animal studies which did not reveal any adverse effects at a dose of 6.88×10^{10} cfu (spores)/kg body weight [9,20,26]. In another animal study, *B. coagulans* containing 5×10^9 cfu (spores)/g was administered by gavage to male mice at dose levels of 1, 3 or 5 g/kg body weight and no deaths occurred, nor was there any abnormality such as diarrhea. Hence, the results of the study suggested that the LD50 of a powder containing *B. coagulans* was greater than 5 g/kg body weight [9,26]. From the animal studies, the current double-blinded, placebo-controlled two arm study was conducted to evaluate the safety and tolerability of *B. coagulans* MTCC 5856 at a dose of 2×10^9 cfu (spores)/day in healthy adults over 30 days supplementation period. The treatment compliance was 99% for the *B. coagulans* MTCC 5856 group and 97% for the placebo group. There were no statistically significant differences in the laboratory parameters between participants in the *B. coagulans* MTCC 5856 group and those in the placebo after a 30 day supplementation with *B. coagulans* MTCC 5856. The baseline hemoglobin and hematocrit levels were statistically significantly higher in participants randomized to the placebo group compared to those randomized to the *B. coagulans* MTCC 5856 group. However, this difference did not translate into a statistically significant difference between groups after the 30 day supplementation. Within groups, participants supplemented with *B. coagulans* MTCC 5856, showed no differences in weight, BMI, heart rate and systolic and diastolic blood pressure from baseline to Day 30. Further, there were no significant differences in the anthropometric measurements between *B. coagulans* MTCC 5856 and placebo groups. To the best of our knowledge, this is the first study demonstrating clinical safety (blood hematology, clinical chemistry parameters and anthropometric measures) of *B. coagulans* MTCC 5856 probiotic at a dose of 2×10^9 cfu (spores)/day in healthy adults over 30 days supplementation period. However, there are many other strains of *Bacillus coagulans* consumed worldwide and well-studied for their clinical efficacy and safety [10,27-32].

Adverse events were rigorously monitored in the study in order to document all events that occurred during the 30 day supplementation with *B. coagulans* MTCC 5856. Special emphasis was directed to any gastrointestinal related symptoms such as vomiting, diarrhea and abdominal pain. Participants receiving *Bacillus coagulans* MTCC 5856 did not report any adverse events such as vomiting and diarrhea. Participants on placebo reported two adverse events classified as abdominal pain and those on *B. coagulans* MTCC 5856 reported one adverse event classified as abdominal pain. Therefore, abdominal pain was not limited to the *B. coagulans* MTCC 5856 group. *B. coagulans* MTCC 5856 and placebo tablets were reported by the participants to be tolerable, easy to swallow and had minimal effects on the stomach during the 30 days of supplementation. The number of bowel movements was similar between the placebo group and *B. coagulans*

MTCC 5856 group during the baseline week and during the 30 days of supplementation. BSS were also similar between placebo and *B. coagulans* MTCC 5856 during the 30 day supplementation period. The results from the current study are in the agreement with the published literature [10,27-32]. For the first time, we report a detailed safety and tolerability of *B. coagulans* MTCC 5856 at a dose of 2×10^9 cfu (spores)/day in healthy individuals during the 30 days of supplementation. However, in another study, 36 subjects were randomized into two groups who received either *B. coagulans* MTCC 5856 or placebo. *B. coagulans* MTCC 5856 treatment revealed a significant change/decrease in the clinical symptoms such as bloating, vomiting, diarrhea, abdominal pain and stool frequency towards end of the study [33].

Ugba, a fermented African OIlbean seeds (*Pentaclethra macrophylla*, Benth) is a popular protein-rich solid, flavorful alkaline food in the Ibo ethnic group of Nigeria. *B. coagulans* was reported to be major organism responsible for the fermentation of Ugba [34]. This validates the traditional safe use of *B. coagulans*. Several clinical studies on the safety aspects of *B. coagulans* have been reported. However, it is essential to evaluate the safety of every probiotic strains which is intended for human consumption [8]. Additionally, *B. coagulans* has been granted Qualified Presumption of Safety (QPS) status since 2008 by the European Food Safety Authority [35] and the Japanese Ministry of Health and Welfare has also approved *B. coagulans* for improvement in symptoms caused by abnormalities in the intestinal flora or in dysbiosis [17, 20]. In addition to the above approved uses, USFDA had also issued a "no questions" letter to the GRAS notices on the use of *B. coagulans* spores preparations to be used at a maximum level of approximately 2×10^9 cfu/serving in several food categories.

In conclusion, this study has verified that *B. coagulans* MTCC 5856 at a dose of 2×10^9 cfu (spores)/day in healthy individuals was safe and tolerable in healthy participants supplemented for 30 days. *B. coagulans* MTCC 5856 was also easy to swallow, tolerable and had no statistically significant effects on the stomach during the 30 days of supplementation. The results of the study suggested that oral administration of *B. coagulans* MTCC 5856 at a dose level of 2×10^9 cfu (spores)/day for 30 days was safe and well tolerated in healthy subjects.

Acknowledgements

We thank the clinical trial investigators Dr. Dale Wilson, KGK Synergize Inc. Canada and their team members in conducting this clinical trial. These investigators and team had no influence on any aspect relevant to this study.

The authors also recognize the following intellectual property rights for ingredients used in the current clinical study.

LactoSpore® stable probiotic is a registered logo (U.S Trademark Registration No.4068336) of Sabinsa Corporation, 20 Lake Drive, East Windsor, NJ, USA 08520.

LACTOSPORE is a registered brand name (U.S Trademark Registration No. 17013661) of Sabinsa Corporation, 20 Lake Drive, East Windsor, NJ, USA 08520.

References

1. Cebra JJ (1999) Influences of microbiota on intestinal immune system development. Am J Clin Nutr 69: 1046S-1051S.

2. Noverr MC, Huffnagle GB (2004) Does the microbiota regulate immune responses outside the gut? Trends Microbiol 12: 562-568.

3. De Moreno de LeBlanc A, LeBlanc JG (2014) Effect of probiotic administration on the intestinal microbiota, current knowledge and potential applications. World J Gastroenterol 20: 16518-16528.

4. Macpherson AJ, Uhr T (2004) Induction of protective IgA by intestinal dendritic cells carrying commensal bacteria. Science 303: 1662-1665.

5. Koning CJ, Jonkers D, Smidt H, Rombouts F, Pennings HJ, et al. (2010) The effect of a multispecies probiotic on the composition of the faecal microbiota and bowel habits in chronic obstructive pulmonary disease patients treated with antibiotics. Br J Nutr 103: 1452-1460.

6. Tuohy KM, Probert HM, Smejkal CW, Gibson GR (2003) Using probiotics and prebiotics to improve gut health. Drug Discov Today 8: 692-700.

7. Högenauer C, Hammer HF, Krejs GJ, Reisinger EC (1998) Mechanisms and management of antibiotic-associated diarrhea. Clin Infect Dis 27: 702-710.

8. Joint Food and Agriculture Organization of the United Nations (2002) World Health Organization Working Group report on drafting guidelines for the evaluation of probiotics in food. WHO.

9. Endres JR, Clewell A, Jade KA, Farber T, Hauswirth J, et al. (2009) Safety assessment of a proprietary preparation of a novel Probiotic, *Bacillus coagulans*, as a food ingredient. Food Chem Toxicol 47: 1231-38.

10. Kalman DS, Schwartz HI, Alvarez P, Feldman S, Pezzullo JC, et al. (2009) A prospective, randomized, double-blind, placebo-controlled parallel-group dual site trial to evaluate the effects of a *Bacillus coagulans*-based product on functional intestinal gas symptoms. BMC Gastroenterol 9: 85.

11. Hun L (2009) *Bacillus coagulans* significantly improved abdominal pain and bloating in patients with IBS. Postgrad Med 121: 119-124.

12. Kimmel M, Keller D, Farmer S, Warrino DE (2010) A controlled clinical trial to evaluate the effect of GanedenBC(30) on immunological markers. Methods Find Exp Clin Pharmacol 32: 129-132.

13. Mandel DR, Eichas K, Holmes J (2010) *Bacillus coagulans*: a viable adjunct therapy for relieving symptoms of rheumatoid arthritis according to a randomized, controlled trial. BMC Complement Altern Med 10:1.

14. Clarke G, Cryan JF, Dinan TG, Quigley EM (2012) Review article: probiotics for the treatment of irritable bowel syndrome--focus on lactic acid bacteria. Aliment Pharmacol Ther 35: 403-413.

15. Baron M (2009) A patented strain of *Bacillus coagulans* increased immune response to viral challenge. Postgrad Med 121: 114-118.

16. Jensen GS, Benson KF, Carter SG, Endres JR (2010) GanedenBC30 cell wall and metabolites: anti-inflammatory and immune modulating effects in vitro. BMC Immunol 11: 15.

17. Majeed M, Prakash L (1998) LactoSpore®: The Effective Probiotic. Piscataway, NJ: NutriScience Publishers pp. 1-56.

18. [No authors listed] (2002) *Lactobacillus sporogenes*. Altern Med Rev 7: 340-342.

19. Jurenka JS (2012) *Bacillus coagulans*: Monograph. Altern Med Rev 17: 76-81.

20. Majeed M, Kamarei R (2012) *Bacillus coagulans*: Probiotic of choice. NutraCos 19-21.

21. Majeed M, Majeed S, Nagabhushanam K, Natarajan S, Sivakumar A et al. (2016) Evaluation of the stability of *Bacillus coagulans* MTCC 5856 during processing and storage of functional foods. Int J Food Sci Technol, doi:10.1111/ijfs.13044.

22. Majeed M, Nagabhushanam K, Natarajan S, Sivakumar A, et al. (2016) Evaluation of genetic and phenotypic consistency of *Bacillus coagulans* MTCC 5856: a commercial probiotic strain. World J Microbiol Biotechnol 32: 60.

23. Majeed M, Majeed S, Nagabhushanam K, Natarajan S, Sivakumar A, et al. (2016) Evaluation of anti-diarrhoeal activity of *Bacillus coagulans* MTCC 5856 and its effect on gastrointestinal motility in wistar rats. Int J Pharma Bio Sci 7: 311-16.

24. ICH-GCP Guideline (1997) International Conference on Harmonisation, Good Clinical Practice. E6 (R1), Federal Register 62: 25691-25709.

25. Lewis SJ, Heaton KW (1997) Stool form scale as a useful guide to intestinal transit time. Scand J Gastroenterol 32: 920-924.

26. Endres JR, Qureshi I, Farber T, Hauswirth J, Hirka G, et al. (2011) One-year chronic oral toxicity with combined reproduction toxicity study of a novel probiotic, *Bacillus coagulans*, as a food ingredient. Food Chem Toxicol 49: 1174-1182.

27. Sudha RM, Sunita M, Sekhar BM (2011) Safety studies of *Bacillus coagulans* Unique IS-2 in rats: Morphological, biochemical and clinical evaluations. Int J Probiotics Prebiotics 6: 43-48.

28. Mohan JC, Arora R, Khalilullah M (1990) Preliminary observations on effect of *Lactobacillus sporogenes* on serum lipid levels in hypercholesterolemic patients. Indian J Med Res 92: 431-432.

29. Chandra PK (2002) Effect of Lactobacillus on the incidence and severity of acute rotavirus diarrhoea in infants. A prospective placebo-controlled double-blind study. Nutr Res 22: 65-69.

30. Astegiano M, Pellicano R, Terzi E, Simondi D, Rizzetto M (2006) Treatment of irritable bowel syndrome. A case control experience. Minerva Gastroenterol Dietol 52: 359-363.

31. Ratna Sudha M, Yelikar KA, Deshpande S (2012) Clinical Study of *Bacillus coagulans* Unique IS-2 (ATCC PTA-11748) in the Treatment of Patients with Bacterial Vaginosis. Indian J Microbiol 52: 396-399.

32. Urgesi R, Casale C, Pistelli R, Rapaccini GL, de Vitis I (2014) A randomized double-blind placebo-controlled clinical trial on efficacy and safety of association of simethicone and *Bacillus coagulans* (Colinox®) in patients with irritable bowel syndrome. Eur Rev Med Pharmacol Sci 18: 1344-53.

33. Majeed M, Kalyanam N, Sankaran N, Vaidyanathan P, Karri S, et al. (2014) Process for the therapeutic management of Diarrhea predominant irritable bowel syndrome using *Bacillus coagulans* SBC-37-01, MTCC 5856 US patent application 14536701, PCT application PCT/US16/12409.

34. Isu NR, Njoku HO (1997) An evaluation of the microflora associated with fermented African oil bean (Pentaclethra macrophylla Bentham) seeds during ugba production. Plant Foods Human Nutr 51: 145-157.

35. EFSA, European Food Safety Authority (2012) Panel on Biological Hazards (BIOHAZ); Scientific Opinion on the maintenance of the list of QPS biological agents intentionally added to food and feed. EFSA Journal 10: 3020.

Claudin 5 Transcripts Following Acrolein Exposure Affected by Epigenetic Enzyme

Kuk-Young Moon[1#], Pureun-Haneul Lee[1#], Byeong-Gon Kim[1], Moo-Kyun Park[2] and An-Soo Jang[1*]

[1]*Genome Research Center for Allergy and Respiratory Diseases Soonchunhyang University Bucheon Hospital, Republic of Korea*

[2]*Otolaryngo Rhinology, Seoul National University, Korea*

[#]*These authors equally contributed to this work.*

[*]**Corresponding author:** An Soo Jang, Division of Allergy and Respiratory Medicine, Department of Internal Medicine, Soonchunhyang University Bucheon Hospital,170 Jomaru-ro, Wonmi-gu, Bucheon, Gyeonggi-Do, 420-767, South Korea, E-mail: jas877@schmc.ac.kr

Abstract

Background and objective: Acrolein is a highly reactive α, β-unsaturated aldehyde and a respiratory irritant that is ubiquitously present in the environment but that can also be generated endogenously at sites of inflammation. Apical junctional protein claudin 5 can be affected by acrolein. This study aimed to determine the impact of aberrant expression of DNMT1, DNMT3b, MBD3, and MeCP2 on acrolein induced claudin 5.

Methods: EA.hy926 cell lines were exposed to acrolein 30 nm for 1 h, 2 h, and 4 h. Epigenetic enzyme such as DNMT1, DNMT3b, MBD3 and MeCP2 were quantified in the cell line using real time PCR. Claudin 5 methylation was checked by methtyl specific PCR.

Results: After acrolein 30 nm exposure, MBD3 and MeCP2 transcript were decreased at 1 h and increased at 2 h and 4 h compared to control. DNMT3b transcript was decreased at 1 h, 2 h, and 4 h following acrolein 30 nm exposure. DNMT1 transcript was not different between control and acrolein 30 nm exposure. Claudin 5 methylation transcript /total Claudin 5 transcript was decreased at 1 h, 2 h and 4 h following acrolein 30 nm exposure.

Conclusion: These findings demonstrate that acrolein exposure modify epigenetic enzyme leading to Claudin 5 methylation change, suggesting that acrolein contribute to enzyme pathway involved in epigenetic regulation.

Keywords Acrolein; Epigenomics; Methylation; Claudin 5

Introduction

Acrolein (2-propenal) is a highly reactive α, β-unsaturated aldehyde and a respiratory irritant that is ubiquitously present in the environment but that can also be generated endogenously at sites of inflammation [1,2] . Acrolein is abundant in tobacco smoke, which is the major environmental risk factor for asthma and chronic obstructive pulmonary disease (COPD), and elevated levels of acrolein are found in the lung fluids of asthma and COPD patients [1-3]. Because of its reactivity with respiratory-lining fluid or cellular macromolecules, acrolein alters gene regulation, inflammation, mucociliary transport, and alveolar–capillary barrier integrity [1].

An integral membrane protein, Claudin 5 (CLDN5), is a critical component of endothelial tight junctions that control pericellular permeability [2]. Acrolein can induce ALI with perivascular edema in mice, accompanying by a compensatory increase in CLDN5 transcript and protein, which was more evident in a resistant than a sensitive mouse strain [2].

Epigenetics is the study of stable modifications of fixed genomes that direct which genes are expressed and silenced [4,5]. Although heritable from parent to child, and potentially stable between cell cycles, epigenetic regulation of DNA transcription can also be modified by a number of external factors to allow flexible responses to a changing environment such as air pollution, tobacco smoke, and other sources of oxidant stress, along with the microbial environment, pesticides, and toxins [4]. A number of different disease processes among them cancer, atherosclerosis, mental retardation syndromes, autoimmune, and allergic processes are in part controlled by epigenetic processes [4,6]. DNA methylation is accomplished by several subtypes of the DNA methyl transferases (DNMT). DNMT1 is considered the maintenance methyltransferase because this isoform acts to maintain methylation states during mitosis and in the daughter cells. DNMT3A and DNMT3B initiate de-novo methylation [7], although the triggers for this activity are only partly identified. Age, sex, genetic polymorphisms, and environmental exposures are some factors associated with altered methylation [8]. Histones can be modified by a number of processes including by acetylation, phosphorylation, methylation, ubiquitination or sumoylation [5]. This study aimed at examining the effect of epigenetic enzyme on claudin 5 expresion exposed to acrolein.

Materials and Methods

Cell culture and acrolein treatment

(No. CRL 2922; ATCC, Manassas, VA), Confluent cells were washed in D-PBS, incubated for 30 min, and then exposed to 30 nm acrolein (<4 h) in D-PBS.

Total RNA extraction and real-time PCR to measure methylation enzymes expression levels

Total RNA was extracted using a TRI REAGENT (Molecular Research Center, Cincinnati, OH, USA) according to the manufacturer's instructions. We quantified RNA and reverse transcribed cDNA from 3 µg of total RNA. RNA was reverse-transcribed by incubation with 0.5 mM dNTP, 2.5 mM MgCl$_2$, 5 mM DTT, 1 ul of Oligo DT(0.5 ug/ul) and SuperScript II RT (200 unit/ul) at 42°C for 50 min, and heat inactivated at 70°C for 15 min. About 50 ng cDNA was amplified using Applied Biosystems Step One TM Real-Time PCR System. The PCR mixture (20 µl) contained 1ul of cDNA, 1 µl of 10 pmol forward and reverse primers and 10 µl of 2X SYBR Green Supermix (Applied Biosystems). The reaction was carried out in a two-step procedure: denaturation at 95°C for 10 min and 40 cycles with denaturation at 95°C for 15 s, 60°C for 1 min and melt curve stage was performed at 95 for 15 s, 60 for 1 min and 90°C for 15 s. The comparative cycle number threshold (CT) method ($\Delta\Delta$CT) was used to quantify the transcript expression levels. The change in CT value (ΔCT=CT gene of interest -CTPGK1) was calculated for each sample. The comparative $\Delta\Delta$CT calculation involved finding the difference between each sample's ΔCT and the mean ΔCT for the control samples. These values were transformed to absolute values using the formula: comparative expression level (fold change)=2-$\Delta\Delta$CT. The conditions and primers designed for detected genes were listed in Table 1.

Gene		Sequences (5'-3')	Annealing temperature (°C)	PCR products size (bp)
PGK1	F	GACCTAATGTCCAAAGCTGAGA	58	127
	R	A		
		CAGCAGGTATGCCAGAAGCC		
DNMT1	F	AACCTTCACCTAGCCCCAG	58	125
	R	CTCATCCGATTTGGCTCTTTCA		
DN MT3b	F	CCAATCCTGGAGGCTATCCG	60	152
	R	ACTGGGGTGTCAGAGCCAT		
MeCP2	F	TGACCGGGGACCCATGTAT	58	145
	R	CTCCACTTTAGAGCGAAAGGC		
MBD3	F	CAGCCGTGACCAAGATTACC	59	135
	R	CTCCTCAGCAATGTCGAAGG		

Table 1: Primer sets for real time PCR.

Claudin-5 CpG methylation in vitro by methylation-specific PCR (MSP) and real-time MSP

Total genomic DNA from the EA.hy 926 cells was extracted using a mini DNeasy Kit (Qiagen, Tokyo, Japan). Bisulfite conversion of genomic DNA was performed using a Zymo EZ DNA Methylation Gold kit (Zymo Research Corp, Orange, CA). MSP was performed to determine the methylation status of the CLDN5 gene. Specific methylated or unmethylated sequences of the primers: Human Claudin-5-M methylated primers forward:

GTAAGGTGTTTTTGGAATGATTTC reverse: ATCCAACCACCAATCTTAATACG Human Claudin-5-U unmethylated primers forward: GTAAGGTGTTTTTGGAAATGATTTT revers: ATCCAACCACCAATCTTAATACAAC. These primers designed using the Methprimer tool.

Methyl amplification used hot start premix (bionner, Daejeon, Republic of Korea) and conditions were as follows: initial denaturation at 95°C for 10 min, denaturation at 94°C for 30 s, annealing at 58°C for 30s, and extension at 72°C for 30 s for 35 cycles, followed by a stabilization for 7 min at 72°C. Unmethyl amplification followed the same procedure. Amplification products were separated by gel electrophoresis and stained with ethidium bromide. The density (intensity 3 square millimeters) of each band specific for methyl and unmethyl primers was measured under UV light and promoter methylation status was expressed by percent density of methyl band / [methyl band+unmethyl band].

Statistical analysis

All data were analyzed using the SPSS version 7.5 for Windows. Data are expressed as mean ± SEM. Inter-group comparisons were assessed by non-parametric method using Mann-Whitney U test. A p-value of less than 5% was regarded as statistically significant.

Results

DNMT3b transcript decrease after exposure to acrolein

EA.hy926 cell lines were exposed to acrolein 30 nm for 1 h, 2 h, and 4 h. Epigenetic enzyme such as DNMT1, DNMT3b, MeCP2 and MBD3 were quantified in the cell line using real time PCR. DNMT3b transcript was decreased at 1 h, 2 h, and 4 h following acrolein 30 nm exposure (Figure 1A). DNMT1 transcript was not different between control and acrolein 30 nm exposure (Figure 1B).

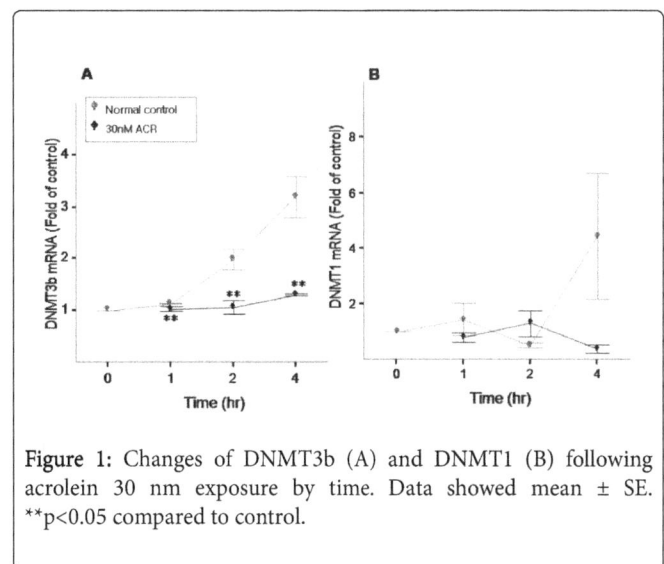

Figure 1: Changes of DNMT3b (A) and DNMT1 (B) following acrolein 30 nm exposure by time. Data showed mean ± SE. **p<0.05 compared to control.

Changes of MeCP2 and MBD3 transcript exposed to acrolein

After acrolein 30 nm exposure, MeCP2 (Figure 2A) and MBD3 (Figure 2B) transcript were decreased at 1 h and increased at 2 h and 4 h compared to control.

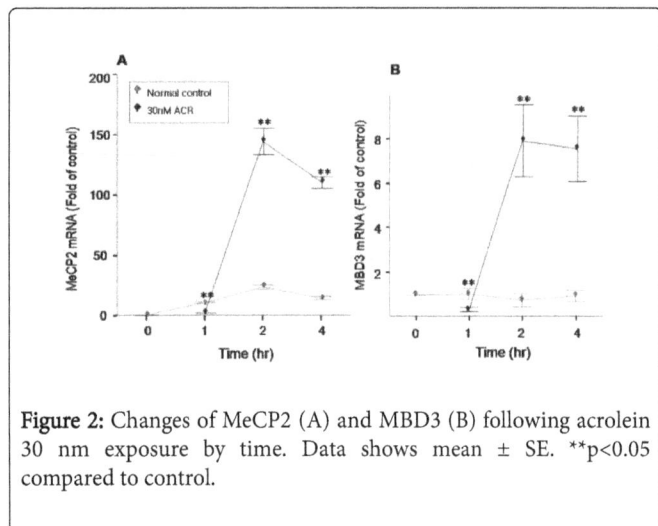

Figure 2: Changes of MeCP2 (A) and MBD3 (B) following acrolein 30 nm exposure by time. Data shows mean ± SE. **p<0.05 compared to control.

Claudin 5 methylation transcript decrease after exposure to acrolein

Claudin 5 methylation was checked by methtyl specific PCR. Claudin 5 methylation transcript/total Claudin 5 transcript was decreased at 1 h, 2 h, and 4 h following acrolein 30 nm exposure (Figure 3).

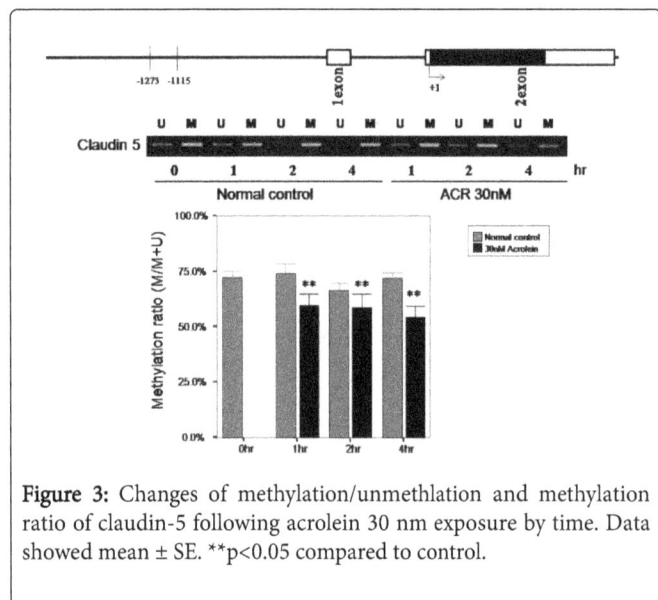

Figure 3: Changes of methylation/unmethlation and methylation ratio of claudin-5 following acrolein 30 nm exposure by time. Data showed mean ± SE. **p<0.05 compared to control.

Discussion

This study adds to novel information that acrolein exposure modify differently epigenetic enzyme by time windows. Acrolein (an α, β-unsaturated 2-alkenal) is highly reactive in biological systems and can be extremely irritating [9-11]. Acrolein levels are elevated in second-hand smoke compared with mainstream smoke because side-stream smoke is generated at lower combustion temperatures [12-14].

Epigenetics refer to inheritable changes beyond DNA sequence that control cell identity and morphology and play key roles in development and cell fate commitments and highly impact the etiology of many human diseases such as respiratory diseases [4]. DNA methylation, histone modification, and miRNAs represent coordinated processes that regulate gene silencing or expression by architectural remodeling of the genome [4].

Epigenetic changes are modulated by environmental exposures such as air pollutants, making epigenetics the interface between genes and environment [4]. With more knowledge about acrolein effect on human effects, it may be the window through which we can control exposures to protect patients from environmental exposure. In our study claudin 5 methylation ratio (methylation/unmethylation plus methylation) was decreased at 1 h, 2 h, and 4 h following acrolein 30 nm exposure indicating that methylation of claudin-5 gene decrease gene expression.

DNA methylation has been shown to be a key contributor to epigenetic regulation of gene expression. Its mechanism of action can be mediated through direct inhibition of transcription factors or DNA interactions modulated by methylation of specific regions of promoters [15-19], recognition of methylated DNA sequences by transcriptional repressors associated with the recruitment of corepressors [20,21], or binding of methylated DNA binding proteins (MBPs) to nucleosomes leading to chromatin compaction, as shown with methyl-CpG-binding protein 2 (MeCP2) [22].

Understanding how the methylome is affected by environmental signals that do not affect methyl donor levels is more challenging. Aging [23], smoking [24,25], and heavy metal exposure [26,27], acrolein [28,29] have all been associated with changes in the DNA methylome, and with changes in DNMT expression, but the mechanisms by which these changes occur are largely unknown. DNA methyltransferases (DNMTs) such as DNMT1, DNMT3A and DNMT3B contribute to various physiologic and pathologic conditions including embryo implantation [30], cytomegalovirus infection [31], radiation [32], cancer, aging, neural cell differentiation [33]. In this study although DNMT3b was increased at 1 h, 2 h, and 4 h, and DNMT1 was not changed compared to control in acrolein 30 nm exposure. Those results suggest that acrolein exposure affect DNMTs enzymes according to acrolein concentration.

MeCP2 (Methyl-CpG-binding protein 2) was the first MBP discovered to selectively recognize and bind methylated DNA sequences [34]. Since the discovery of MeCP2, 4 additional members of the MBP family (MBD1, MBD2, MBD3, and MBD4) have been identified through bioinformatic analysis of the polypeptide sequence of the methylated DNA binding domain (MBD) shared by these proteins [35].

MeCP2 was also the first MBP found to interact with HDAC-containing complexes, linking two epigenetic repression mechanisms: DNA methylation and histone deacetylation [36]. After acrolein 30 nm exposure, MBD3 and MeCP2 were decreased compared to control at 1 h and increased at 2 h and 4 h, indicating that MBD and MeCP2 differently function by time and dose following acrolein exposure.

In conclusion our study demonstrate that acrolein exposure modify MBD 3 and DNMTs and MeCP2 related to epigenetics, suggesting that acrolein contribute to enzyme pathway involved in epigenetic regulation. Further studies will be needed to explain the role of specific gene related to acrolein exposure.

Acknowledgement

This subject is supported by Korea Ministry of Environment (2012001360001) as "The Environmental Health Action Program" and Soonchunhyang University.

References

1. Bein K, Leikauf GD (2011) Acrolein a pulmonary hazard. Mol Nutr Food Res 55: 1342-1360.

2. Jang AS, Concel VJ, Bein K, Brant KA, Liu S, et al. (2011) Endothelial dysfunction and claudin 5 regulation during acrolein-induced lung injury. Am J Respir Cell Mol Biol 44: 483-490.

3. Moretto N, Volpi G, Pastore F, Facchinetti F (2012) Acrolein effects in pulmonary cells: relevance to chronic obstructive pulmonary disease. Ann N Y Acad Sci 1259: 39-46.

4. Pacheco KA (2012) Epigenetics mediate environment: gene effects on occupational sensitization. Curr Opin Allergy Clin Immunol 12: 111-118.

5. North ML, Ellis AK (2011) The role of epigenetics in the developmental origins of allergic disease. Ann Allergy Asthma Immunol 106: 355-361.

6. Klose RJ, Bird AP (2006) Genomic DNA methylation: the mark and its mediators. Trends Biochem Sci 31: 89-97.

7. Liang G, Chan MF, Tomigahara Y, Tsai YC, Gonzales FA, et al. (2002) Cooperativity between DNA methyltransferases in the maintenance methylation of repetitive elements. Mol Cell Biol 22: 480-491.

8. Cookson WO, Moffatt MF (2011) Genetics of complex airway disease. Proc Am Thorac Soc 8: 149-153.

9. Andre E, Campi B, Materazzi S, Trevisani M, Amadesi S, et al. (2008) Cigarette smoke-induced neurogenic inflammation is mediated by alpha,betaunsaturated aldehydes and the TRPA1 receptor in rodents. J Clin Invest 118: 2574-2582.

10. Steinhagen WH, Barrow CS (1984) Sensory irritation structure-activity study of inhaled aldehydes in B6C3F1 and Swiss-Webster mice. Toxicol Appl Pharmacol 72: 495-503.

11. Weber A, Jermini C, Grandjean E (1976) Irritating effects on man of air pollution due to cigarette smoke. Am J Public Health 66: 672-676.

12. Faroon O, Roney N, Taylor J, Ashizawa A, Lumpkin MH, et al. (2008) Acrolein health effects. Toxicol Ind Health 24: 447-490.

13. Leikauf GD (2002) Hazardous air pollutants and asthma. Environ Health Perspect 110: 505-526.

14. Leikauf GD (2009) Formaldehyde and other aldehydes. In: Lippmann M (ed.) Environmental toxicants: human exposures and their health effects. John Wiley and Sons, pp. 257-316.

15. Hashimoto H, Vertino PM, Cheng X (2010) Molecular coupling of DNA methylation and histone methylation. Epigenomics 2: 657-669.

16. Bell AC, Felsenfeld G (2000) Methylation of a CTCF-dependent boundary controls imprinted expression of the Igf2 gene. Nature 405: 482-485.

17. Hark AT, Schoenherr CJ, Katz DJ, Ingram RS, Levorse JM, et al. (2000) CTCF mediates methylation-sensitive enhancer-blocking activity at the H19/Igf2 locus. Nature 405: 486-489.

18. Holmgren C, Kanduri C, Dell G, Ward A, Mukhopadhya R, et al. (2001) CpG methylation regulates the Igf2/H19 insulator. Curr Biol 11: 1128-1130.

19. Szabó PE, Pfeifer GP, Miao F, O'Connor TR, Mann JR (2000) Improved in vivo dimethyl sulfate footprinting using AlkA protein: DNA-protein interactions at the mouse H19 gene promoter in primary embryo fibroblasts. Anal Biochem 283: 112-116.

20. Jones PA, Gonzalgo ML, Tsutsumi M, Bender CM (1998) DNA methylation in bladder cancer. Eur Urol 33: 7-8.

21. Nan X, Ng HH, Johnson CA, Laherty CD, Turner BM, et al. (1998) Transcriptional repression by the methyl-CpG-binding protein MeCP2 involves a histone deacetylase complex. Nature 393: 386-389.

22. Georgel PT, Horowitz-Scherer RA, Adkins N, Woodcock CL, Wade PA, et al. (2003) Chromatin compaction by human MeCP2. Assembly of novel secondary chromatin structures in the absence of DNA methylation. J Biol Chem 278: 32181-32188.

23. Li Y, Liu Y, Strickland FM, Richardson B (2010) Age-dependent decreases in DNA methyltransferase levels and low transmethylation micronutrient levels synergize to promote overexpression of genes implicated in autoimmunity and acute coronary syndromes. Exp Gerontol 45: 312-322.

24. Liu H, Zhou Y, Boggs SE, Belinsky SA, Liu J (2007) Cigarette smoke induces demethylation of prometastatic oncogene synuclein-gamma in lung cancer cells by downregulation of DNMT3B. Oncogene 26: 5900-5910.

25. Zhang S, Zhou M, Jiang G, Gong C, Cui D, et al. (2015) Expression and DNA methylation status of the Rap2B gene in human bronchial epithelial cells treated by cigarette smoke condensate. Inhal Toxicol 27: 502-509.

26. Jiang G, Xu L, Song S, Zhu C, Wu Q, et al. (2008) Effects of long-term low-dose cadmium exposure on genomic DNA methylation in human embryo lung fibroblast cells. Toxicology 244: 49-55.

27. Brown TA, Lee JW, Holian A, Porter V, Fredriksen H, et al. (2015) Alterations in DNA methylation corresponding with lung inflammation and as a biomarker for disease development after MWCNT exposure. Nanotoxicology .

28. Helling BA, Yang IV (2015) Epigenetics in lung fibrosis: from pathobiology to treatment perspective. Curr Opin Pulm Med 21: 454-462.

29. Wang HT, Weng MW, Chen WC, Yobin M, Pan J, et al. (2013) Effect of CpG methylation at different sequence context on acrolein- and BPDE-DNA binding and mutagenesis. Carcinogenesis 34: 220-227.

30. Ding YB, He JL, Liu XQ, Chen XM, Long CL, et al. (2012) Expression of DNA methyltransferases in the mouse uterus during early pregnancy and susceptibility to dietary folate deficiency. Reproduction 144: 91-100.

31. Esteki-Zadeh A, Karimi M, Straat K, Ammerpohl O, Zeitelhofer M, et al. (2012) Human cytomegalovirus infection is sensitive to the host cell DNA methylation state and alters global DNA methylation capacity. Epigenetics 7: 585-93.

32. Armstrong CA, Jones GD, Anderson R, Iyer P, Narayanan D, et al. (2012) DNMTs are required for delayed genome instability caused by radiation. Epigenetics 7: 892-902.

33. Liu L, van Groen T, Kadish I, Li Y, Wang D, et al. (2011) Insufficient DNA methylation affects healthy aging and promotes age-related health problems. Clin Epigenetics 2: 349-360.

34. Lewis JD, Meehan RR, Henzel WJ, Maurer-Fogy I, Jeppesen P, et al. (1992) Purification, sequence, and cellular localization of a novel chromosomal protein that binds to methylated DNA. Cell 69: 905-914.

35. Hendrich B, Bird A (1998) Identification and characterization of a family of mammalian methyl-CpG binding proteins. Mol Cell Biol 18: 6538-6547.

36. Nan X, Ng HH, Johnson CA, Laherty CD, Turner BM, et al. (1998) Transcriptional repression by the methyl-CpG-binding protein MeCP2 involves a histone deacetylase complex. Nature 393: 386-389.

3

Clinical Analysis in Chronic Alcoholic Encephalopathy: A Retrospective Study of 43 Subjects

Honghong Li, Lei He, Shuwei Qiu, Yi Li and Ying Peng*

Department of Neurology, Sun Yat-Sen Memorial Hospital, Sun Yat-Sen University, Guangzhou 510120, China

*Corresponding author: Ying Peng, M.D., Ph.D., Professor, Department of Neurology, Sun Yat-Sen Memorial Hospital, Sun Yat-Sen University, Guangzhou, China, Email: 2353352460@qq.com

Abstract

Background and purpose: Chronic alcoholic encephalopathy (CAE) refers to the effects of chronic alcohol consumption on cerebral structure and function in human. The diagnosis is frequently missed for its atypical clinical presentation. Here, we performed this retrospective study to analyze clinical manifestations, neuroimaging findings and electroencephalography (EEG) alterations in CAE patients, with the aim to highlight the importance of recognition or diagnosis of CAE.

Patients and methods: We analyzed the clinical manifestations, neuroimaging findings and EEG alterations of 43 patients (42 males and 1 female) with CAE diagnosed in Sun-Yat Sen Memory Hospital, Guangzhou from 1998 to 2013.

Results: Mental impairment (25.58%), limbs tremor (25.58%), and dizziness (25.58%) were the most frequent clinical manifestations. Other less common presentations including memory impairment (16.28%), ataxia (13.95%), dysarthria (13.95%), consciousness disturbance (11.63%), epileptic seizure (11.63%), ocular motor dysfunction (0.11%), dementia (0.11%), and headache (0.05%) were also observed. Neuroimaging findings showed brain atrophy, ischemia, and demyelinated changes. Among 14 patients who undertwent EEG examination, diffuse slow wave or theta rhythm (3-4 Hz, 10-40 uV) was found in 10 patients. Most patients with CAE showed good response to abstinence and vitamin B supplement.

Conclusion: For the alcoholic patients, detailed medical history and close follow-up with MRI scan and EEG are valuable tools to detect CAE. Abstinence combined with vitamin B supplement usually obtain a gratifying clinical improvement.

Keywords Alcoholic encephalopathy; Manifestation; Magnetic resonance imaging; Electroencephalography

Introduction

Alcoholism is an addictve disorder due to excessive consumption of alcohol. Frequent concomitants of alcoholism are liver disease, including hepatitis, steatosis and cirrhosis [1]. Chronic alcoholic encephalopathy (CAE) refers to the effects of chronic alcohol consumption on cerebral structure and function in human. The extent of injury to the brain and effects of alcohol abuse vary from person to person. CAE is associated with several risk factors, such as direct toxicity of alcohol, malnutrition, thiamine deficiency and family history of alcoholism [2].

Alcoholic encephalopathy covers a wide range of alcohol related intellectual and neurological syndrome, including Wernicke's encephalopathy (WE), Korsakoff's syndrome (KS), alcohol demetia, and other disorders affecting many structures in the brain [3]. WE is an acute neuropsychiatric syndrome associated with thiamine deficiency due to chronic alcoholism [3]. This disorder is characterized by a classical clinical triad of ocular motor dysfunction, ataxia (cerebellar dysfunction), and mental impairment [4]. However, the classical presentation of the syndrome is rare. Incidence rates of WE in patients with alcoholism can be as high as 12.5%, but noly 0.1-2.8% in general population [5]. KS, developed from undiagnosed and untreated WE, is a typically permanent neurological disorder characterized by anterograde amnesia [6].

Though chronic alcoholic encephalopathy is an effectivelly preventable and treatable disease, we often missed the diagnosis in daily medical practice for its atypical clinical manifestations. Hence, we carried out this retrospective study to analyze clinical manifestations, neuroimaging findings and electroencephalography (EEG) alterations, with the aim to highlight the importance of recognition, diagnosis and management of CAE (Table 1).

Methods

This retrospective study was approved by the Ethical committee of the Sun Yat-Sen Memory Hospitan, Sun Yat-Sen University. The study comprised 43 CAE patients, who were admitted to Sun-Yat Sen Memory Hospital of Sun-Yat Sen University between 1998 and 2013. We excluded patients with acute alcoholism or peripheral neuropathy due to chronic alcoholism. Diagnosis of CAE was based on the patient's detailed history, clinical presentation, neuroimaging and EEG alterations. After identification of patients, clinical and neuroimaging features, EEG alterations and treatment were collected. All diagnosed patients were educated to quit alcohol and treated with vitamin B.

Results

Individual characteristics

The study consisted of 42 males and 1 female with the age rangeing from 29 to 73 years. Thirty one patients had received MRI/CT examination, and 14 patients underwent EEG examination. Abdominal color Doppler ultrasound was performed in 15 patients.

Clinical characteristics

Various clinical manifestations were found in patients with CAE, which were summarized in Figure 1. Mental impairment (25.58%), limbs tremor (25.58%), and dizziness (25.58%) were the most frequent clinical manifestations. Other less common presentations including memory impairment (16.28%), ataxia (13.95%), dysarthria (13.95%), consciousness disturbance (11.63%), epileptic seizure (11.63%), ocular motor dysfunction (0.11%), dementia (0.11%), and headache (0.05%) were also observed. Fifteen patients underwent abdominal color Doppler ultrasound examination, and hepatic steatosis were found in 12 cases.

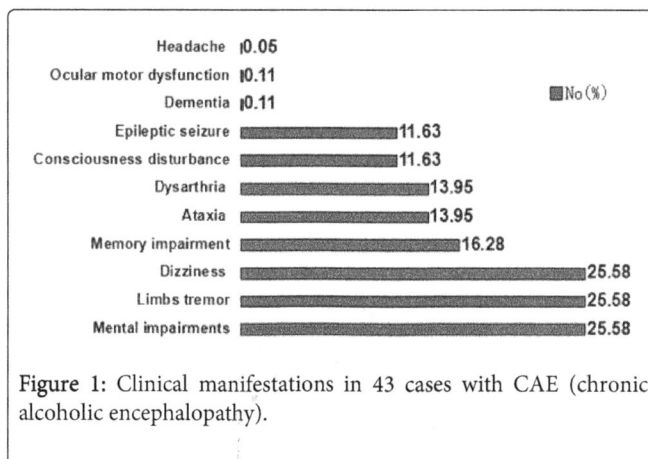

Figure 1: Clinical manifestations in 43 cases with CAE (chronic alcoholic encephalopathy).

Clinical signs	Number of patients	No (%)
Ocular motor dysfunction	2	0.11
Ataxia	6	13.95
Mental impairments	11	25.58
Dementia	2	0.11
Memory impairment	7	16.28
Consciousness disturbance	5	11.63
Limbs tremor	11	25.58
Epileptic seizure	5	11.63
Dysarthria	6	13.95
Dizzy	11	25.58
Headache	1	0.05

Table 1: Clinical signs of the CAE in 43 diagnosed cases.

Neuroimaging features

Nine cases of the 43 CAE patients received brain CT examination. Ischemic lesions in white matter were observed in four patients, as well as brain atrophy in one patient. As CT is not sensitive to the early change of brain, especially demyelinated change, so we mainly focus on MRI findings. Twenty two patients underwent MRI examination. Eleven patients showed ischemic lesions on corpus callosum, fornices, and frontal-parietal cortex. Cortical volume deficits and expanded ventricle were found in nine patients (Figure 2). Three patients showed remarkable demyelinated changes (Figure 3). Hypointensity on T1-weighted images (T1WI), and hyperintensity on T2-weighted images (T2WI) and fluid-attenuated inversion recovery (FLAIR) images were found in bilateral basal ganglia, insular lobes, right-side frontal lobe and temporal lobe.

EEG

EEG were performed in 14 cases. Abnormal EEG record were found in ten patients, including diffuse slow wave and theta rhythm (3-4Hz, 10-40uV) in the background rhythm of EEG (Figure 4).

Treatment

All cases accepted abstinence and vitamin B supplement. Patients were divided into four categories according to the curative effects. The main symptoms and signs disappeared by more than 85%, 60%, and 30%, were respectively classified as cure, marked improvement and slight improvement. No improvement was considered when the disappeared symptoms and signs were less than 30%. Among the outcome of the 43 CAE patients, 23.26% patients had been totally cured, 25.58% clinical manifestations had been markedly improved, 41.86% had been only slightly improved, and 9.30% of the cases had no improvements.

Discussion

Alcohol can cause a spectrum of structural and functional change in the brain, including shrinkage and sometimes permanent death cells. The brain structures most vulnerable to the effects of alcoholism are neocortex, limbic system, and the cerebellum [7]. The molecular basis is still not clear. Peng Ying found decreased expression of several neural genes (xPax6, xOtx2, xSox3, xSox2, and xNCAM) in alcohol-induced microcephaly [8]. In addition, alcohol could interfere with the thiamine absorption, which may contribute to the acute neurological disorder WE. WE may lead to Kosakoff's syndrome (KS), a severe neurological disorder characterized by anterograde amnesia [9]. As clinical manifestations are often atypical, the neuroimaging and electrophysiology play an important role in the detection of CAE. Hence, we analyzed the characteristics of CAE with the aim to improve the diagnosis and management of this disease.

The present study showed variability in clinical features of CAE. The most frequent clinical manifestations in patients with CAE were mental impairment, limbs tremor, and dizziness. However, mental impairment was rarely observed in Pitel's study [10], and ataxia of gait was more common in Damsgaard's study [11]. Patients with mental impairment were usually misdiagnosed as psychosis. Thus, clinicians should attach more importance to detailed history of alcoholism and some assistant examination. Most studies were focused on WE [11-14], however, not all patients with WE have classical triad syndrome. Similarly, not all KS patients exhibit permanent amnesia [15]. When the presentations limited clinical assessment, the diagnosis can be made from the history, CT/MRI findings, EEG, as well as a good response to thiamine supplement.

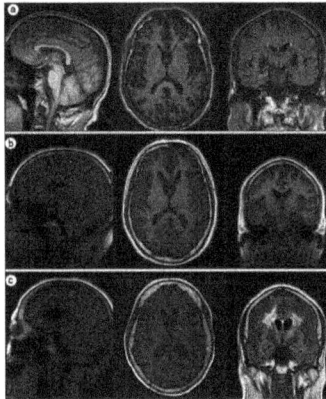

Figure 2: Brain-volume deficits in alcoholism and its sequelae. Sagital (left column), axial (middle column) and coronal (right column) brain T1-weighted MRI are shown. (a) a 65-year-old healthy control male, (b) a 64-year-old man with alcoholism, and c. a 50-year-old man with alcoholism. Enlargement of the ventricles (b, c) can be observed compared with the healthy control (a), which indicating shrinkage of the surrounding tissue. Leukoaralosis around the ventricles can be observed in picture c The abnormal signal around the ventricles (c) was leukoaralosis.

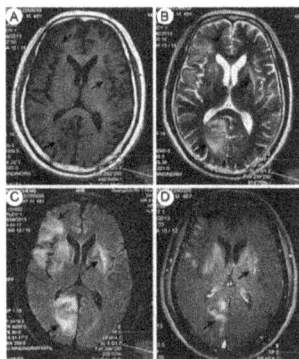

Figure 3: Demyelinated changes and its sequelae in a 50-year-old man with alcoholism. Hypointensity (arrow) on T1-weighted images (A), and hyperintensity (arrow) on T2-weighted images (B), fluid-attenuated inversion recovery (C) images, and post-contrast T1 (D) can be observed in bilateral basal ganglia, insular lobes, right-side frontal lobe and temporal lobe.

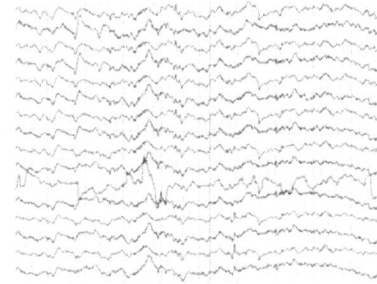

Figure 4: Abnormal EEG record in a 70-year-old with CAE. Theta rhythm (3-4 Hz, 10-40 uV) can be observed in EEG record.

Abstinence and vitamin B supplement are the key to the treatment. It can be explained by the fact that alcohol related brain damage is partialy reversible [9]. Most patients were good respond to treatment with abstinence and vitamin B. About 23% of the 43 patients obtained well recovery, and 90% received mild to moderate improvement in our study. In addition, eliminating the oxide and free radicals also exert valuable role in CAE. Because metabolites induced by ethanol can lead to oxidative damage [16,17]. Reports showed that oxidative and nitrosative stresses can contribute to alcohol-induced fetal ocular injury [18-20].

The CT and MRI have enabled more detailed insights into brain structure and function. The European Federation National Societies (EFNS) recommend MRI to support the diagnosis of WE in the published Guidelines for diagnosis, therapy and prevention of WE [21]. In our study, hypointensity on T1WI, and hyperintensity on T2WI, FLAIR images, and post-contrast T1 were observed in some cases (Figure 3). Cortical volume deficits and expanded ventricle were found in nine patients (Figure 2). These findings were consistent with the early studies [22,23]. Chronic alcohol abuse causes gross morphological change and result in individual differences in gray matter density or volume [24]. This is probably due to that gray matter is more heavily vascularied than white matter in brain [25]. Furthermore, eleven patients' MRI showed ischemic lesions in bilateral basal ganglia, insular lobes, right-side frontal lobe and temporal lobe. Because excessive alcohol might lead to stroke via reduction of cerebral blood flow and induction of cardiac arrthythmias and cerebral embolism [26].

EEG provides a noninvasive measure of brain function by recording the electrical signals from the brain. Report showed that the EEG record is different in alcoholics and nonalcoholics [27]. Fourteen cases underwent EEG examination in this study. Diffuse slow wave or theta rhythm (3-4 Hz, 10-40 uV) was found in 10 patients (Figure 4). These abnormalities were consistent with Rangaswamy's study [26], which implied decreased cognitive activity and the imbalance of excitatory and inhibitory neurons in the cortex [27]. Therefore, EEG is a valuable assistant examination to support the diagnosis of CAE.

Limitations of the study

The main limitation of our study is its retrospective design and the data have been collected during a 15-year period. In addition, some patients with CAE may not have been identified due to the absence of predefined criteria and atypical clinical characteristics. However, in spite of this limitation, we have still collected enough information to allow meaningful analysis of the clinical characteristics with CAE patients.

Conclusion

CAE are life-threatening conditions with atypical neurological presentation. The clinical diagnosis of CAE and even WE can be difficult to make, and many cases of this conditions have been missed. As shown in this paper, the most common clinical manifestations in patients with CAE were mental impairments, limbs tremor, and dizziness. These clinical signs are abnormal in some other central nervous systemic disease and even other systemic disorders. Therefore, clinicians must maintain a high index of suspicion in order to make the early diagnosis of CAE, and large dose of vitamin B should be given. Furthermore, MRI and EEG are valuable tools for the diagnosis. Patients with CAE were usually finely responsed to treatment with abstinence and vitamin B supplementation. In addition, public education program should be recommended to help alcoholic individuals to recognize that components of the structural and functional changes associated with alcoholism are partially reversible after several weeks of abstinence [27].

References

1. Lieber CS (2004) Alcoholic fatty liver: its pathogenesis and mechanism of progression to inflammation and fibrosis. Alcohol 34: 9-19.

2. Pessione F, Gerchstein JL, Rueff B (1995) Parental history of alcoholism: a risk factor for alcohol-related peripheral neuropathies. Alcohol Alcohol 30: 749-754.

3. Schmidt KS, Gallo JL, Ferri C, Giovannetti T, Sestito N, et al. (2005) The neuropsychological profile of alcohol-related dementia suggests cortical and subcortical pathology. Dement Geriatr Cogn Disord 20: 286-291.

4. Zahr NM, Kaufman KL, Harper CG (2011) Clinical and pathological features of alcohol-related brain damage. Nat Rev Neurol 7: 284-294.

5. Harper C (2006) Thiamine (vitamin B1) deficiency and associated brain damage is still common throughout the world and prevention is simple and safe! Eur J Neurol 13: 1078-1082.

6. Butters N, (1981) The Wernicke-Korsakoff syndrome: a review of psychological, neuropathological and etiological factors. Curr Alcohol 8: 205-232.

7. Peng Y, Yang PH, Ng SS, Wong OG, Liu J, et al. (2004) A critical role of Pax6 in alcohol-induced fetal microcephaly. Neurobiol Dis 16: 370-376.

8. Pitel AL (2011) Signs of preclinical Wernicke's encephalopathy and thiamine levels as predictors of neuropsychological deficits in alcoholism without Korsakoff's syndrome. Neuropsychopharmacology 36: 580-588.

9. Damsgaard L, Ulrichsen J, Nielsen MK (2010) Wernicke's encephalopathy in patients with alcohol withdrawal symptoms. Ugeskr Laeger 172: 2054-2058.

10. Lough ME (2012) Wernicke's encephalopathy: expanding the diagnostic toolbox. Neuropsychol Rev 22: 181-194.

11. Thomson AD, Marshall EJ, Bell D (2013) Time to act on the inadequate management of Wernicke's encephalopathy in the UK. Alcohol Alcohol 48: 4-8.

12. Nilsson M, Sonne C (2013) [Diagnostics and treatment of Wernicke-Korsakoff syndrome patients with an alcohol abuse]. Ugeskr Laeger 175: 942-944.

13. Nakamura K, Iwahashi K, Furukawa A, Ameno K, Kinoshita H, et al. (2003) Acetaldehyde adducts in the brain of alcoholics. Arch Toxicol 77: 591-593.

14. Alcohol's effects on brain and behaviour.

15. Bora PS, Lange LG (1993) Molecular mechanism of ethanol metabolism by human brain to fatty acid ethyl esters. Alcohol Clin Exp Res 17: 28-30.

16. Peng Y, Yang PH, Guo Y, Ng SS, Liu J, et al. (2004) Catalase and peroxiredoxin 5 protect Xenopus embryos against alcohol-induced ocular anomalies. Invest Ophthalmol Vis Sci 45: 23-29.

17. Peng Y, Kwok KH, Yang PH, Ng SS, Liu J, et al. (2005) Ascorbic acid inhibits ROS production, NF-kappa B activation and prevents ethanol-induced growth retardation and microencephaly. Neuropharmacology 48: 426-434.

18. Peng Y, Yang PH, Ng SS, Lum CT, Kung HF, et al. (2004) Protection of Xenopus laevis embryos against alcohol-induced delayed gut maturation and growth retardation by peroxiredoxin 5 and catalase. J Mol Biol 340: 819-827.

19. Galvin R, Bråthen G, Ivashynka A, Hillbom M, Tanasescu R, et al. (2010) EFNS guidelines for diagnosis, therapy and prevention of Wernicke encephalopathy. Eur J Neurol 17: 1408-1418.

20. Zuccoli G, Siddiqui N, Cravo I, Bailey A, Gallucci M, et al. (2010) Neuroimaging findings in alcohol-related encephalopathies. AJR Am J Roentgenol 195: 1378-1384.

21. Jernigan TL, Butters N, DiTraglia G, Schafer K, Smith T, et al. (1991) Reduced cerebral grey matter observed in alcoholics using magnetic resonance imaging. Alcohol Clin Exp Res 15: 418-427.

22. Estruch R, Nicolás JM, Salamero M, Aragón C, Sacanella E, et al. (1997) Atrophy of the corpus callosum in chronic alcoholism. J Neurol Sci 146: 145-151.

23. Srivastava V, Buzas B, Momenan R, Oroszi G, Pulay AJ, et al. (2010) Association of SOD a mitochondrial antioxidant enzyme, with gray matter volume shrinkage in alcoholics. Neuropsychopharmacology 35: 1120-1128.

24. Kim SG, Ogawa S (2012) Biophysical and physiological origins of blood oxygenation level-dependent fMRI signals. J Cereb Blood Flow Metab 32: 1188-1206.

25. Gorelick PB (1987) Alcohol and stroke. Stroke 18: 268-271.

26. Porjesz B Begleiter H (2003) Alcoholism and human electrophysiology. Alcohol Res Health 27: 153-160.

27. Rangaswamy M, Porjesz B, Chorlian DB, Choi K, Jones KA, et al. (2003) Theta power in the EEG of alcoholics. Alcohol Clin Exp Res 27: 607-615.

4

Comparative Analysis of Heavy Metal Profile of *Brassica campestris* (L.) and *Raphanus sativus* (L.) Irrigated with Municipal Waste Water of Sargodha City

Imran Khan[1*], **Abdul Ghani**[2], **Abd-Ur-Rehman**[1], **Samrah Afzal Awan**[1], **Attia Noreen**[2] and **Imran Khalid**[2]

[1]*Department of Botany, PMAS-Arid Agriculture University, Rawalpindi, Pakistan*

[2]*Department of Botany, University of Sargodha, Sargodha, Pakistan*

*Corresponding author: Imran Khan, Department of Botany, PMAS-Arid Agriculture University, Rawalpindi, Pakistan, E-mail: Friendsstrength4@gmail.com

Abstract

The recent study was carried out for the comparative analysis of heavy metals in *Brassica campestris* and *Raphanus sativus* irrigated with municipal waste water of Sargodha city. Field surveys were done for this experiment. Three experimental sites i.e Bhalwal road, Ajnala road and Faisalabad road were selected in Sargodha city for field surveys. Vegetables samples were collected from these sites which were grown in municipal waste water. These Samples were used for the analytical comparison of heavy metals i.e Copper, Chromium, Lead, Cadmium, Nickel, Zinc, Cobalt, Arsenic, Manganese, Iron, Magnesium and Molybdenum, accumulated in *Brassica campestris* and *Raphanus sativus* at three life stages.

Keywords: Comparative; Municipal; Chromium; Arsenic; Accumulated

Introduction

There is water shortage in the country and farmers use waste water to irrigate their vegetable fields. These irrigation practices give very good crop yields because waste water contains large amounts of organic material and some inorganic elements essential for plant growth. But it may also contain large amounts of non-essential heavy metals which can be transferred to animal and human beings through food chain [1].

Pakistan is an agrarian country of Southeast Asia. Increased urbanization and industrialization have resulted in discharge of effluents of toxic nature, polluting the water bodies and making them unfit for consumption in agriculture sector [2].

Heavy metals are generally present in agricultural soils at low levels but due to their cumulative behavior and toxicity they have potential hazardous effects on plants and human health [3].The main problem is increasing amount of heavy metals in our environment by industrialization use of fertilizers in agricultural and domestic activities, this leads harmful effects on the human beings and ecosystem [4].

Farmers use wastewater for irrigation with an objective of being a rich source of nutrient and economically sufficient, as it saves a lot of fertilizer costs [5] particularly in agricultural lands located near cities or in the vicinity of an industrial area [1].

Continuous irrigation with wastewater could lead to the accumulation of heavy metals in soils beyond crop tolerance levels [6]. The uptake of metals from the soil depends on different factors such as their soluble content in it, soil pH, plant growth stages types of species, fertilizers and soil [7]. Consequently, the usage of wastewater for irrigation ends to soil contamination and heavy metals accumulation both in soil and crops [8,9].

Uptake of trace metals from soil differs from plant to plant and from site to site. Thus, there is need of careful studies in order to fully analyze and understand the long term environmental impacts of the use of sewage water for crop irrigation [10]. The impact of anthropogenic activities on urban and suburban soil has also increased. The original structure and properties of soil have been deeply modified, and new soils with particular characteristics, have been created [11].

Waste water has deleterious effects on soil and it cannot be properly used for agricultural practices due to salinity and sodicity problems which impose harmful effects on seedlings of plants [12]. Most of the leafy vegetables which were grown in contaminated soil accumulate higher amount of heavy metals in their leaves [13].

Plants grown in contaminated soils or irrigated with municipal wastewater when consumed by people can result in health problems like diarrhea, mental retardation, liver and kidney damage [14]. The practice of using industrial and sewage wastewater has become common to irrigate fields in countries which are developing [15-18].

The widespread heavy metal contamination has raised public and scientific interest hence special attention is given to them throughout the world due to their effects even at very low concentrations [19]. Industrial and domestic liquid wastes are frequently channeled either into the same sewerage system (if a sewerage system exists) or into the same open drains. The number and types of livestock the household owns will influence the type of wastewater-related activities in which they engage [20].

Dietary intake of heavy metals through contaminated vegetables may cause various diseases. Heavy metal concentrations such as Cd, Cu, Zn and Pb in surface soils have been a focus of investigation over the past decade [21].

The aim of this research work is to investigate the heavy metal profile of *Brassica campestris* and *Raphanus sativus* irrigated with municipal wastewater of Sargodha city.

Materials and Methods

Collection of samples

The vegetables (*Brassica campestris* and *Raphanus sativus*) samples were randomly collected from the fields irrigated with municipal wastewater of Sargodha city at three growth stages (seedling, vegetative and maturity stages). Leafy vegetables were preferred for sampling because previous researches indicate that they accumulate heavy metals at a greater capacity than other vegetables [13].

Study area

Three different sites were selected to determine the sewage water effects on vegetables

i) Bhalwal road, ii) Ajnala road, iii) Faisalabad road

Washing of samples

The collected vegetable samples were washed with distilled water to remove dust particles. The samples were then cut to separate the roots/stems and leaves. After washing the fresh weight of samples were taken and then places in an oven at 100°C for one week to dry samples. When samples dried these were ground into fine powder, stored and used for acidic digestion.

Preparation of samples/Wet digestion

Samples (0.2 g) of leaves of each vegetable were weighed on electric balance and treated with 10 ml of concentrated HNO_3. A sample was prepared applying 10 ml of HNO_3 into empty digestion flask. The flasks were kept for a night at room temperature.

After that the samples were digested against 2 ml H_2O_2 on Hot plate. H_2O_2 was further added to the sample (2 ml of each was added occasionally) and digestion continued until a colorless solution was obtained.

After cooling, the solution was filtered with Whatman No. 42 filter paper and it was then transferred quantitatively to a 50 ml volumetric flask by adding distilled water up to 50 ml volume. Soil digestion was also carried out in the same way as above. Water was filtered and then subjected to analysis.

Preparation of standards and analysis of samples

Working standard solutions of Lead (Pb), Copper (Cu), Chromium (Cr), Zinc (Zn), Cadmium (Cd), Iron(Fe), Arsenic (As), Cobalt (Co), Aluminum (Al), Mercury (Hg),Manganese (Mn), Nickel (Ni), Magnesium (Mg) and Molybdenum (Mo) were prepared from the stock standard solutions containing 1000 ppm of element and measurement of elements were done on atomic absorption spectrophotometer.

The calibration curves were prepared for each element individually applying linear correlation by least square method. A blank reading was also taken and necessary correction was made during the calculation of concentration of various elements.

Statistical analysis

Three samples of leaves of each vegetable were analyzed individually. Data were reported as significant and non-significant.

One way SPSS analysis of variance (ANOVA) was used to determine significant difference between groups (Tables 1 and 2).

Parameters	Seedling stage	Vegetative stage	Maturity stage
Mn	0.000***	0.000***	0.000***
Fe	0.000***	0.000***	0.000***
Cd	0.000***	0.000***	0.001**
Co	0.003**	0.003**	0.000***
Zn	0.001***	0.004***	0.006***
Ni	0.001**	0.003**	0.003**
Mg	0.003**	0.000***	0.004**
Cu	0.000***	0.004**	0.008**
Cr	0.001**	0.000***	0.006**
Pb	0.000***	0.002**	0.002**
As	0.000***	0.000***	0.000***
Hg	0.000***	0.000***	0.000***
Mo	0.001**	0.000***	0.000***
Al	0.000***	0.000***	0.001**

Table 1: Heavy metal profile of *Brassica campestris* at three growth stages. The table shows p-values, results are significant at (p<0.05-P<0.001), where *=0.05, **=0.01 and ***=0.001.

Parameters	Seedling stage	Vegetative stage	Maturity stage
Mn	0.000***	0.000***	0.000***
Fe	0.000***	0.000***	0.000***
Cd	0.000***	0.002***	0.004***
Co	0.000***	0.000***	0.000***
Zn	0.002***	0.003***	0.004***
Ni	0.000***	0.001**	0.002**
Mg	0.000***	0.000***	0.000***
Cu	0.123	0.000***	0.000***
Cr	0.000***	0.000***	0.000***
Pb	0.000***	0.000***	0.000***
As	0.000***	0.000***	0.000***
Hg	0.000***	0.000***	0.000***
Mo	0.123	0.001**	0.000***
Al	0.000***	0.000***	0.000***

Table 2: Heavy metal profile of *Raphanus sativus* at three growth stages. The table shows p-values, results are significant at (p<0.05-P<0.001), where *=0.05, **=0.01 and ***=0.001

Results and Discussion

The surveyed data showed variation in heavy metals concentrations of different water sources, soil and vegetable samples. All the sewage water samples by which vegetables were irrigated showed the safe limits of heavy metals accumulation. The field experimental data showed that due to sewage application, Zn content was much higher in leaves of *Brassica campestris* ranging from 0.001 to 0.006 mg.Kg^{-1}. Cadmium accumulation in the vegetables irrigated with sewage water was also much higher ranging from 0.001 to 0.004 mg.Kg^{-1}. Nickel also showed the similar trend for its accumulation in the vegetables ranging from 0.001 to 0.002 mg.Kg^{-1}.

Rests of the elements are not toxic to human unless they are present in high concentrations. The present study provides baseline data on trace metal concentrations of Lead (Pb), Copper (Cu), Chromium (Cr), Zinc (Zn), Cadmium (Cd), Iron (Fe), Arsenic (As), Cobalt (Co), Aluminum (Al), Mercury (Hg),Manganese (Mn), Nickel (Ni), Magnesium (Mg), and Molybdenum (Mo), in *Brassica campestris* and *Raphanus sativus*, their proximate analysis and nutritional composition (Figure 1).

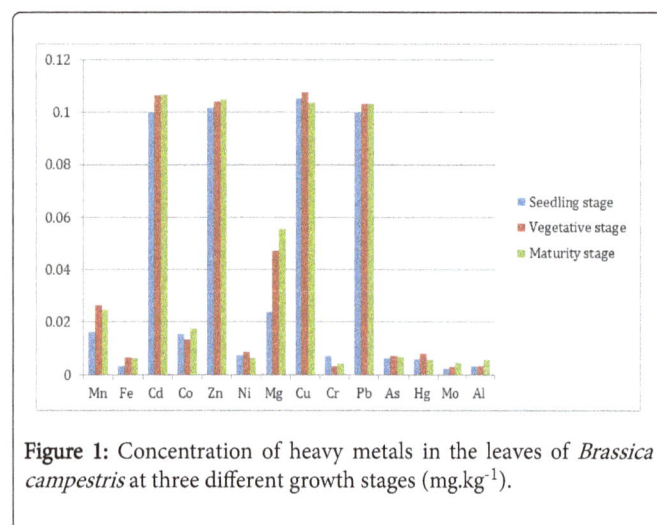

Figure 1: Concentration of heavy metals in the leaves of *Brassica campestris* at three different growth stages (mg.kg^{-1}).

Manganese (Mn) Concentration was maximum at vegetative stage and minimum concentration was examined at initial stage of *Brassica campestris*. Iron (Fe) concentration in *Brassica campestris* was minimum in seedling stage but nearly equal at vegetative and maturity stage. Cadmium (Cd) concentration in *Brassica campestris* was maximum at maturity stage but minimum at seedling stage. Cobalt (Co) concentration in *Brassica campestris* leaves was maximum at maturity stage and minimum at vegetative stage. Zinc (Zn) concentration in *Brassica campestris* leaves was in order as maturity>vegetative>seedling. Nickel (Ni) concentration in *Brassica campestris* was maximum at vegetative stage but minimum at maturity stage. Magnesium (Mg) concentration in *Brassica campestris* leaves was in order as maturity>vegetative>seedling. Copper (Cu) concentration in *Brassica campestris* was maximum at vegetative stage but minimum at final stage. Chromium (Cr) concentration in *Brassica campestris* leaves was maximum at seedling stage but minimum at vegetative stage. Lead (Pb) concentration in *Brassica campestris* leaves were minimum at seedling stage and almost equal at vegetative and maturity stage. Arsenic (As) concentration in *Brassica campestris* leaves was maximum at vegetative stage and minimum at seedling stage.

Mercury (Hg) concentration in *Brassica campestris* was maximum at vegetative stage but minimum at maturity stage. Molybdenum (Mo) concentration in *Brassica campestris* leaves was in order as maturity>vegetative>seedling. Aluminium (Al) Concentration was maximum at maturity stage but nearly equal at seedling and vegetative stage.

Mostly higher concentration was examined at maturity stage which may be due to Bioaccumulation or Biomagnification. These results are in accordance with results of [22]. Some of these metals are even not essential for plant growth and after accumulating in the soil could be transferred to food chain (Figure 2).

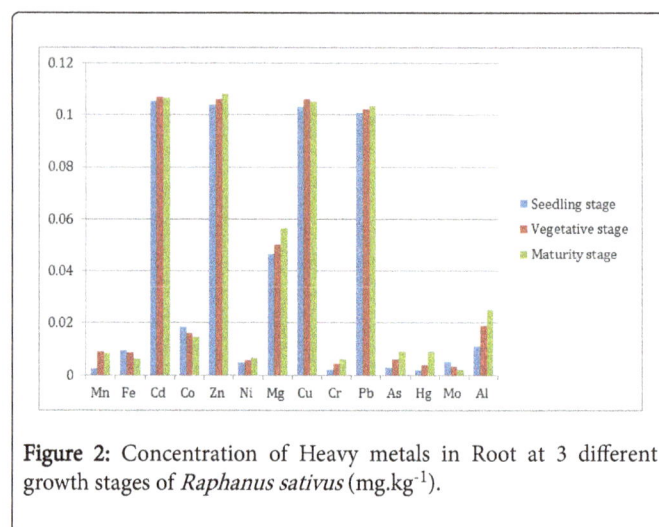

Figure 2: Concentration of Heavy metals in Root at 3 different growth stages of *Raphanus sativus* (mg.kg^{-1}).

Concentration of Mn was maximum at vegetative stage and minimum concentration was examined at initial stage. Fe concentration in *Raphanus sativus* was maximum at seedling stage but minimum at final stage. Cd concentration in *Raphanus sativus* was maximum at maturity stage but minimum at seedling stage. Co concentration in *Raphanus sativus* leaves was maximum at seedling stage and minimum at final stage. Zn concentration in *Raphanus sativus* leaves was in order as final>middle>initial. Ni concentration in *Raphanus sativus* was maximum at maturity stage but minimum at seedling stage and intermediate at middle stage. Mg concentration in *Raphanus sativus* leaves was in order as middle>final>initial. Cu concentration in *Raphanus sativus* was maximum at vegetative stage but minimum at initial stage. Cr concentration in *Raphanus sativus* leaves was minimum at initial stage but maximum at maturity stage. Pb concentration in *Raphanus sativus* leaves was in order as maturity>vegetative>seedling. As concentration in *Raphanus sativus* leaves was in order as maturity>vegetative>seedling. Hg concentration in *Raphanus sativus* was maximum at maturity stage but minimum at seedling stage. Mo concentration in *Raphanus sativus* leaves was in order as seedling> vegetative>maturity. Al Concentration was maximum at maturity stage and minimum concentration was examined at seedling stage.

Concentrations of metals vary greatly at three different stages of studied vegetables. Same results were reported by Y. Latif [23]. Soils irrigated with wastewater had higher concentrations of metals as compared to canal or underground water/other sources. However, the concentration of metals varied with soil texture, depth and concentration of metals in polluted water [23].

Conclusion

The survey data revealed variation in heavy metals concentrations of different water sources. All water samples in sewage water irrigated vegetables were within the safe limits. As comparison the leaves of *Brassica campestris* accumulated higher concentration of heavy metals at three different growth stages while the roots of *Raphanus sativus* have least significant lower concentration of heavy metals. The field experimental data showed that due to sewage application, Zn content was much higher in leaves of *Brassica campestris*. Cadmium accumulation in the vegetables irrigated with sewage water was also much higher. Like all the heavy metals, Nickel also showed the similar trend for its accumulation in the vegetables.

References

1. Murtaza G, Ghafoor A, Qadir M, Owens G, Aziz MA (2010) Disposal and use of sewage on agricultural lands in Pakistan: A review. Pedosphere 20: 23-34.

2. Ahmad K, Ejaz A, Azam M, Khan ZI, Ashraf M (2011) Lead, cadmium and chromium contents of canola irrigated with sewage water. Pakistan journel of Botany 43: 1403-1410.

3. Das P, Samantaray S, Rout GR (1997) Studies on cadmium toxicity in plants: a review. Environ Pollut 98: 29-36.

4. Mataka LM, Henry EMT, Masamba WRL, Sajidu SM (2006) Lead remediation of contaminated water using Moringa Stenopetala and Moringa oleifera seed powder. International Journal of Environmental Science & Technology 3: 131-139.

5. Lone MI, He ZL, Stoffella PJ, Yang XE (2008) Phytoremediation of heavy metal polluted soils and water: progresses and perspectives. J Zhejiang Univ Sci B 9: 210-220.

6. Rusan MJM, Hinnawi S, Rousan L (2007) Long term effect of wastewater irrigation of forage crops on soil and plant quality parameters. Desalination 215: 143-152.

7. Ismail BS, Farihah K, Khairiah J (2005) Bioaccumulation of heavy metals in vegetables from selected agricultural areas. Bull Environ Contam Toxicol 74: 320-327.

8. Bigdeli M, Seilsepour M (2008) Investigation of metals accumulation in some vegetables irrigated with waste water in Shahre Rey-Iran and toxicological implications. American-Eurasian Journal of Agricultural & Environmental Sciences 4: 86-92.

9. Zulfqar S, Wahid A, Farooq M, Maqbool N, Arfan M (2012) Phytoremediation of soil cadmium using Chenopodium species. Pakistan journal of Agricultural sciences. 49: 435-445.

10. Nabulo G, Origa HO, Nasinyama GW, Cole D (2007) Assessment of Zn, Cu, Pb, and Ni contamination in wetland soils and plants in the lake basin. International Journal of Environmental Science and Technology 5: 65-74.

11. Marcotullio PJ, Onishi T (2008) The impact of urbanization on soils. In Land use and soil resources 201-250.

12. Ansari MI, Malik A (2007) Biosorption of nickel and cadmium by metal resistant bacterial isolates from agricultural soil irrigated with industrial wastewater. Bioresour Technol 98: 3149-3153.

13. Al Jassir MS, Shaker A, Khaliq MA (2005) Deposition of heavy metals on green leafy vegetables sold on roadsides of Riyadh City, Saudi Arabia. Bull Environ Contam Toxicol 75: 1020-1027.

14. Uzair M, Ahmad M, Nazim K (2009) Effects of industrial waste on seed bank and growth of wild plants in Dhabeji area, Karachi, Pakistan. Pakistan Journal of Botany, 41: 1659-1665.

15. Kumar Sharma R, Agrawal M, Marshall F (2007) Heavy metal contamination of soil and vegetables in suburban areas of Varanasi, India. Ecotoxicol Environ Saf 66: 258-266.

16. Pandey S, Parvez S, Ansari R A, Ali M, Kaur M (2008) Effects of exposure to multiple trace metals on biochemical, histological and ultrastructural features of gills of a freshwater fish, Channa punctata Bloch. Chemico-biological interactions 174: 183-192.

17. Nath K, Singh D, Shyam S, Sharma YK (2009) Phytotoxic effects of chromium and tannery effluent on growth and metabolism of Phaseolus mungo Roxb. J Environ Biol 30: 227-234.

18. Nagajyothi PC, Dinakar N, Suresh S, Udaykiran Y, Suresh C, et al. (2009) Effect of industrial effluent on the morphological parameters and chlorophyll content of green gram (Phaseolus aureus Roxb). J Environ Biol 30: 385-388.

19. Islam Eu, Yang XE, He ZL, Mahmood Q (2007) Assessing potential dietary toxicity of heavy metals in selected vegetables and food crops. J Zhejiang Univ Sci B 8: 1-13.

20. Buechler S, Devi G (2003) Household food security and wastewater-dependent livelihood activities along the Musi River in Andhra Pradesh, India. Report submitted to the World Health Organization (WHO), Geneva, Switzerland.

21. Tumuklu A, Yalcin M, Sonmez M (2007) Detection of Heavy Metal Concentrations in Soil Caused by Nidge City Garbage Dump. Polish Journal of Environmental Studies 16: 651.

22. Qadir M, Ghafoor A, Hussain SI, Murtaza G, Mahmood T (1999) Copper concentration in city effluents irrigated soils and vegetables. Pakistan Journal Soil Sciences 97-102.

23. Latif MI (2009) Quantitaive assessment of heavy metals in soils and vegetables irrigated with sewage In rawalpindi area.

5

Critical Score as a Predictor for Progression of Tramadol Intoxication

Seham Fouad[1], Nahla Hassan[1], Nabil Nassief[1], Fathia El- Halawany[2] and Rania Hussien[1*]

[1]Department of Forensic Medicine and Clinical Toxicology, Faculty of Medicine, Ain Shams University, Egypt

[2]Statistics Department, Cairo University, Egypt- King Abdulaziz University, Faculty of Science for Girls, Jeddah

*Corresponding author: Rania Hussien, Department of Forensic Medicine and Clinical Toxicology, Faculty of Medicine, Ain Shams University, E-mail: rania_8887@yahoo.com

Abstract

The rate of tramadol abuse in Egypt is becoming disastrous in spite of adding it to the narcotics list by the Egyptian government in the recent years. This study aims to construct a predictive model for acute tramadol intoxicated cases. This study was conducted on tramadol intoxicated patients attending the emergency department of the Poison Control Center (PCC), Ain Shams University hospitals during the period from 1/10/2010 to 30/9/2011. All the patients were subjected to history taking, clinical examination, laboratory investigations, electrocardiography (ECG) and calculation of the APACHE II score. The current study constructs and assesses a new score for prediction of prognosis of tramadol intoxicated patients from clinical and laboratory results obtained from the most predictive parameters affecting the APACHE II score and the most important variables that differentiate best between the studied groups. The area under the ROC curve for the predictive score was 0.996, the best cut-off point was 26 with a sensitivity of 98.46% and specificity of 95.62%.Conclusion: patients with predictive score >26 on admission considered as mild cases while patients with predictive score<26 on admission considered as moderate or severe cases.

Keywords: Critical; Score; Predictor; Progression; Tramadol; Intoxication

Introduction

Tramadol is a widely used, synthetic centrally acting opioid analgesic for the treatment of moderate to severe pain. It has a weak μ-receptor agonist activity that blocks the pain pathways as well as the inhibition of the reuptake of the biogenic amines especially serotonin and norepinephrine in central nervous system [1]. It was approved for marketing as a non controlled analgesic in 1995 under the trade name of Ultram® [2]. Although tramadol was generally considered to be devoid of any serious adverse effects of traditional opioid receptor agonists, such as respiratory depression and drug dependence; recently, abuse and dependence as well as toxicity and deaths have been increasingly reported as it is the only clinically available nonscheduled opioid in most countries [3-5]. Tramadol overdose became one of the most common causes of drug poisoning in the recent years, especially in male young adults with history of substance abuse [6]. Oral route is the most common route of toxicity due to its availability in pharmacies. Toxicity can happen to those who take therapeutic doses of the drug as well as those who abuse it [7,8]. Several deaths have been reported when tramadol was ingested alone in overdose or with others drugs, particularly the central nervous

system (CNS) depressants like benzodiazepine and also in ultrarapid metabolizers. The usual causes of death related to tramadol ingestion include cardiorespiratory depression, refractory shock, asystole and even severe hepatic failure [9-11]. The clinical manifestations of tramadol toxicity can vary from person to person. It depends on many factors including how an individual's body responds to the drug, how much was taken and whether it was taken in combination with any other substances or not [12]. The main signs of tramadol intoxication include seizures which may be followed by extreme drowsiness progressing to coma with respiratory depression, cold clammy skin, cardiac arrest and death [8]. The recently published data have shown an important increase in tramadol poisoning which is still constitutes a major challenge for hospitals and poisoning centers [13]. Standardized diagnostic pathways may be helpful in reducing the risk of false or delayed admissions to the ICU in tramadol intoxicated patients [14].The overall prognosis of patients admitted to ICU directly from emergency departments is better than the prognosis for those admitted to the ICU from general wards and the delayed recognition of critically ill patients increases the risk of cardiopulmonary arrests and death in the intensive care unit (ICU) [15,16]. Patients with intoxication are seen first in the emergency departments (ED) so evaluation of these patients and assessment of their status are mandatory and this needs a good scoring system for analyzing patient status to be beneficial in predicting their prognosis [13].

	Group I (n=73)	Group II (n=64)	Group IIIa (n=56)	Group IIIb (n=9)	F-value	p-value
	M ± SD	M ± SD	M ± SD	M ± SD		
Delay time (hr)	3.44 ± 1.96[a]	3.72 ± 2.18[a]	4.69 ± 0.54[ab]	6.00 ± 1.67[b]	3.115	0.027*

Dosage (mg)	837.67 ± 568.35[a]	1350.78 ± 954.97[a]	1439.29 ± 804.49[a]	2856.25 ± 826.23[b]	10.88	0.000*
Systolic blood pressure (mmHg)	142.05 ± 22.91[b]	134.22 ± 29.64[b]	130.89 ± 31.23[b]	92.50 ± 13.72[a]	7.93	0.000*
Diastolic blood pressure (mmHg)	92.6 ± 14.72[b]	88.13 ± 19.75[b]	86.43 ± 19.39[b]	57.50 ± 9.59[a]	9.07	0.000*
Mean artereial pressure (mmHg)	109.05 ± 17.27[b]	104.16 ± 22.55[b]	101.20 ± 22.95[b]	69.78 ± 23.45[a]	9.24	0.000*
Respiratory rate (breath/minute)	16.74 ± 1.99[b]	17.33 ± 1.92[b]	11.71 ± 5.60[a]	32.11 ± 2.14[c]	49.236	0.000*
Temperature (°C)	37.32 ± 0.29[a]	37.37 ± 0.35[a]	37.34 ± 0.837[a]	38.56 ± 1.45[b]	11.27	0.000*

M: Mean; SD: Standard Deviation

*There is a significant difference by using One Way ANOVA at p<0.05

The same letter means that there is no significant difference between the two groups by using Duncan multiple comparison test at p<0.05

The different letters mean that there is a significant difference between the two groups by using Duncan multiple comparison test at p<0.05

Group I: Patients in Emergency Room (ER) and discharged

Group II: Patients admitted to inpatient unit

Group IIIa: Patients admitted to intensive care unit (ICU) and survived

Group IIIb: Patients admitted to intensive care unit (ICU) and died

Table 1: Comparison between studied groups as regards delay time (hours), dosage of tramadol taken (mg) and vital data.

Material and Methods

This prospective study was conducted on tramadol intoxicated patients attending the emergency department of the Poison Control Center (PCC), Ain Shams University hospitals during the period from 1/10/2010 to 30/9/2011. An informed consent was obtained from each patient or from his/her relatives for inclusion in the study.

ABG	Group I (n=73)	Group II (n=64)	Group IIIa (n=56)	Group IIIb (n=9)	F-value	p-value
	M ± SD	M ± SD	M ± SD	M ± SD		
pH	7.39 ± 0.03[d]	7.29 ± 0.06[c]	7.19 ± 0.19[b]	7.11 ± 0.20[a]	40.59	0.000*
PaCO₂ (mmHg)	38.69±0.04[a]	40.9 ± 10.14[a]	44.20 ± 13.69[a]	57.00 ± 12.93[b]	10.45	0.000*
HCO₃⁻ (mmol/L)	23.13 ± 1.68[c]	19.68 ± 5.18[b]	16.41 ± 7.62[a]	16.72 ± 7.25[a]	18.47	0.000*
Glucose (mg/dl)	89.10 ± 18.89[a]	86.19 ± 26.77[a]	142.86 ± 68.8[b]	159.00 ± 35.08[b]	19.38	0.000*
Na (meq/l)	137.34 ± 3.72[a]	138.39 ± 26.50[a]	138.20 ± 5.78[a]	135.78 ± 12.90[a]	0.80	0.495
K (meq/l)	3.66 ± 0.30[b]	3.53 ± 0.39[b]	2.97 ± 0.24[a]	4.42 ± 1.75[c]	37.158	0.000*
Aspartate Aminotransferase (AST) (U/l)	20.38 ± 6.87[a]	21.83 ± 8.26[a]	36.09 ±10.97[b]	86.22 ± 29.45[c]	76.56	0.000*

Alanine transaminase (ALT) (U/l)	9.37 ± 4.50^a	10.63 ± 5.54^a	24.11 ± 9.54^b	72.56 ± 23.43^c	104.12	0.000*
Bilirubin (mg/dL)	0.78 ± 0.86^a	0.66 ± 0.15^a	0.68 ± 0.25^a	0.82 ± 0.46^a	0.69	0.554
Urea (mg/dL)	27.42 ± 7.21^a	28.63 ± 7.66^a	31.59 ± 12.68^a	92.78 ± 27.35^b	105.23	0.000*
Creatinine (mg/dl)	0.73 ± 0.27^a	0.76 ± 0.26^a	0.91 ± 0.25^b	2.11 ± 0.43^c	71.22	0.000*
Creatine phosphokinase (CPK) (IU/L)	59.88 ± 4.98^a	58.95 ± 5.91^a	130.91 ± 10.41^b	525.33 ± 186.72^c	142.29	0.000*
Creatine kinase MB (CK-MB) (U/L)	16.46 ± 7.86^a	13.94 ± 7.51^a	31.00 ± 10.85^b	123.56 ± 10.40^c	440.366	0.000*
Hematocrit value (%)	38.23 ± 2.77^a	39.978 ± 5.10^{ab}	42.06 ± 5.64^b	48.06 ± 9.57^b	14.63	0.000*
Total leucocyte count (10^3/mm)	8.593 ± 2.96^a	9.283 ± 3.55^a	16.25 ± 6.54^b	17.58 ± 4.07^b	44.30	0.000*

Table 2: Laboratory parameters of studied groups.

Exclusion criteria: Age under 15 years of both sexes was excluded as APACHE II has not been validated for use in children or young people aged under 15 due to difference in its parameters. Patients with renal, hepatic, cardiovascular or respiratory diseases were excluded from the study to avoid the effect of these diseases on the results obtained. This was known from detailed history obtained from patients and was confirmed by clinical examination. The patients with history of epilepsy were also excluded. Co-administration of benzodiazepines, barbiturates, alcohol, cannabis or opiates with tramadol was excluded from the study. Pregnant females were also excluded to avoid the effect of pregnancy on the laboratory parameters obtained.

Groups	Group I (n=73)	Group II (n=64)	Group IIIa (n=58)	Group IIIb (n=9)	F-value	p-value
	M ± SD	M ± SD	M ± SD	M ± SD		
APACHE II Score	3.38 ± 1.32^a	8.06 ± 1.78^b	16.23 ± 3.99^c	35.67 ± 6.1^d	498.51	0.000*
M: Mean; SD: Standard Deviation						
*There is a significant difference by using One Way ANOVA at p<0.05						
The same letter means that there is no significant difference between the two groups by using Duncan multiple comparison test at p<0.05						
The different letters means that there is a significant difference between the two groups by using Duncan multiple comparison test at p<0.05						
Group I: Patients in Emergency Room (ER) and discharged						
Group II: Patients admitted to inpatient unit						
Group IIIa: Patients admitted to intensive care unit (ICU) and survived						
Group IIIb: Patients admitted to intensive care unit (ICU) and died						

Table 3: Comparison between studied groups as regards the APACHE II score.

The patients were classified according to their pattern of management in the Poison Control Center (PCC) of Ain Shams University Hospital into three groups: Group I (Emergency department cases): Patients discharged from the hospital after clinical assessment and observation for 4-6 hours. Group II (Inpatient cases): Patients admitted to the inpatient unit. Group III {Intensive Care Unit (ICU) cases}: this group represents patients admitted to the Intensive Care Unit. Patients of this group are subdivided according to their outcome into two subgroups: Group IIIa: Patients admitted to Intensive Care Unit (ICU) and survived. Group IIIb: Patients admitted to Intensive Care Unit (ICU) and died.

Independent variables	Coeffecients B	Std.Error	T-test		F-test		R²%
			Value	p-value	Value	P value	
Constant	9.930	17.948	0.553	0.581			
Mean arterial pressure	0.023	0.007	3.217	0.002			
Glasgow coma score (GCS)	-1.481	0.093	-15.942	0.000	211.198	0.000*	88.50
pH	-5.802	2.206	-2.630	0.009			
Serum creatinine	2.977	0.574	5.185	0.000			
Total leukocyte count	0.118	0.044	2.660	0.008			
*p<0.05							

Table 4: The multiple linear regression model for the dependent variable (APACHE II score) with different independent variables.

Every selected patient was subjected to the following: a) History taking including personal history. b) Clinical examination including general and systemic examination. c) Investigations include Electrocardiography (ECG), arterial blood gases (pH, HCO3⁻, PaO2 and PaCO2), routine investigations (Serum glucose, Na, K), renal profile (BUN, serum creatinine), hepatic profile {Aspartate Aminotransferase (AST), Alanine transaminase (ALT) and serum bilirubin}, CBC {white blood cells (WBCs), hematocrit value}, Creatine phosphokinase (CPK) and Creatine kinase MB (CK-MB) levels. d) Calculation of APACHE II score for all patients was done.

	Eigenvalue	% of Variance	Canonical Correlation	Wilks' Lambda	Chi-square	df	P-value
Function	35.648	71.9	0.986	0.188	1469.50	39	0.000

Table 5: Summary of canonical discriminant function.

Statistical analysis: Data were collected, checked, revised and analyzed by SPSS statistical package version 19. Excel computer program was used to tabulate the results, and represent it graphically. One Way ANOVA was used to declare the significant difference between groups at p<0.05 for the quantitative variables. Variables required for calculating the APACHE II score were collected for each patient and entered into a computer program designed to provide an estimate. Qualitative variables were expressed as count and percentages. Chi-square test for distribution was used to show the significant difference between study groups at p<0.05. Multiple linear Regression was used for getting the most predictive parameters affecting the APACHE II score. Discriminant analysis was done to identify the variables (clinical and laboratory) in tramadol intoxication that best discriminate patients in ER, patients in inpatient unit and patients in ICU (survived and none survived).A new score for prediction of prognosis of tramadol intoxicated patients was constructed from clinical and laboratory results obtained from the most predictive parameters affecting the APACHE II score by the multiple linear regression in addition to the most important variables that differentiate best between the studied groups obtained from the discriminant analysis. The ability and the accuracy of this score to predict the prognosis of tramadol intoxicated patients was assessed and evaluated by the ROC curve analysis.

Results

In this prospective study, a total of 202 patients met our inclusion criteria and were enrolled into the study. Group I (Emergency department cases) was 73 patients who were assessed clinically and observed for 4-6 hours then discharged from the hospital. Group II (Inpatient cases) was 64 patients. Group III {Intensive Care Unit (ICU) cases} consisted of 65 patients who were subdivided according to their outcome into two subgroups: Group IIIa (56 patients): Patients admitted to Intensive Care Unit (ICU) and survived. Group IIIb (9 patients): Patients admitted to Intensive Care Unit (ICU) and died.

Age and sex

Age of the patients ranged from 16 to 69 years with mean age between 28.84 and 34.97 years with non-significant difference between studied groups. Males represented the majority of cases (78.7%) while females represented (21.3%).

Delay time, dosage taken, manner of poisoning and vital data

Table (1) shows that the mean delay time for reaching hospital was between 3.44 hours and 3.72 hours in group I and II while it was between 4.69 hours and 6.00 hours in group IIIa and IIIb. The mean dosage of tramadol taken ranged between 837.67 mg (group I) and 2856.25 mg (group IIIb). The majority of patients (81.7%) were addict on tramadol and showed accidental toxicity, 15.8% attempted suicide and only 2.5% due to iatrogenic manner. Duration of hospitalization of patients ranged between 1 to 6 days with most of them discharged within 1-2 days. Regarding vital data, almost all studied patients had tachycardia. There was non-significant difference between group I, II and IIIa regarding systolic and diastolic blood pressure as well as the mean arterial pressure while there was significant decrease in group IIIb. Respiratory rate was within normal range in patients of group I and II while it was decreased in patients of group IIIa and increased in patients of group IIIb. Group IIIb showed significant increase in body temperature when compared with group I, II and IIIa.

	Group I	Group II	Group IIIa	Group IIIb
	(n=73)	(n=64)	(n=58)	(n=9)
Manner of poisoning	16.339	19.601	17.892	19.493
Respiratory rate	1.326	1.22	-1.846	-2.275
Cyanosis	-2.088	2.461	34.335	37.338
Respiratory Failure	76.065	83.579	158.732	172.147
Pulmonary oedema	-17.5	-21.211	-12.361	-21.351
Shock	-13.609	-10.278	2.873	27.773
Cardiac arrest	141.146	132.046	127.259	233.208
Seizure	-49.094	-19.704	-12.998	-16.039
Coma	-11.506	-2.573	8.586	6.653
ST segment changes	49.829	66.426	87.721	121.984
pH	623.242	607.869	606.527	608.071
HCO3$^-$	0.235	-0.031	0.321	0.668
K	25.061	23.154	18.848	25.04
Alanine transaminase (ALT)	-0.174	-0.136	-0.127	0.279
Creatine kinase MB (CKMB)	-1.1	-1.159	-0.897	0.145

| (Constant) | -2367.5 | -2275.8 | -2305.2 | -2541.7 |

Table 6: Classification function coefficients of discriminant analysis.

General manifestations

As regards skin examination, sweating was found in more than half of patients of group I (54.8%), 46.9% of group II and most of patients of group IIIa and IIIb (75% and 66.7% respectively). Cyanosis was seen in about all patients of group IIIa and IIIb while it was not observed in any patient of group I or II. Regarding the pupil size, miosis was observed in most of patients of group IIIa and IIIb while mydriasis was observed in less than half of patients of group II (45.3%) and IIIb (44.4%).

Systemic manifestations

Examination of the respiratory system revealed respiratory failure which occurs in most of patients of group III a (94.6%) and all patients of group IIIb (100%). Pulmonary oedema was observed in all patients of group IIIb (100%) and 21.4% of group IIIa. Regarding the cardiovascular system, most of the studied patients had minor cardiovascular effects such as palpitation which occurred in 47.94% of patients of group I, 75% of group II and 41.1% of group IIIa. On the other hand, severe cardiovascular effects such as shock and cardiac arrest occurred in patients of group IIIa and IIIb as 7.1% of group IIIa and 77.8% of group IIIb suffered shock while 33.3% of patients of group IIIb presented with cardiac arrest.

Concerning the gastrointestinal manifestations, almost all cases of group I, II and about half of cases of group IIIa suffered nausea. Vomiting occurred in all patients of group II and most of patients of group I, IIIa and IIIb. Regarding the neurological manifestations, headache occurred in near half of patients of group I, II and IIIa. Dizziness was observed in 24.7% of group I and 45.3% of group II. Agitation was noticed in most of patients of group I, II and about half of group IIIa. All patients of group II (100%), 85.7% of group IIIa and 44.4% of group IIIb had seizures. As regards coma, none of patients of group I presented with it which was seen in more than half of patients of group II and all patients of group IIIa and IIIb and it was commonly grade I. The mean glascow coma score (GSC) was between 13.91 and 14.95 in group I and II while it was between 3.00 and 8.76 in group IIIa and IIIb.

Parameter	Score
Manner of poisoning	
Therapeutic error	3
Addiction	2
Suicidal	1
Blood pressure	
Normal (110-135/65-85 mmHg)	3
Hypertension (>140/90 mmHg)	2
Hypotension (BP<90/60 mmHg)	1
Respiratory rate	2

Normal (12-24breath/min)	
Bradypnea (<12 breath/min) or Tachypnea>24 breath/min)	1
Cyanosis	
Absent	2
Present	1
CNS manifestations	
a)Seizure	
Absent	2
Present	1
b)Coma	2
Absent	
Present	1
Cardiovascular complications	
a)Shock	
Absent	2
Present	1
b)Cardiac arrest	
Absent	2
Present	1
Pulmonary complications	
a)Respiratory failure	
Absent	2
Present	1
b) Pulmonary edema	
Absent	2
Present	1
Ischemic changes	
Absent	2
Present(elevated or depressed ST segment, flat or inverted T wave, deep Q)	1
pH	
7.35-7.45	3
7.23-7.34	2
<7.23	1
HCO3⁻	
22-24 mmol/l	3
15-21.9 mmol/l	2

<15 mmol/l	1
Serum K	
3.5-5 meq/l	2
<3.5 meq/l or >5 meq/ l	1
Serum createnine	
0.6-1.4 mg/dl	2
>1.4 mg/dl	1
Alanine Aminotransferase (ALT)	
5-56 U/L	2
>56 U/L	1
White blood cell count	
4,500 - 10,000 mm3	2
>10000 mm3	1
Creatine kinase MB (CK-MB)	
Up to 24 U/L	2
>24 U/L	1
Total Maximum	**40**
Minimum	**18**

Table 7: predictive Score for progression of tramadol intoxication.

Laboratory parameters

Table (2) shows the values of laboratory parameters of studied groups. Arterial blood gas analysis (ABG) revealed metabolic acidosis in patients of group I and II while mixed metabolic and respiratory acidosis was observed in severe cases (group IIIa and IIIb).Serum glucose was within the normal range for patients of group I and group II while it was slightly increased in patients of group IIIa and IIIb where half of studied patients (50%) had normal glucose level, 31.2% had hyperglycemia and only 18.8% of patients had hypoglycemia. As regards serum Na, it was within the normal range in almost all studied patients. On the other hand, serum potassium was within the normal range in patients of group I and II while it was decreased in patients of group IIIa and increased in patients of group IIIb. As regards liver function tests, Aspartate Aminotransferase (AST) and Alanine transaminase (ALT) were within the normal range for patients of group I and II while they were increased in patients of group IIIa and IIIb. Regarding kidney function tests, serum urea was within the normal range for patients of group I, II and IIIa while it was increased in patients of group IIIb. Serum creatinine was within the normal range for patients of group I and II while it was increased in patients of group IIIa and IIIb. Creatine phosphokinase (CPK) and Creatine kinase MB (CK-MB) levels were within normal levels in patients of group I and II while they were slightly increased in patients of group IIIa and markedly increased in group IIIb. The total leukocyte count was within the normal range for patients of group I and II while it was increased in patients of group IIIa and IIIb. The hematocrit value was within normal value in patients of group I and II while it was slightly increased in patients of group IIIa and IIIb.

Electrocardiographic changes (ECG)

Most of patients had sinus tachycardia (56.9%), 37.1% had prolonged QTc, 1.5% had elevated ST segment, 3% had depressed ST segment and 3% of patients had inverted T wave.

APACHE II score: It was calculated to all studied patients as an emergency score. Table (3) shows the APACHE II score of studied groups. Group IIIb showed statistically significant nadir score (recorded to be 35.67) when compared with group I, II and IIIa.

Multiple linear Regression analysis: Multiple linear Regression analysis was used for getting the most predictive parameters affecting the APACHE II score. Table (4) shows that out of the 14 parameters which constituted the APACHE II score, mean arterial pressure, serum creatinine, pH, total leukocyte count and glascow coma score (GSC) were more often disturbed in patients who had a complicated outcome by multiple linear regression statistical analysis.

Discriminant Analysis: It determines which variables (clinical and laboratory) discriminate best between the studied groups. Table (5) shows the summary of the discriminant function. The discriminant function has Eigenvalue of 35.648 and accounts for 71.9 percent of the variance. The Wilks' Lambda which evaluates the statistical significance of the discriminatory power of the discriminant function was 0.188 with canonical correlation of 0.986, Chi-square of 1469.50 and degree of freedom (df) of 39. The discriminant function is statistically significant in differentiating between the four studied groups.

Table (6) shows that by using discriminant analysis, the current study has discovered 15 variables, which best discriminate between the four studied groups. These variables are manner of poisoning, respiratory rate, cyanosis, respiratory failure, pulmonary oedema, shock, cardiac arrest, seizures, coma, ST segment changes, pH, HCO3⁻, K, Alanine transaminase (ALT) and Creatine kinase MB (CK-MB).

Construction of a predictive score: The current study constructs and assesses a new score for prediction of prognosis of tramadol intoxicated patients from clinical and laboratory results obtained from the most predictive parameters affecting the APACHE II score by the multiple linear regression and the most important variables that differentiate best between the studied groups obtained from the discriminant analysis.

Table (7) shows The predictive score which depends on manner of poisoning, blood pressure, respiratory rate, skin manifestations (cyanosis), CNS manifestations (coma and seizures), cardiovascular manifestations (shock and cardiac arrest), pulmonary manifestations (respiratory failure and pulmonary edema) and ECG findings (ischemic changes as elevated or depressed ST segment, flat or inverted T wave, deep Q). In addition to investigational parameters which are simple, routine and readily available in most hospitals {pH, HCO3³⁻, serum K, creatinine, Alanine transaminase (ALT), total leukocyte count and Creatine kinase MB (CK-MB)}.

The ability and the accuracy of this score to predict the prognosis of tramadol intoxicated patients was assessed and evaluated by the ROC curve analysis. The area under the ROC curve for the predictive score was 0.996, the best cut-off point was 26 with a sensitivity of 98.46% and specificity of 95.62%. It means that if the patient has score <26, the patient condition is moderate or severe and if it was ≥26, the patient condition is mild.

Discussion

Tramadol abuse became a disastrous problem in the Egyptian community in spite of adding it to the narcotics list by the Egyptian government. This problem is increasing due to its lower price, illegal transactions and availability without prescription either with fake prescriptions from pharmacies or on the black market [10,17]. Several fatal incidents have drawn attention toward its underestimated toxicity despite of the general attitude about its safety [18].

According to records from the Poison Control Center of Ain Shams University Hospitals (PCC) of Egypt; 190, 376 and 691cases of tramadol toxicity were admitted in the years 2008, 2009 and 2010 respectively. This crescendo highlights the rising of this type of toxicity (records from PCC).The incidence of tramadol poisoning has over increased during the time of the current study. In the period between October 2010 and September 201, 1020 patients presented to PCC with tramadol intoxication of which 202 cases met our inclusion criteria were enrolled in the study [19-24].

As regards the results of the current study, the mean APACHE II Score in group III b showed statistically significant highest worse score (recorded to be 35.67) when compared with group I, II and III a. This significantly higher mean APACHE II score with 100% deaths agrees with Abbott et al., 1991; Chen et al., 1993; Chiavone & Sens, 2003 and Gupta& Arora, 2004; as these studies reported nonavailability of

survivors above APACHE II score of 40 and patients with APACHE II scores of 35 or higher in ICUs had a 100% hospital mortality rate. A study by Chen et al., 2007 found that the post-ICU non survivors had greater severity of illness on admission with a mean admission APACHE II score of 22.9 ± 5.5, compared to 18.6 ± 6.1 for post-ICU survivors. Haidri et al., 2011 demonstrated that the mean APACHE II score of patients who were successfully discharged from ICU has lower score as compared to patients who died.

Out of the 14 parameters which constituted the APACHE II score, mean arterial pressure, serum createnine, pH, total leukocytic count and Glasgow coma score were more often disturbed in patients who had a complicated outcome. The Glasgow coma score and serum createnine had the maximum significance clearly indicating that glascow coma score (GCS) and serum createnine played an important role in mortality prediction for the patients in this study.

The severity scoring systems are needed to assess quality of care, treatment efficacy, reducing health care cost, providing better care, and improving outcomes. The prediction of patient outcome was useful in prognosis, decision making for treatment withdrawal, cost benefit analysis, comparison between different centers, monitoring and assessment of new therapies [15,25,26]. A major limitation of scoring system is their dependence on sophisticated investigations. Such investigations may not be easily available in any hospital therefore there is a need for a simple prognostic scoring system which can be used easily for patients with tramadol intoxication [27].

From the current study, it could be noticed that the clinical course of tramadol intoxication may vary from a mild self-limiting to a life-threatening. Patients whose condition progresses to severe may require intensive therapy and such treatment may require admission to ICU. Therefore determination of the severity for patients with acute tramadol intoxication is critical. Previous clinical approaches to this problem have required the collection of a large amount of clinical and laboratory data to derive prognostic scores such as the APACHE II score. Such a system would require the collection and storage of a large number of data points, which might limit its practical use. Recent modifications to the scoring systems have explored approaches in which fewer data points are used [16].

It is necessary for every intensive care unit to have a prediction system which is validated for its specific kind of patients because of the differences between intensive care unit patients [21].

The aim of the present study is to construct a score able to accurately predict a severe outcome in tramadol intoxicated patients on admission (in the Emergency Department), using routine and easily measured parameters which are available in any hospital. This score can be a useful tool to select on admission the patients with a high risk of developing severe manifestations and who need to be hospitalized in the Intensive Care Unit (ICU). The current study constructs and assesses a new score for prediction of prognosis of tramadol intoxicated patients from clinical and laboratory results obtained from the most predictive parameters affecting the APACHE II score by the multiple linear regression and the most important variables that differentiate best between the studied groups obtained from the discriminant analysis.

This predictive score depends on manner of poisoning, blood pressure, respiratory rate, skin manifestations (cyanosis), CNS manifestations (coma and seizures), cardiovascular manifestations (shock and cardiac arrest), pulmonary manifestations (respiratory failure and pulmonary edema) and ECG findings (ischemic changes as elevated or depressed ST segment, flat or inverted T wave, deep Q). In addition to investigational parameters which are simple, routine and readily available in most hospitals {pH, HCO3⁻, serum K, createnine, Alanine transaminase (ALT), total leukocyte count and Creatine kinase MB (CK-MB)}.The area under the ROC curve for the predictive score was 0.996, the best cut-off point was 26 with a sensitivity of 98.46% and specificity of 95.62%.

Conclusion

The predictive score of the present study is considered to be specific and sensitive and it can be used for prediction of outcome and rapid initiation of appropriate therapy in the emergency department for lowering hospital morbidity and mortality in tramadol intoxicated patients and it may be helpful in reducing the risk of false or delayed admissions to the ICU in these patients. It can be assessed soon at emergency department, is quick and easy to use and applicable even in small hospitals.

References

1. Emamhadi M, Sanaei-Zadeh H, Nikniya M, Zamani N, Dart RC (2012) Electrocardiographic manifestations of tramadol toxicity with special reference to their ability for prediction of seizures. Am J Emerg Med 30: 1481-1485.

2. Marquardt KA, Alsop JA, Albertson TE (2005) Tramadol exposures reported to statewide poison control system. Ann Pharmacother 39: 1039-1044.

3. Brinker A, Bonnel RA, Beitz J (2002) Abuse, dependence, or withdrawal associated with tramadol. Am J Psychiatry 159: 881.

4. Tjäderborn M, Jönsson AK, Hägg S, Ahlner J (2007) Fatal unintentional intoxications with tramadol during 1995-2005. Forensic Sci Int 173: 107-111.

5. Elkalioubie A, Allorge D, Robriquet L, Wiart JF, Garat A, et al. (2011) Near-fatal tramadol cardiotoxicity in a CYP2D6 ultrarapid metabolizer. Eur J Clin Pharmacol 67: 855-858.

6. Ahmadi H, Rezaie M, Hoseini J (2012) Epidemiology Analysis of Poisonings with Tramadol. J Forensic Res 3: 151.

7. Gholami K, Shalviri G, Zarbakhsh A, Daryabari N, Yousefian S (2007) New guideline for tramadol usage following adverse drug reactions reported to the Iranian Pharmacovigilance Center. Pharmacoepidemiol Drug Saf 16: 229-237.

8. Shadnia S, Soltaninejad K, Heydari K, Sasanian G, Abdollahi M (2008) Tramadol intoxication: a review of 114 cases. Hum Exp Toxicol 27: 201-205.

9. Ripple MG, Pestaner JP, Levine BS, Smialek JE (2000) Lethal combination of tramadol and multiple drugs affecting serotonin. Am J Forensic Med Pathol 21: 370-374.

10. Daubin C, Quentin C, Goullé JP, Guillotin D, Lehoux P, et al. (2007) Refractory shock and asystole related to tramadol overdose. Clin Toxicol (Phila) 45: 961-964.

11. Pothiawala S, Ponampalam R (2011) Tramadol Overdose: A Case Report. Proceedings of Singapore Healthcare 20: 219-223.

12. Clarot F, Goullé JP, Vaz E, Proust B (2003) Fatal overdoses of tramadol: is benzodiazepine a risk factor of lethality? Forensic Sci Int 134: 57-61.

13. Taghaddosinejad F, Sheikhazadi A, Yaghmaei A, Mehrpour O, Schwake L (2012) Epidemiology and Treatment of Severe Poisoning in the Intensive Care Unit: Lessons from a One-Year Prospective Observational Study. J Clinic Toxicol S1:00

14. Mahmoudin GA, Solhi H, Afzali S (2008) Epidemiological study on poisoned patients who were admitted in the ICU ward of Shohadaie Ashaier and Tamine- Ejtemaii hospitals of Khoram Abad, Iran from Oct 2006 until Oct 2007. Iran J Toxicol 2: 173-177.

15. Subbe CP, Slater A, Menon D, Gemmell L (2006) Validation of physiological scoring systems in the accident and emergency department. Emerg Med J 23: 841-845.

16. Bouch DC, Thompson JP (2008) Severity scoring systems in the critically ill. Continuing Education in Anaesthesia, Critical Care & Pain 8: 181-85.

17. Ismaiel OA, Hosny MM (2012) Development and Validation of a Spectrophotometric Method for the Determination of Tramadol in Human Urine Using Liquid-Liquid Extraction and Ion Pair Formation. International Journal of Instrumentation Science 1: 34-40.

18. Gheshlaghi F, Eizadi-Mood N, Fazel K, Behjati M (2009) An unexpected sudden death by oral tramadol intoxication: a case not reported earlier. Iranian Journal of Toxicology 2: 292-294.

19. Abbott RR, Setter M, Chan S, Choi K (1991) APACHE II: prediction of outcome of 451 ICU oncology admissions in a community hospital. Ann Oncol 2: 571-574.

20. Chen FG, Koh KF, Goh MH (1993) Validation of APACHE II score in a surgical intensive care unit. Singapore Med J 34: 322-324.

21. Chiavone PA, Sens YA (2003) Evaluation of APACHE II system among intensive care patients at a teaching hospital. Sao Paulo Med J 121: 53-57.

22. Gupta R, Arora VK (2004) Performance evaluation of APACHE II score for an Indian patient with respiratory problems. Indian J Med Res 119: 273-282.

23. Chen YC, Lin MC, Lin YC, Chang HW, Huang CC, et al. (2007) ICU discharge APACHE II scores help to predict post-ICU death. Chang Gung Med J 30: 142-150.

24. Haidri FR, Rizvi N, Motiani B (2011) Role of APACHE score in predicting mortality in chest ICU. J Pak Med Assoc 61: 589-592.

25. Teres D1 (2004) The value and limits of severity adjusted mortality for ICU patients. J Crit Care 19: 257-263.

26. Le Gall JR1 (2005) The use of severity scores in the intensive care unit. Intensive Care Med 31: 1618-1623.

27. Mishra A, Sharma D, Raina VK (2003) A simplified prognostic scoring system for peptic ulcer perforation in developing countries. Indian J Gastroenterol 22: 49-53.

6

Cytotoxicity Studies of Functionalized Gold Nanoparticles using Yeast Comet Assay

Saritha Suvarna[1], **Rajesha Nairy**[2], **Sunil K C**[1] **and Narayana Y**[1*]

[1]*Department of Studies in Physics, Mangalore University, Mangalagangotri, India*

[2]*Department of Physics, P.A College of Engineering, Mangalore, India*

[*]**Corresponding author:** Narayana Y, Department of Studies in Physics, Mangalore University, India, E-mail: narayanay@yahoo.com

Abstract

In the present study gold nanoparticles and glucose capped gold nanoparticles are synthesized by chemical route method and characterized using UV-SPR, FTIR and TEM analysis. Single cell gel electrophoresis (SCGE) assay was used to study DNA damage. Studies show that glucose capped gold nanoparticles are less toxic as compare to gold nanoparticles at DNA level. Somewhat larger gold nanoparticle used to monitor endocytosis in log-phase *S. cervisiae* spheroplasts at 10 to 30 µM was not reported to cause growth inhibition. It shows that glucose capped gold nanoparticles are nontoxic to yeast strain D7. DNA damage was observed by using standard method called Yeast comet assay, which provides a very sensitive method for detecting strand breaks and repair kinetics in single cells. Studies showed that 5 µM-30 µM having very less sign of DNA damage in case of Glucose capped gold nanoparticles and it also shows toxic effect for without glucose capped gold nanoparticles. OTM for different concentration as shown in the image and OTM with respect to different concentration shows the DNA damage, these studies also correlated with survival studies.

Keywords: Gold nanoparticles; Glucose capped gold nanoparticles; Yeast Comet assay; DNA damage

Introduction

In recent years, most of the metal nanoparticles, particularly gold nanoparticles are very attractive from their property such as bio-applications, therapeutics and diagnostics. Synthesis of nanoscale structures of inert metals like gold is of great interest for the current day researchers as gold possess certain physical properties, which are suitable for several biomedical applications. Thus gold nanoparticles (AuNps) having unique physicochemical features show significant future promise in the fields of biomedical imaging and therapy [1-5]. Studies also lay special emphasis on the uniqueness of the gold nanoparticles for treatment of life threatening diseases like cancer [6]. Available reports show potential of gold nanoparticles as explored in the field of photodynamic therapy due to their ability of producing heat to kill the tumors [7]. However although gold is biologically inert and thus shows much less toxicity, as compared to other metal nanoparticles, gold has a relatively lower rate of clearance from circulation and hence can pose serious deleterious effects on health[8]. Recent studies showed them AuNPs could cross the blood-brain barrier, interact with the DNA and even produce genotoxic effects [9]. As such surface modifications of AuNps are gaining attention in current day research programs where attaching a ligand, capping of the AuNps could help making the particles more biocompatible so as to achieve specific targeting of diseased cells and tissues [10-14]. Synthesizing AuNps with lesser toxicity is now one of the primary interests in the field of nanotechnology for its applicability in biomedical sciences. Based on this perspective the present work has been designed to formulate a synthesis of a novel glucose capped gold nanoparticle as a better theranostic candidate. The glucose analog 2-deoxy-D-glucose(2DG),an inhibitor of glycolytic ATP production and glucose transport is the most widely reported, metabolic inhibitor for targeting glucose metabolism . 2-deoxy-D-glucose labeled gold nanoparticles have been shown to provide high-resolution metabolic and anatomic information of tumor in a single CT scan [15,16]. Studies showed that glucose capped gold nanoparticles has been specially choosen to target cancer cells as such capped nanoparticles show faster cellular uptake in cancer cells. Additionally, larger number of glucose molecules are internalized via glucose transporter (GLUT) receptors present on the cancer cell surface [17]. These types of gold nanoparticles are incorporated into numerous technologies and applications widely used in case of Therapeutics and biomedical because of their conjugation with various bio molecules due to the presence of 6s free electrons in conduction band of nano-Gold [18,19]. Moreover, Yeast Comet assay is a new, fast and easily developing assay for detection of environmental genotoxic agents without using higher organisms. *Saccharomyces cerevisiae*, which is a fast growing organism and easy to handle. This simple eukaryote possesses homologues or functional analogues of almost all factors involved in these processes. *S. cerevisiae* is one of the most thoroughly studied model systems whose full genome sequence is now available. For these reasons, the yeast has become a valuable tool for studying the eukaryotic cell and it has also been used as a test organism for estimating the mutagenic potential of different chemicals [20,23]. Yeast comet assay also used to study DNA damage in case of food additives. Zymolose-20T did not open the cell wall, therefore zymolose-100T used to achieve degradation of cell wall [24]. DNA damaging agent was used as Glucose-gold nanoparticles. Gold nanoparticles having tremendous properties in the field of biomedical application due their wider range of properties. Bio molecular capping gold nanoparticles shows very less toxicity, Because of their metabolic properties. Main Purpose of the studies is showing level of DNA damage caused due to gold nanoparticles. These studies are more compatible for biomedical application due to their easy availability.

Materials and Methods

Chemicals

HAuCl4.3H2O (Sigma), β-D glucose, Sodium hydroxide, Agarose normal and low melting powder form, EDTA sodium salt, Tris base, Triton X – 100, Di methyl sulphoxide, Ethidium bromide, Sodium chloride, Methanol were procured from Alpha.

Synthesis of gold nanoparticles

Gold nanoparticles are synthesized by using citrate reduction method and Glucose-capped AuNPs were synthesized by chemical route method [18] using $HAucl_4.3H_2O$ and β-D-Glucose. The aqueous solution of 0.05M $HAuCl_4.3H_2O$ was added to β-D-glucose (0.03M) and stirred for 30 minutes. Subsequently, 0.5 M sodium hydroxide (NaoH) was added for completing reduction of gold salt. This resulted in a red colored solution of Glu-AuNPs. β-D-glucose acted as both reducing as well as capping agent in the AuNp synthesis. Capping was confirmed by FTIR and TEM analysis.

Characterization of Glucose capped gold nanoparticles

Synthesis of glucose-capped gold nanoparticles and gold nanoparticles are observed by UV-visible absorption spectrometer (model HU-1090) which shows a surface plasma resonance(SPR) at a wavelength 540 nm FTIR analysis was carried out to study the elemental chemical bonding, and Transmission electronic microscopic (TEM) analysis shows dimension of gold nanoparticles.

Samples preparation

A mutant type diploid yeast strain, *S. cerevisiae* D7 was used for the present study. The single cell stationary-phase cultures were obtained by growing the cells in Yeast extract: Peptone: Dextrose (YEPD) (1:2:2%) medium for several generations in stationary phase to a density of approximately 3×10^8 cells/ml. Cells were washed thrice by centrifugation (2000 for 5 min) using double distilled water and re-suspended to a cell concentration of 1000 cells/ml (by counting in heamocytometer) in a polypropylene vial for treatment with gold nanoparticles and without capped gold nanoparticles for 1hr.

Survival assay

Treated and untreated samples were suitably diluted and plated in quadruplicate on YEPD agar medium. Plates were incubated for 2-3 days at 30°C in dark and normal atmospheric conditions and the colonies were counted. The data points in all figures in the survival results are the means from at least three independent experiments. The error bars in all figures indicate the standard error of the mean. The statistical analysis was carried out using origin 8.0 software.

Yeast comet assay

Yeast comet assay was performed by using *Saccharomyces cerevisiae* D7 strains. Five milliliters of YEPD (Yeast extract: Peptone : Dextrose) (1:2:2%) are inoculated with D7 strain and incubated overnight at 30°C, 200 rpm. At 1×10^6 cells were harvested by centrifugation at 4°C, after washing, the pellet was re suspended in 10 ml ice-cold S buffer (1 M sorbitol, 25 mM KH_2PO_4, pH-6.5). Cells were distributed by aliquots containing 4×10^6 cells and centrifuged at 4°C, 18000 rpm. These cells are treated with nanoparticles for 1 h in the concentration

range of 5 μM-30 μM. The cells was re suspended in 80 μl of 1.5% (w/v) LMA (Low Melting Agarose) containing 2 mg/ml zymolyase 100 T at 35°C (LMA was previously melted with S buffer at 50°C, cooled to 35°C and zymolyase was added, mixed and maintained at 35°C until use). The suspension was transferred to a glass slide and covered immediately with the cover slip before solidification. Glass slides were incubated at 30°C for 60-90 min and cover slips were removed gently. All subsequent manipulations were done at 4°C. The toxic was removed by incubating the glass slides in S buffer for 5 mins and cells were lysed with lysis buffer (30 mM NaoH, 1 M NaCl, 0.05%, w/v, laurylsarcosine, 50 mM EDTA, 10 mM Tris-HCl, pH 10) for 20 min. After lysis, cells were washed three times with electrophoresis buffer (30 mM NaOH, 10 mM EDTA, 10 mM Tris-Hcl, pH10) for 20 min. Glass slides were placed in an electrophoresis tank immersed in electrophoresis buffer and electrophoresis was done at 0.7 V/cm for 10 min. After electrophoresis cells were neutralized with incubation in 10 mM Tris-Hcl, pH 7.4 for 10 min and treated with 76% ethanol 10 min and, subsequently with 96% ethanol for 10 min. DNA was stained with 10 μg/ml ethidium bromide (10 μl), covering the area of the cells in the glass slide, without the cover slip, and overlaying with a new one and visualization was done immediately or after several days (slides were stored at 4°C). Observation of comets was done with a fluorescence microscope with 100x magnification. Comets were analyses using the Comet score software.

Gold nanoparticles are treated with Yeast strains: Yeast strain D7 was treated with different concentration of with and without capped gold nanoparticles of the range of 10 μM, 20 μM, 30 μM and 40 μM. D7 strains are treated with different concentration of nanoparticles for 1hr.

Result and Discussions

UV-Visible spectroscopy shows absorbance peak at 545 nm as shown in the Figure 1, FTIR spectrum shows the –OH stretching at 3332.5 cm^{-1} due to the presence of glucose on the surface of gold nanoparticles (Figure 2).

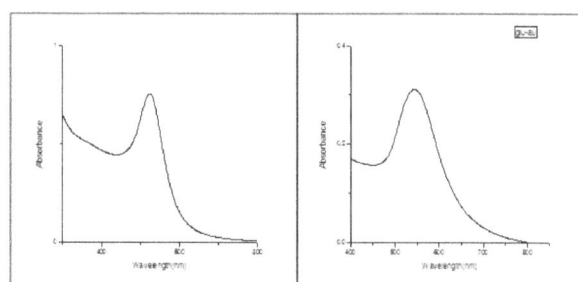

Figure 1: Shows the UV-absorbance spectrum of 545 nm Glu-capped gold nanoparticles.

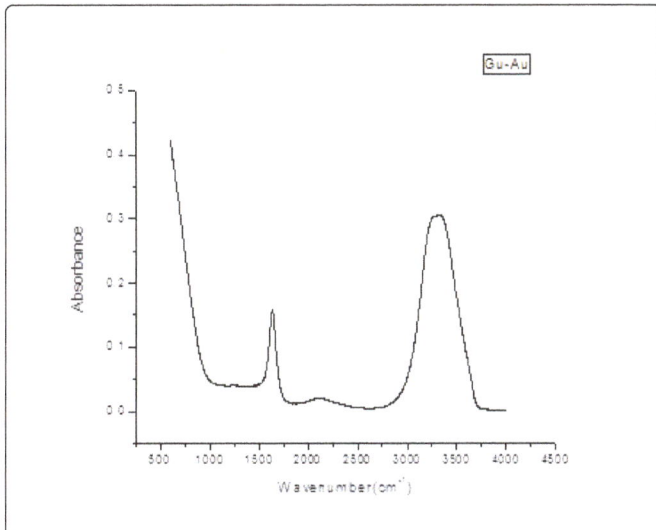

Figure 2: Shows the FTIR Spectrum of Glucose-capped gold nanoparticles.

Morphology of gold nanoparticles is analyzed from TEM analysis. It shows the triangular shape of the gold nanoparticles and also shows the size distribution plot as shown in Figures 3 and 4.

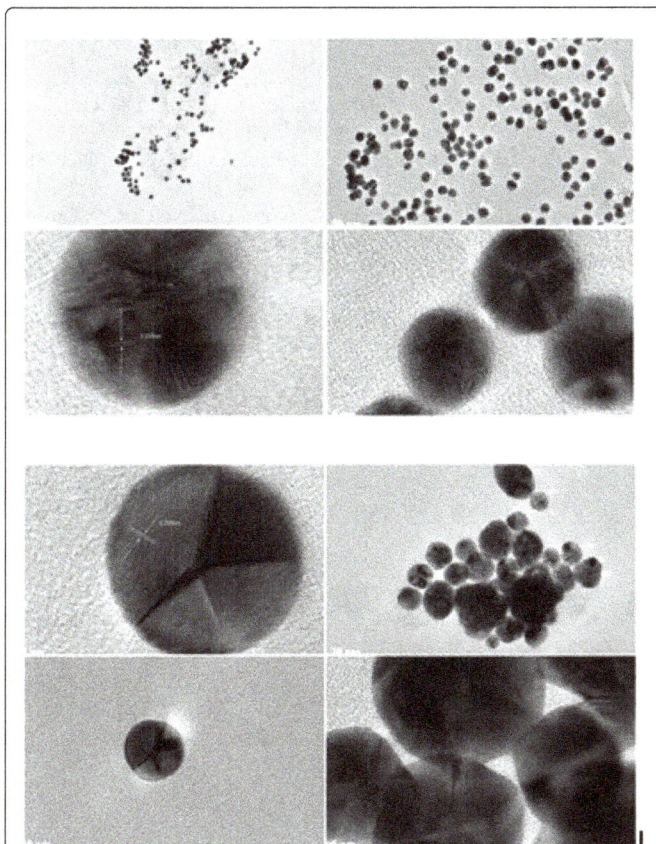

Figure 4: Shows that diameter of glucose-capped gold nano particles are 19.04 ± 1.13 nm.

Glucose capped gold nanoparticles are treated yeast strain D7 with different concentration in the range of 10 μM-30 μM. The increasing use of nanoparticles in industrial processes and commercial products has generated a need for systematic assessment of potential biological and environmental risks. A related but somewhat larger gold nanoparticle used to monitor endocytosis in log-phase *S. cervisiae* spheroplasts at 10 to 30 μM was not reported to cause growth inhibition Survival plot as shown in the Figure 5.

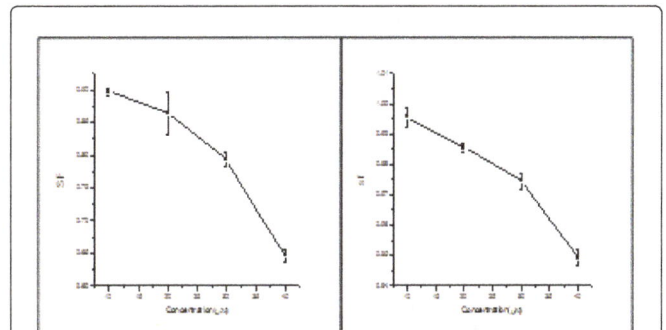

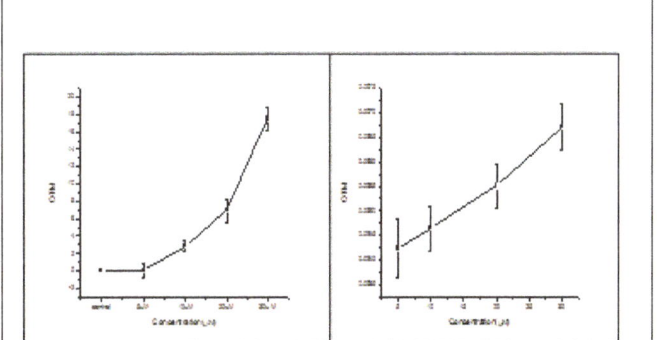

Figure 3: Shows the TEM image of glucose-capped gold nanoparticles: i) d spacing 0.236nm was calculated by using J-image software. ii) Shows the images of glucose-capped gold nanoparticle

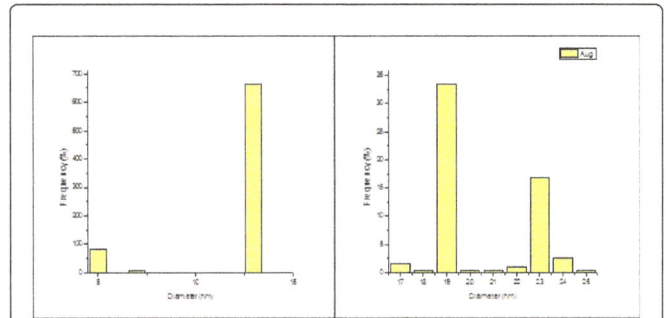

Figure 5: Shows OTM increases with increase in concentration of Glu-Au.

A related but somewhat larger gold nanoparticle used to monitor endocytosis in log-phase *S. cervisiae* spheroplasts at 10 to 30 μM was not reported to cause growth inhibition, from the graph it shows that 90% of the viability at concentration 10 μM and upon increasing the concentration to 30 μM, viability was reduced to 70 %. It shows that glucose capped gold nanoparticles are nontoxic to yeast strain D7. DNA damage was observed by using standard method called Yeast comet assay, OTM for different concentration as shown in the image and OTM with respect to different concentration shows the DNA damage. Correlation plot between OTM and Survival Fraction gives R 2 value is about -0.99 as shown in the Figure 6. Results shows that gold nanoparticles are toxic as compare to glucose capped gold nanoparticles, Because of the metabolic properties (Figure 7).

Figure 6: Images shows DNA damage when treated with glucose capped gold nanoparticles in 100X resolution.

Figure 7: Images shows DNA damage captured using fluorescent microscopy using 100X resolution treated with citrate gold nanoparticles

Conclusion

Concluded that, Gold nanoparticles and Glucose capped gold nanoparticles are characterized by using UV, FTIR and TEM analysis. Yeast strain D7, are treated with different concentration of with and without capped gold nanoparticles, to check the DNA damage using Single-cell gel electrophoresis (yeast comet assay), which provides a very sensitive method for detecting strand breaks and repair kinetics in single cells. Studies showed that 5 μM-30 μM having very less sign of DNA damage in case of Glucose capped gold nanoparticles and it also shows toxic effect for without glucose capped gold nanoparticles.

Acknowledgment

The authors thankfully acknowledge Prof. P.V. Satyam for the use of HRTEM facility at Institute of Physics, Bhubaneswar, India. The authors also acknowledge use of the facilities at Microtron center, Mangalore University.

References

1. Pradeep T (2001) A Textbook of Nanoscience and Nanotechnology. Pub: Tata McGraw Hill Education Private Limited, USA.

2. Che H, Li XY (2012) In Integrated Biomaterials for Biomedical technology. Wiley 1184: 1-34.

3. Sanjay SS, Singh R, Tiwari A, Pandey AC (2012) In Intelligent Nanomaterials. APE (Edn) Wiley 978: 625-648.

4. Qingfeng Z, Nicolas L, Peter N, Hui W (2014) Porous Au Nanoparticles with tunable Plasmon resonances and intense field enhancements for single-particle SERS. J Phys Chem Lett 5: 370-374.

5. Pedro Pedrosa, Raquel Vinhas, Alexandra Fernandes, Pedro V Baptista (2015) Gold Nanotheranostics: Proof-of-concept or clinical tool? Nanomaterials 5: 853-887.

6. Jyothi M, Parth J, Pranjali T, Khanh V, Baohong Y, et al. (2013) Nanomaterials for photo-based diagnostic and therapeutic applications. Theranostics 3: 152-166.

7. Carlo M, Dora B, Renzo V, Marzia B, Elena F, et al. (2013) One-step synthesis of star-like gold nanoparticles for surface enhanced Raman spectroscopy. Materials chemistry and Physics 143: 1215-1221.

8. Zhang X (2015) Gold Nanoparticles: Recent Advances in the Biomedical Applications. Cell Biochem Biophys 72: 771-775.

9. Hyangah C, Sangyeop L, Sang W, Hwan C, Jaebum C (2009) Highly Sensitive Immunoassay of Lung Cancer Marker Carcinoembryonic Antigen using Surface-Enhaced Raman Scattering of Hollow Gold nanospheres. Anal chem 81: 3029-3034.

10. Wang X, Yang DP, Huang P, Li M, Li C, et al. (2012) Hierarchically assembled Au micro spheres and sea-urchin-like architectures: formation mechanism and SERS study. Nanoscale 4:7766-7772.

11. Lanlan S, Dongxu Z, Meng D, Haifeng Z, Binghui Li (2013) One-step synthesis of shape-controllable Gold Nanoparticles and their application in surface-enhanced Raman scattering. J Mater Sci Technol 29: 613-618.

12. Mohammed S, Gowda D, Siddaramaiah H (2013) Gold nanoparitcles, A paradigm shift in biomedical applications. Adv coll inter scie 200: 44-58.

13. Chunyuan S, Zhuyuan W, Ruhuo Z, Jing Y, Xueb T, et al. (2014) Highly sensitive immunoassay based on Raman reporter-labeled immune-Au aggregates and SERS-active immune substrate. J Bios 25: 826-831.

14. Tatsuo M, Yuhei F, Tetsuya M (2015) Synthesis of gold nanoparticles using various amino acids. J Colld Inter Sci 447: 254-257.

15. Ji L, Ahmed C, Steven JC, Charles P, Tijana R, et al. (2010) A novel functional CT contrast agent for molecular imaging of cancer. Phys Med Biol 55: 4389-4397.

16. Wilson R, Xiaojing Z, Linghong G, Andrew S, Xiuying H, et al. (2009) Gold nanoparticle sensitize radiotherapy of Prostate cancer cells by regulation of the cell cycle. Nanotechnology 9: 9.

17. Chenxia H, Martin N, Daniel Y, Steven C, Jie C (2015) Treating cancer stem cells and cancer metastasis using glucose-coated gold nanoparticles. Int J Nanomed 10: 2065-2077.

18. Juncheng L, Gaown Q, Poovathinthodiyil R, Yukata R (2006) Facile "Green" Synthesis, characterization, and catalytic Function of β-D-glucose Stabilized Au Nanocrystals. A European Journal 12: 2131-2138.

19. Turkevich J, Stevenson PC, Hillier J (1951) A study of the nucleation and growth processes in the synthesis of colloidal gold. Disss Farad Sol 11: 55-75.

20. Tice RR, Agurell E, Anderson D, Burlinson B, Hartmann A, et al. (2000) Single Cell Gel/Comet assay: Guidelines for in vitro and invivo genetic toxicology testing. EnviroMol mtagenss 35:206-201.

21. Jette R, Kristian S, Klara J (2009) Comet assay on tetraploid yeast cells. Mutation Research 673: 53-58.

22. George M, Ivailo M, Boyka A (2002) Application of the single cell gel electrophoresis on yeast cells. Mutation Research 513: 69-74.

23. Ekaterina P, Radostina A, George M (2014) Application of the yeast comet assay in testing of food additives for genotoxicity. Fd Sci Technolo 59: 510-517.

24. Anna L, Beata M, Wneek M (2014) Assessment of Yeast Chromsome comet assay. Fung gencs biol 63: 9-16.

25. Saritha Suvarna, Ujjal Das, Sunil K C, Snehasis Mishra, Sudarshan M, et al. (2017) Synthesis of novel glucose capped gold nanoparticles are better candidate for theranostic. PLOS ONE.

7

Development of a Medical Toxicology Curriculum in Spanish with Content Informed by a Population Survey for Medical Trainees in the Dominican Republic

Cynthia Santos[1,2*]**, Reynolds Kairus**[3]**, Ziad Kazzi**[4]**, Suzanne Bentley**[5] **and Ruben Olmedo**[6]

[1]*Emory University School of Medicine, Centers for Disease Control, Atlanta, GA, USA*

[2]*Icahn School of Medicine at Mount Sinai, New York, NY, USA*

[3]*Pontificia Universidad Católica Madre y Maestra, Santiago, Dominican Republic*

[4]*Director International Postdoctoral Fellowship in Medical Toxicology, Emory University School of Medicine, Atlanta, GA, USA*

[5]*Assistant Professor of Medical Education, Mount Sinai School of Medicine, New York, NY, USA*

[6]*Director of the Division of Toxicology, Mount Sinai School of Medicine, New York, NY, USA*

Corresponding author: Cynthia Santos, Emory University School of Medicine, Centers for Disease Control, Atlanta, GA, USA, E-mail: cynthia.d.santos@emory.edu

Abstract

Introduction: The aim of this study is to develop a curriculum based on the American Board of Emergency Medicine (ABEM) core content toxicology category with emphasis on exposures prevalent in the Dominican Republic (DR) as informed by a population survey.

Methods: A survey was designed to identify common toxicological exposures, practices, and perceptions in community members and medical trainees in Santiago, DR. A toxicology curriculum was taught to medical residents using a curriculum made available online through the Global Educational Toxicology Uniting Project (GETUP).

Results: 175 people completed the survey and 34 medical residents completed the course.

The average percent of students/residents and community members reported the following, respectively: frequent substance abuse (12.2%, 44.0%), safe storage practices (21.7%, 13.7%), and traditional remedy use (15.2%, 21.8%). Community members answered 44%, medical students answered 61%, and residents answered 73% of the basic knowledge questions correctly. The mean pretest and posttest scores in the medical residents who took the toxicology course were 61% and 83%, respectively.

Conclusions: The results suggest this population would benefit from education regarding safe-storage practices, the potential dangers of traditional remedy use, as well as education on the sources and effects of common exposures like lead and pesticide poisoning. Many practice high risk behaviors including substance abuse, unsafe remedy use, as well as the use of products that are either illegal or improperly labeled/handled. The long-term goals of this project are to raise awareness and implement expanded toxicology training in this country.

Keywords: Education; Survey; Curriculum; Caribbean; Public health

Introduction

Substance abuse is a leading cause of death and disability in the Dominican Republic (DR), [1] yet there are no formal training in toxicology, no poison centers, and relatively little access to laboratory testing, antidotes, and specialty referral centers. Illicit drug abuse and drug trafficking in the DR is on a steep rise, with an 800% increase in the past two years [2]. Also the DR has a high rate of fatalities from alcohol-related road traffic accidents [3]. In addition to substance abuse certain toxins poste a particular public health threat in this region for a variety of reasons. Dominicans area increased risk for certain toxicological exposures due to insufficient or improperly enforced regulations, lack of public awareness campaigns or expert knowledge, insufficient toxicological training in the medical community, lack of poison control centers, and the popularity of certain traditional remedies or risky behavioral practices.

For example, poisonings from pesticides [4-6], lead [7,8], and camphor [9,10] are particularly common in Dominican communities. One notable example of pesticide poisoning occurred in 2002 when 153 textile workers in the DR were admitted to several hospitals throughout Santiago after paraquat was sprayed on nearby grounds [11]. A notable example for lead poisoning occurred in Haina, DR which according to the United Nations, was considered to have the highest level of lead contamination in the world, a determinant made after results of testing revealed that its entire population carried indications of lead poisoning due to the improper disposal practices of a battery recycling plant that potentially exposed a population of 80,000 [12]. In the DR camphor is used for homeopathic healing purposes as well as spiritual purposes and its potentially toxic effects are not well appreciated by the public [13]. In the US, over the counter products are not allowed to contain more than 11% camphor, while it is common to find pure camphor sold in many Dominican stores [13].

In recognition of the impact of toxicological exposures on the public health of this region a survey and curriculum were designed in order to mitigate this problem. We performed a needs assessment survey to define future educational needs regarding toxicological exposures in this region. The 2nd part of this project was the creation of a toxicology curriculum written in Spanish for medical students and resident physicians. The long-term goal of this project is to raise both public awareness and medical training standards in toxicology, create community outreach programs, and implement more formal training in toxicology in the DR.

Methods

We developed the questionnaire guided by a methodological review of recent literature. It contains 8 sections consisting of 84 items (Table 1). The first section includes demographic data from the participants. The second section consists of substance abuse history and patterns of use. The third section lists a history of previous medical encounters either at a clinic, emergency room (ER), or pharmacy. The fourth section includes a history of traditional home remedies for overdose. The fifth section consists of storage practices of potentially hazardous substances. The sixth, seventh and eighth sections assess fund of knowledge and use of lead, camphor, and pesticide, respectively. Questions were asked using primarily closed-end questions; however open-end questions were also included in each section in order to capture responses not included in the closed-end answer choices. Questions regarding fund of knowledge used a 3-point rating scale, range being "1-Yes", "2-No", "3-Not Sure. Questions regarding history of substance use, history of medical encounters, and storage practices used a 2-point rating scale, with "1-Yes" and "2-No." Questions regarding substance abuse were taken from the Alcohol, Smoking and Substance Involvement Screening Test (ASSIST), which was available also in Spanish by the World Health Organization (WHO) [14]. Questions regarding the use of certain pesticides were adopted from a USAID report list of toxic pesticides [15] and from a list of pesticides banned from the Agricultural Ministry of Dominican Republic [16]. No validated questions regarding the use of traditional home remedies in the Dominican Republic or similar populations were available. The list of traditional home remedies were adopted from previously published cross-sectional survey of patients visiting a general practioner in Europe, however many of the remedies were excluded and others included based on the primary author's discretion [17]. There were no validated survey tools regarding the fund of knowledge regarding camphor, lead, or pesticide exposure so questions pertaining to these subjects were created by the primary author. There was also no validated tool regarding storage practices of potentially hazardous substances that would be relevant for this population so these questions were also created by the primary author.

Survey Section	Topic
1	Demographic data
2	Substance abuse history and patterns of use
3	History of previous medical encounters either at a clinic, emergency room (ER), or pharmacy
4	History of traditional home remedies for overdose
5	Storage practices of potentially hazardous substances
6	Fund of knowledge and use of lead
7	Fund of knowledge and use of camphor
8	Fund of knowledge and use of pesticides

Table 1: Eight survey topics covered in the questionnaire.

Eligible survey respondents were either 1) patients in the waiting room areas of the Emergency Departments (EDs) and clinics of Hospital Juan XXIII and Hospital Regional Universitario José María Cabral y Baez (HRUJMCB), 2) community members participating in a basic responder noncertification training course for lay persons held at Hospital Juan XIII 3) medical students enrolled in Pontificia Universidad Católica Madre y Maestra (PUCMM) 4) family medicine residents at Juan XXIII Hospital or 5) emergency medicine residents at HRUJMCB. PUCMM is a private medical school in Santiago, DR whereas Hospital Juan XXIII and HRUJMCB are both public hospitals in Santiago. Hospital Juan XXIII is considered more of a community hospital, whereas HRUJMCB is a main referral center for patients requiring intensive care, cardiac, head trauma, and orthopedic care. Respondents less than 18 years of age were excluded from participating in the survey. Written consent was obtained in Spanish. Institutional Review Board approval was obtained through both the Icahn School of Medicine at Mount Sinai and through PUCMM in Santiago, DR. None of the participants who completed the basic responder course declined participation in the survey. The lay person basic responder course was taught by the Dominican medical student volunteer who is a medical student at PUCMM and a NYC trained paramedic. None of the basic responder participants had formal medical training or medical certifications. Patients in the waiting rooms were approached by the medical student study volunteer and were asked to participate in a voluntary survey. Patients who declined study participation did so for many reasons. Cited reasons for declining participation included not having sufficient time to fill out the form, or feeling too unwell to fill out the survey. The survey was distributed by the primary author and the medical student volunteer who assisted the survey respondents fill out the forms as needed. For example, participants who either had visual impairments or were illiterate had the survey read out loud and filled out by the medical student volunteer. The survey respondents who were medical students, family medicine residents, or emergency medicine residents were chosen based on convenience (i.e. if they were physically present in the ER or clinic and if they had time to fill out the survey).

A 72-page curriculum was created by the primary author with Spanish translation assistance from Dominican medical students, a Spanish speaking medical toxicologist, and a Spanish language teacher. A written copy of the curriculum was distributed to all students and the course was made available online at http://www.acmt.net/Links.html. The content of the curriculum was based on the toxicology category of the American Board of Emergency Medicine (ABEM) core content [18] as well as the results from the survey described above. The survey was used to identify common exposures, perceptions, and assess the fund of knowledge of community members and medical trainees in Santiago, DR. Informal interviews and an informal literature search were also used to guide curriculum development. The coursework of the curriculum was taught over 15 days (Monday to Friday for 3 weeks) through morning rounds, lectures and PowerPoint presentations at the 2 hospital sites. The lectures and presentations were the same at both hospital sites. The content covered during morning rounds varied depending on the patients who were physically present in the ERs. Nineteen emergency medicine residents at HRUJMCB and 15 family medicine residents at Hospital Juan XXIII completed the course. All the family medicine and emergency medicine residents from Hospital Juan XXIII and HRUJMCB, respectively, who were physically rotating in the ER during the 15 day study period, completed the course. A pretest and posttest was distributed to all residents who completed the course.

Results

Pre-hoc determination of sample size was determined by using previously published estimates of substance abuse in similar populations. The incidence of daily heavy drinking has been estimated to be 33.9% in Hispanics in a National Institutes of Health (NIH) Study [19]. The incidence of daily alcohol consumption in a study published by the American Medical College Association in 4 U.S medical schools was found to be 8.9% [20]. The minimum sample size was calculated to be 96 (24 group 1, 72 group 2) for a study with a group 1 incidence rate of 33.9% and a group 2 incidence rate of 8.9% with an enrollment ratio of 3:1 (3 community members/lay persons: 1 medical student/ resident), alpha of 0.05, and power of 80%. The total sample size in the current study was 175, which met the minimum sample size of 96 to sufficiently power this study. Post-hoc analysis of the study showed that the sample size was adequately powered in medical students/ residents and patients/lay persons, respectively for the incidence of frequent substance abuse (12.2%, 44%: calculated post-hoc power 98.8%).

Demographics

175 surveys were completed from 134 community individuals, 22 medical resident physicians, and 19 medical students (Table 2). In the students/residents group the age range was 20-32 (average=25) years; 56.1% were female, 43.9% were male; 54.7% were medical students, 46.3% were residents; 26.8% live in suburban areas, 73.2% in an urban apartment or home, none lived on rural farms or ranches. In the patients/community group the age range was 20-54 (average=37) years; 59.0% were female, 41.0% were male; 32.1% never completed high school, 44.0% were in the process of completing a college or other advanced degree, 23.9% had completed a college or advanced degree (Figure 1); 21.6% live in suburban areas, 47.0% live in an urban apartment or home, 31.4% live in a rural area or ranch.

Survey Item	Students/ Residents (n=41)	Patients/Lay Persons (n=134)
Age	range 20-32	range 20-54
	(mean=25 years)	(mean=37years)
Gender	Female 56.1%,	Female 59.0%, Male 41.0%
	Male 43.9%	
Education Level		
Never completed high school	0%	32.10%
High school graduate or college/medical school/ advanced degree in process	54.70%	44.00%

College/medical school/ advanced degree completed	46.30%	23.90%
Residence		
Suburban apartment or home	26.80%	21.60%
Urban apartment or home	73.20%	47.00%
Rural or ranch dwelling	0%	31.40%

Table 2: Survey responses to demographic questions.

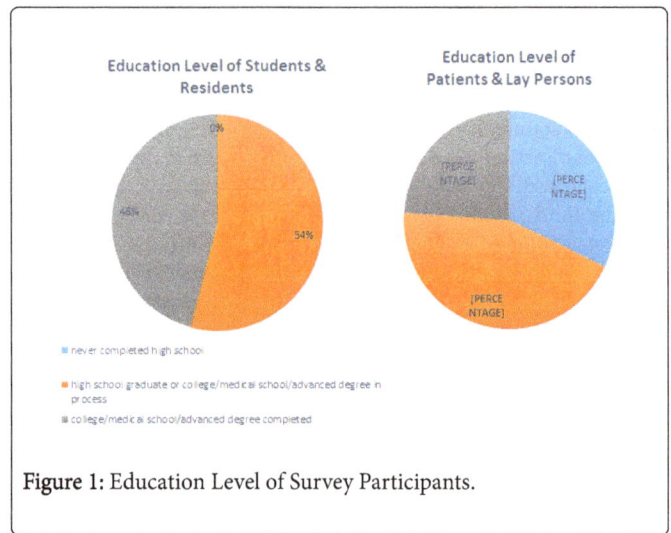

Figure 1: Education Level of Survey Participants.

Alcohol, illicit substances, and prescription pain or sedative medication abuse

In the previous year the use of alcohol was reported in 82.9% of students/residents, 62.7% of patients/lay persons (Table 3a). The annual use of prescription pain medications was 4.9% in students/ residents and 22.4% in patients/lay persons. The annual use of illicit drugs was 7.3% in students/residents and 9.9% in patients/lay persons. A total of 12.2% of students/residents and 44.0% of patients/ community members reported having regular (daily or almost daily) substance abuse. The percentage of students/residents and patients/ community members that have had frequent substance abuse defined as daily or almost daily exposure to the following substances, respectively are: heavy alcohol use (more than 2 drinks per day or more than 7 drinks per week) 4.9%, 23.1%; prescription sedative or pain medication use 2.4%, 13.4%; illicit drug use (e.g. cannabis, cocaine, amphetamine, hallucinogens, opioids, other) 4.9%, 7.5% (Table 3b). None of the survey respondents reported past use or present abuse of inhalants (nitrous, glue, petrol, paint thinner, etc.) (Figure 2).

History of Any Substance Use in the Previous Year		
Survey Item	Students/ Residents	Patients/Lay Persons
Alcohol use	82.90%	62.70%
Prescription pain medication use	4.90%	22.40%

Illicit drug use (marijuana, cocaine, heroin, ecstasy, LSD, acid, PCP, opioids, amphetamines etc)	7.30%	9.90%
Total sum of respondents who reported use of alcohol, prescription pain medications, or illicit drug use at any point in the previous year	95.10%	95.00%

History of Frequent (Daily or Almost Daily) Substance Abuse

Survey Item	Students/ Residents	Patients/Lay Persons
Heavy alcohol use (more than 2 drinks per day or more than 7 drinks per week)	4.90%	23.10%
Prescription pain medication use	2.40%	13.40%
Illicit drug use (marijuana, cocaine, heroin, ecstasy, LSD, acid, PCP, opioids, amphetamines etc)	4.90%	7.50%
Total sum of respondents who reported frequent alcohol, prescription pain medications, or illicit drug use	12.20%	44.00%

Table 3a and 3b: Survey responses to history of substance use in the past year or daily use.

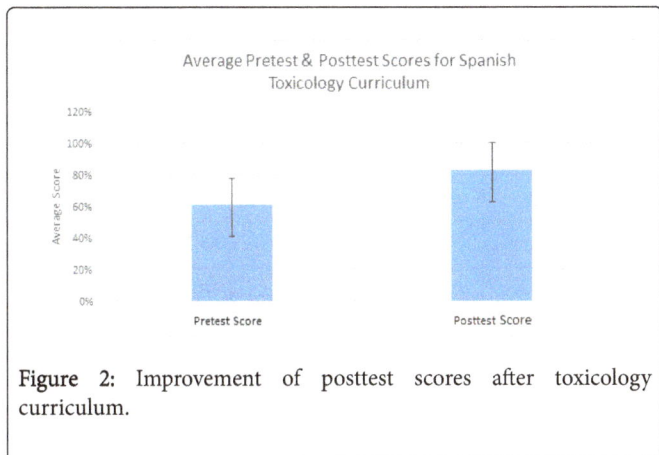

Figure 2: Improvement of posttest scores after toxicology curriculum.

Use and storage practices of potential household toxins

An average of 21.7% of students/residents and 13.7% of patients/community members practice safe storage practices of potential household toxins (Table 4). The percentage of students/residents and patients/community members that practice safe storage practices of the following products, respectively are: cosmetics: 2.4%, 3.7%; over the counter medications or prescriptions: 36.6%, 17.2%; cleaning products: 4.9%, 4.5%; automobile products: 7.3%, 3.0%; water filtration products: 7.3%, 2.2%; roach or insect spray: 43.9%, 31.3%; rat venom, powder, pellets or other traps 41.4%, 26.9%; weed killer or other

gardening/farming products: 31.7%, 21.6%; and anti-mold products 19.5%, 12.7%.

Safe Storage Practices (locked cabinets, high location out of reach for children, hidden, etc)		
Survey Item	Students/ Residents	Patients/Lay Persons
Cosmetics such as nail polish, nail polish remover, makeup remover, hairspray	2.40%	3.70%
Over-the-counter or prescription medications (pain killers, steroids, malaria pills, etc.)	36.60%	17.20%
Disinfectants/cleaning products for the bathroom, kitchen, etc. including bleach	4.90%	4.50%
Automobile Products (anticoagulants, antifreeze, or windshield fluid)	7.30%	3.00%
Water Filtration Products (Pools, Wells)	7.30%	2.20%
Insect repellent (roach or mosquito spray)	43.90%	31.30%
Rat venom, powder, pellets, or other traps	41.40%	26.90%
Herbicides/pesticides-weed killer or other gardening products	31.70%	21.60%
Anti-Mold Products	19.50%	12.70%
*Average Score for Safe Storage Practices	21.70%	13.70%

Table 4: Survey responses to safe storage practices for household products.

Previous medical encounters related to toxic exposures

A total of 7.3% of students/residents and 10.5% of patients/community members reported history of a previous medical encounter associated with a toxic exposure (Table 5a). The percentage of students/residents and patients/community members that have had a previous medical encounter related to the following toxins, respectively are: accidental substance overdose 4.9%, 5.2%; intentional substance overdose 0%, 0.75%; accidental prescription drug overdose 0%, 1.5%; intentional prescription drug overdose 0%, 0%; accidental exposure to household products 2.4%, 3.0%; and intentional exposure to household products 0%, 0%.

Survey Item	Students/ Residents	Patients/Lay Persons
Accidental substance overdose	4.90%	5.20%
Intentional substance overdose	0%	0.80%
Accidental prescription drug overdose	0%	1.50%
Intentional prescription drug overdose	0%	0%

Accidental exposure to household products	2.40%	3.00%
Intentional exposure to household products	0%	0%
Total sum with positive history of medical encounter associated with any substance	7.30%	10.50%

Table 5a: Survey responses to type of previous toxicological medical encounter and location of medical treatment. Positive History of Previous Medical Encounter Associated with Toxic Exposure.

If exposed to a dangerous potential toxin, the percentage of students/residents and patients/community members, respectively, who would seek treatment at the following areas are: clinic: 85.4%, 97.0%; emergency room: 100%, 98.5%; local pharmacy/medicinal store: 2.4%, 17.9% (Table 5b).

Survey Item	Students/ Residents	Patients/Lay Persons
a) clinic	85.40%	97.00%
b) emergency room	100%	98.50%
c) local pharmacy/medicinal store	2.40%	17.90%

Table 5b: Location of medical treatment sought if exposed to a dangerous potential toxin (multiple responses allowed).

Home or traditional remedy practices

An average of 15.2% of students/residents and 21.8% of patients/community members would practice various home or traditional remedies after ingesting a toxin (Table 6). The percentage of students/residents and patients/community members that would practice the following remedies, respectively are: induce vomiting 26.8%, 34.3%; drink water 36.5%, 55.2%; drink milk 14.6%, 21.6%; drink saltwater 31.7%, 36.6%, drink juice 9.8%, 10.4%, drink herbal or spice teas 0%, 9.0%; drink baking soda and water 17.0%, 8.21%; drink camphor and water 12.2%, 16.4%; or consume foodstuffs (oatmeal, rice, bread, etc.) 0%, 8.2%.

Home Remedies Practiced if Exposed to a Potential Toxin		
Survey Item	Students/ Residents	Patients/Lay Persons
Induce vomiting	26.80%	34.30%
Drink water	36.50%	55.20%
Drink milk	14.60%	21.60%
Drink saltwater	19.50%	32.80%
Drink juice	9.80%	10.40%
Drink herbal or spice teas (honey, cinnamon, chamomile, mint, etc.)	0%	9.00%
Drink baking soda and water	17.00%	8.21%

Drink camphor and water	12.20%	16.40%
Consume foodstuffs (oatmeal, rice, bread, etc.)	0%	8.20%
Average use of traditional home remedy	15.20%	21.80%

Table 6: Survey responses to the type of home remedies practiced if exposed to a toxin.

Lead knowledge

An average of 67.5% of students/residents and 44.0% of patients/community members correctly answered questions regarding potential symptoms of lead poisoning (Table 7). An average of 56.9% of students/residents and 52.6% of patients/community members gave correct responses for each source of lead poisoning.

Percentage of Correct Responses Regarding Potential Symptoms of Lead Poisoning		
Survey Item	Students/ Residents	Patients/Lay Persons
Neurological problems or learning impairment	95.10%	73.10%
Cardiovascular damage	70.70%	32.80%
Kidney problems	36.60%	26.10%
Average % answered correctly	67.50%	44.00%
What are potential sources of lead?		
a) Gasoline	85.40%	76.90%
b) Paint	92.70%	67.90%
c) Batteries	19.50%	29.10%
d) Cosmetics	22.00%	20.10%
e) Litargio	46.30%	55.20%
f) Water	90.20%	66.40%
Average % who gave correct responses for each source of lead poisoning	56.90%	52.60%

Table 7: Survey responses to lead knowledge toxicity.

Uses for camphor

The percent of students/residents and patients/community members who use camphor report using it in the following ways, respectively: ritual/spiritual use for camphor (repel evil spirits, spiritual protection, religious practices) 7.3%, 8.2%; aerosol camphor for respiratory infection in infants 4.9%, 15.7%; camphor use topically on infants 4.9%, 26.1%; camphor use in the crib to protect infant 2.4%, 8.2%; camphor dissolved in liquid as medication (e.g. to treat respiratory infection, upset stomach, fever) 9.8%, 24.6%; and camphor used topically as pest repellant 17.1%, 29.1% (Table 8a). An average of 7.7%

of the students/residents and 18.6% of the patients/lay persons use camphor for any of the above methods.

Survey Item	Students/ Residents	Patients/Lay Persons
Ritual/spiritual use for camphor (repel evil spirits, spiritual protection, religious practices)	7.30%	8.20%
Aerosol camphor for respiratory infection in infants	4.90%	15.70%
Camphor use topically on infants	4.90%	26.10%
Camphor use in the crib to protect infant	2.40%	8.20%
Camphor dissolved in liquid as medication for respiratory infection, upset stomach, fever, etc.	9.80%	24.60%
Camphor used topically as pest repellant	17.10%	29.10%
Average % who use camphor for any of the above methods	7.70%	18.60%

Table 8a: Survey responses to camphor use practices and toxicity knowledge. Uses for camphor.

Camphor toxicity knowledge

An average of 71.9% of students/residents and 27.0% of patients/community members correctly answered questions regarding potential symptoms of camphor ingestion (Table 8b). Twenty two percent of students/residents and 11.9% of patients/community members correctly answered that only a small amount of camphor (less than one camphor tablet) can cause poisoning in children.

Survey Item	Students/ Residents	Patients/Lay Persons
a) nausea and vomiting	46.30%	23.10%
b) organ damage (lung, liver, kidney, brain)	90.20%	46.30%
c) neurological effects (delirium, seizures, memory loss)	80.50%	28.80%
d) death	70.70%	9.70%
Average % who correctly answered organ symptoms questions correctly	71.90%	27.00%
% of respondents who correctly answered that less than 1 cube can cause illness in a child	22.00%	11.90%

Table 8b: Percentage of Correct Responses Regarding Potential Symptoms of Camphor Poisoning.

Pesticide use

95.2% of students/residents and 85.0% of patients/lay persons use legal over-the-counter substances as pesticide or insect repellant. The most common types of pesticides or insect repellants used by students/residents and patients/lay persons, respectively, were Essential Oils (36.6%, 12.7%), DEET containing products (22.0%, 18.6%), and Baygon* (19.5%, 24.6%) (Table 9a).

Survey Item	Students/ Residents	Patients/Lay Persons
Baygon®	19.50%	24.60%
DEET containing products (ex. OFF!)	22.00%	18.60%
Camphor (powder, tablet, cube, oil, vapor, etc)	17.10%	29.10%
Essential oils (Citronella, Eucalyptus, Tea Tree, Lemon, Lavender, Rosemary, Clove, Soybean Oil, etc)	36.60%	12.70%
Total % who use either Baygon, DEET, Camphor, or Essential Oils	95.20%	85.00%
Chinese chalk or Miraculous Chalk (deltamethrin, cypermethrin)	2.40%	3.00%
Paraquat (Gramoxone®)	2.40%	6.00%
Tres Pasitos (aldicarb, Temik®)	7.30%	17.90%
Total % who use either Chinese chalk, Paraquat, or Tres Pasitos	12.10%	26.90%

Table 9a: Survey responses to types of insecticide/pesticide/rodenticide used, use of personal protective equipment, and toxicology knowledge. Most common type of insect, pest, or rodent repellant used.

The most commonly reported illegal pesticides used in students/residents and patients/community members, respectively, were: Chinese Chalk or Miraculous Chalk (deltamethrin, cypermethrin) 2.4%, 3.0%; Paraquat (Gramoxone*) 2.4%, 6.0%; and Tres Pasitos (aldicarb, Temik*) 7.3% and 17.9%. The total percent who use illegal pesticides like Chinese Chalk, Paraquat, or Tres Pasitos in students/residents and patients/community members, respectively was 12.1% and 26.9%. The percentage of residents/students and patients/lay persons who immediately was their hands afterwards with soap and water are 80.5% and 66.4%, respectively (Table 9b). The consistent use of personal protective equipment is done in an average of 45.5% of residents/students and 26.9% of patients/lay persons when handling insecticides, pesticides, or rodenticides.

Survey Item	Students/ Residents	Patients/Lay Persons
Wash hands with soap and water immediately afterwards	80.50%	66.40%
Use of gloves	31.70%	17.90%

Wear eyewear while using spray products	26.8.%	14.20%
Use a face mask	24.30%	9.00%
Average % who either wear gloves, eyewear, or mask while handing insecticides, pesticides, or rodenticides	45.50%	26.90%

Table 9b: Consistent use of personal protective equipment with insecticide/pesticide/rodenticides.

Pesticide toxicity knowledge

An average of 69.7% of students/residents and 27.3% of patients/community members correctly answered questions regarding potential symptoms of pesticide ingestion (Table 9c).

Survey Item	Students/ Residents	Patients/Lay Persons
a) gastrointestinal effects (nausea, vomiting)	46.30%	23.10%
b) organ damage (lungs, liver, kidney, CNS, heart)	90.20%	46.30%
c) Cardiovascular effects (irregular rhythms, failure, shock)	61.00%	43.30%
d) Neurological effects (delirium, seizures)	80.50%	14.20%
e) death	70.70%	9.70%
Average % who correctly answered organ symptoms questions correctly	69.70%	27.30%
% of respondents who correctly answered that less than 1 teaspoon of certain pesticides can cause illness in an infant	58.50%	51.50%

Table 9c: Percentage of correct responses regarding potential symptoms of insecticide poisoning. *Baygon contains the pyrethroids cyfluthrin, transfluthrin, prallethrin and the carbamate propoxur and organophosphorus chlorpyrifos, as active ingredients.

Awareness or participation in previous education initiatives

There was a large range in exposure to previous educational campaigns. The following are the percent of students/residents and patients/community members who had previous participation in educational campaigns on the following topics, respectively: alcohol or substance abuse 100%, 73.9%; prescription drug abuse 70.7%, 18.7%; household hazards 46.3%, 12.7%; and traditional/home remedy use 36.6%, 11.9%; lead awareness 75.6%, 62.7%; pesticides 61.0%, 9.0%, and awareness of the disaster that occurred in Haina 9.8%, 3.7%. The average percent with previous exposure of any of the educational campaigns above was 57.1% in students/residents and 27.5% in patients/lay persons (Table 10).

Survey Item	Students/ Residents	Patients/Lay Persons
Alcohol or illicit substance abuse	100%	73.90%
Prescription drug abuse	70.70%	18.70%
Household hazards	46.30%	12.70%
Traditional home remedies	36.60%	11.90%
Lead	75.60%	62.70%
Pesticides	61%	9.00%
Awareness of the disaster that occurred in Haina	9.80%	3.70%
Average percent with previous exposure to any of the educational campaigns above	57.10%	27.50%

Table 10: Survey responses regarding previous exposure to educational campaigns on various toxicological exposures. previous exposure to educational campaigns (school, news, tv, internet, social media, community outreach, etc).

Curriculum assessment

Nineteen emergency medicine residents at HRUJMCB and 15 family medicine residents at Hospital Juan XXIII completed the toxicology course. The mean pretest score was 61% (range 40-88%) and posttest score was 83% (range 63-100%).

Discussion

Our study attempted to fulfill the first step in the development of a medical toxicology curriculum, which is in the Kern model, the identification of a problem through a general needs assessment [21]. The problem we sought to define was the educational needs regarding overdose and toxicological exposures in this study population. The aim of the survey was to characterize this problem in order to develop goals and objectives which in turn may help focus the curriculum's educational and evaluation strategies. The toxicology curriculum we developed for medical trainees was broad and included the essential components as defined by the American Board of Emergency Medicine (ABEM) core content with emphasis on the toxicological exposures that are more particular to this cultural group as identified by the survey. The results of the survey suggest that this community would benefit from education regarding safe-storage practices, when to seek medical attention, the potential dangers of traditional home remedy use, as well as sources, signs and symptoms of common exposures like lead and pesticide poisoning.

A total of 7.3% of students/residents and 10.5% of patients/community members have had a previous medical encounter associated with a toxic exposure. Additionally, after exposure to a potential toxin, more patients/community members (17.9%) would seek treatment at a medicinal store or pharmacy as compared to students/residents (2.4%), which could lead to inappropriate management and delay further definitive care at a medical setting. A total of 12.2% of students/residents and 44.0% of patients/community members have a positive history of frequent (daily or almost daily) alcohol (4.9%, 23.1%), prescription pain medicine (2.4%, 13.4%), or illicit drug use (4.9%, 7.5%), respectively. Other studies in similar populations have yielded roughly similar estimates. For example, the incidence of daily alcohol consumption in a study published by the American Medical College Association in 4 U.S medical schools was found to be 8.9% [20]. The incidence of daily heavy drinking has been estimated to be 33.9% in Hispanics in a National Institutes of Health (NIH) Study [19]. The annual incidence of illicit substance abuse in this study population was slightly above the globally reported average. Globally, it is estimated that in 2010, 3.4-6.6 percent of the world's population in the age group 15-64 years had used an illicit substance at least once in that year [22]. In this study 7.3% of residents/students and 9.9% of patients/community members reported use of any illicit substance in the past year.

The report of practice of traditional home remedies is relatively common in our survey population. Over one-quarter of students/residents and one-third of patients/community would induce vomiting after a potential toxin exposure. More than half of the survey respondents in both groups would try drinking either water, milk, baking soda, camphor, spices, or oatmeal as a remedy for a potential ingestion. In case of ingestion of a household toxin or caustic this could be especially detrimental. Orally ingesting another substance after a caustic ingestion could worsen symptoms by inducing emesis of a caustic chemical. Also in the case of ingestion of a substance with acidic properties, ingesting a basic substance, like baking soda, could result in an exothermic reaction and create more damage.

57.1% of students/residents and 27.5% of patients/community members reported previous exposures to educational campaigns (e.g. school, news, TV, internet, social media, community outreach) on overdose. Students/residents and patients/community members had fewer exposure to educational campaigns on household hazards (46.3%, 12.7%), and traditional/home remedy use (36.6%, 11.9%) as compared to alcohol and illicit substance abuse (100%, 73.9%), respectively. Patients/community members had notably less exposure to educational campaigns on pesticides (9%) as compared to students/residents (61%).

There is room for improvement in both groups regarding the fund of knowledge of various toxicological exposures that are common in the DR. The following are the average percent of correct responses for various exposures in students/residents and patients/community members, respectively: camphor ingestion 71.9%, 27.0%; lead poisoning 67.5%, 44%; and pesticide poisoning 69.7%, 27.3%. There are also a large proportion of individuals who would use dangerous and illegal pesticides like Chinese Chalk, paraquat, or Tres Pasitos; 12.1% of students/residents and 26.9% of patients/community members reported having used these pesticides. A pretest and posttest was given to assess the efficacy of the course. In the students and residents who completed the course there was a considerable improvement in their pretest scores (mean 61%, range 40-88%) and their posttest scores (mean 83%, range 63-100%). Their improvement in test scores is promising and is a positive indicator that the course was effective.

Conclusions

Certain limitations are evident in our survey, which intentionally limited open-ended questions and used either a 3-point or 2-point rating scale for the closed-ended questions. This closed-ended format does not attain outlying response options nor does it allow for qualitative data analysis. The questions that were asked in the survey may not be completely representative of the fund of knowledge or the behaviors practiced by the respondents due to limitations in length of the survey. Due to limitations in time we limited the questions so they could be reasonably answered within 10-15 minutes. Although we did not pilot test the survey instrument in this population, we did informally pilot the survey within the study team itself and extensive edits were made using native Dominican speakers to ensure clarity of the survey language within this study population. It is possible that survey respondents may not have completely understood the questions, although medical students who were native Dominicans and who were familiar with the content of the survey were available to answer any questions during the survey. Respondents also were not randomly selected, instead they were chosen based mainly on convenience. Using survey respondents who were mostly patients or have an interest in first response may impose bias towards people who have underlying medical conditions or who are perhaps related to those who do. The survey itself is novel and has not been previously validated or field tested. The pre-tests and post-tests that were used to evaluate the effectiveness of the curriculum in teaching the residents and medical students were also novel, and not previously validated or tested. Currently the study team is working with the American College of Medical Toxicology (ACMT) in creating new curriculum material including pretests and posttests that have been previously used in both domestic and other international settings.

Future steps in the identification of the problem are to develop a comprehensive definition of the problem, which includes consideration of epidemiology, impact on patients, health care professionals and society. The Kern model for curriculum development [21] highlight 3 requirements as being necessary for developing a comprehensive definition of the problem: 1) review of available information using comprehensive chart reviews, published literature, governmental or public health reports, public health statistics, etc. 2) use of experts in the field through organized societies of health care professionals who have proper training, in this case in toxicology and public health and 3) collection of new information using surveillance programs through governmental public health agencies or in this case, local poison control centers. The ability to develop a comprehensive definition of this problem is at this time still limited due to the lack of published literature, standardized medical records, surveillance programs such as poison control centers, and medical professionals with formal training in toxicology and public health in this region. Future collaborative international efforts and local participation are further needed to support these goals.

References

1. Chestnov O (2014) Dominican Republic. In: Noncommunicable Diseases (NCD) Country Profiles. World Health Organization.

2. Barry L (2007) Hispaniola: The Caribbean's New Big Leaguers in the Drug Trafficking Trade. In: Regions: Dominican Republic. Council on Hemispheric Affairs.

3. Toroyan T (2015) Global Status Report on Road Safety 2015. In: Violence and Injury Prevention. World Health Organization.

4. Tucker A (2006) Health Department reminds New Yorkers to avoid using illegal rat poison tres pasitos and to control pests safely. In: Press Release. NYC Department of Health and Mental Hygiene.

5. Centers for Disease Control and Prevention (CDC) (1997) Poisonings associated with illegal use of aldicarb as a rodenticide -- New York City, 1994-1997. MMWR Morb Mortal Wkly Rep 46: 961-963.

6. Palo W (2010) US AID Report: Dominican Farms Still Use Highly Toxic Pesticides. In: Dominican Republic Today.

7. Centers for Disease Control and Prevention (CDC) (2005) Lead poisoning associated with use of litargirio--Rhode Island, 2003. MMWR Morb Mortal Wkly Rep 54: 227-229.

8. New York City Department of Health and Mental Hygiene (2009) Lead Poisoning in New York City. In: Annual Data Report.

9. Khine H, Weiss D, Graber N, Hoffman RS, Esteban-Cruciani N, et al. (2009) A cluster of children with seizures caused by camphor poisoning. Pediatrics 123: 1269-1272.

10. Peters AL, Dekker E, Michels WM (2011) [Camphor poisoning following ingestion of mothballs 'for headache']. Ned Tijdschr Geneeskd 155: A3676.

11. Olsen A (2002) PANNA: Paraquat Poisons 153 Workers in the Dominican Republic. In: Pesticide Action Network North America.

12. Blacksmith Institute (2006) Haina, Dominican Republic. In: World's Worst Polluted Places Report.

13. Corporan R (2011) La realidad del alcanfor. Hoy.

14. WHO ASSIST Working Group (2008) The ASSIST project - Alcohol, Smoking and Substance Involvement Screening Test. In: Substance Abuse Activities. World Health Organization.

15. United States Agency for International Development (2013) Farmer-to-farmer programmatic PERSUAP (Pesticide Evaluation Report and Safer Use Action Plan). In: US AID.

16. Mereu C (2011) Dominican Republic bans five pesticides, restricts 22 others. In: Agronews.

17. Parisius LM, Stock-Schröer B, Berger S, Hermann K, Joos S (2014) Use of home remedies: a cross-sectional survey of patients in Germany. BMC Fam Pract 15: 116.

18. Counselman FL, Borenstein MA, Chisholm CD, Epter ML, Khandelwal S, et al. (2014) The 2013 Model of the Clinical Practice of Emergency Medicine. Acad Emerg Med 21: 574-598.

19. Chartier KG, Vaeth PAC, Caetano R (2012) Focus On: Ethnicity and the Social and Health Harms From Drinking. In: Alcohol Research: Current Reviews. National Institutes of Health.

20. Schindler BA, Novack DH, Cohen DG, Yager J, Wang D, et al. (2006) The impact of the changing health care environment on the health and well-being of faculty at four medical schools. Acad Med 81: 27-34.

21. Kern DE, Thomas PA, Hughes MT, Chen BY (2009) Curriculum Development for Medical Education - A Six-Step Approach. (2nd eds) Baltimore: The Johns Hopkins Univ Press.

22. United Nations Office of Drugs and Crime (2012) World Drug Report 2012. In: United Nations Publication, Sales No. E.12.XI.1.

8

Echocardiography a Non-Invasive Method for Investigating Preclinical Drug Toxicity and Safety

Gilles Hanton[*]

GH Toxconsulting, Brussels, Belgium

[*]**Corresponding author:** Dr. Gilles Hanton, 27 Avenue Everard, B-1190, Bruxelles, E-mail: gilles.hanton@yahoo.fr

Abstract

Echocardiography (EC) is a method used for investigating cardiac morphology and function. Two-dimensional EC gives a visualization of the morphology of the heart. M-mode EC allows heart function to be monitored. Pulsed Doppler EC is the method of choice for measuring blood flows through valves and large vessels. EC is used in routine in clinic and veterinary practice but is infrequently applied to preclinical evaluation of drug toxicity and safety pharmacology despite a number of advantages. Since similar investigations can be done in laboratory animals and humans, preclinical and clinical findings can easily be transposed to each other. EC is totally non-invasive, it does not induce any suffering to the animals and has no impact on health and physiology. It allows repeated measurements and consequently monitoring of development and evolution of adverse effects. In this way, EC evaluates the functional adverse effects of drugs on the cardiovascular system and the consequences of induced lesions. Moreover, using the different modes of EC it is possible to determine the changes in heart contractility and hemodynamics that are involved in the development of cardiovascular lesions. This is illustrated by an experiment in dogs treated with minoxidil. The development of lesions in the right atrium and left ventricle were considered to be related to changes in the function of these cardiac structures as demonstrated by EC recordings. These findings confirm the usefulness of EC in assessing the pathogenesis of drug-related cardiac toxicity.

Keywords: Echocardiography; Cardiac lesions; Minoxidil; Cardiac function

Introduction

Echocardiography (EC) is a method used for the investigation of cardiac morphology and function.

A transducer is placed on the chest of the subject and emits ultrasounds that are reflected by the cardiac structures and surrounding tissues. The reflected ultrasounds are received by the transducer and then processed by the echographic device in order to form an image on a screen. The fraction of the ultrasounds that are reflected characterizes the echogenicity and depends on the physical properties of the tissues. Bones and air have a strong echogenicity and appear in white on the screen. Liquids such as blood have a weak echogenicity and appear as black areas corresponding to the cardiac cavities and lumen of large vessels. Fibrous tissues and muscles have an intermediate echogenicity and appear as grey structures corresponding to cardiac valves and the wall of heart and main vessels.

Echocardiography can be done in humans and in laboratory animals, in particular dogs and non-human primates.

The methodology of echocardiography and its usefulness in preclinical toxicology are reviewed in the current paper. Then an example of application of echocardiography for the investigation of the pathogenesis of cardiac lesions is given.

The Different Modes of Echocardiography

There are three modes of EC, which are usually performed successively for a complete examination of the cardiac structures, their movements over time and blood flows. Indeed the different modes give pieces of information that complement each other.

Two-dimensional echocardiography

Two-dimensional echocardiography (2-D EC) gives a view of the morphology of the heart on the screen of the echographic device. The transducer emits a planar beam of ultrasounds in which the cardiac structures are visualized.

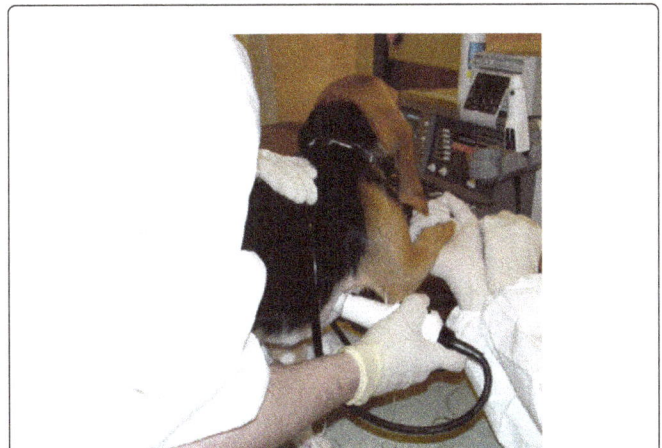

Figure 1: Echocardiography in dogs. Recording in right parasternal incidence.

Depending on the position of the transducer on the chest of the animal, different heart sections are obtained. By changing the orientation of the transducer progressively, the operator can scan the heart in successive sectors from which the walls, the cavities, cardiac valves and main vessels are visualized.

The 2-D EC examination is usually performed in two different incidences.

In parasternal incidence, the transducer is placed on the right side (Figure 1) and the cardiac structures are visualized in two different sections.

A long axis (longitudinal) section is carried out across the left and right ventricles, left atrium and aorta (Figure 2).

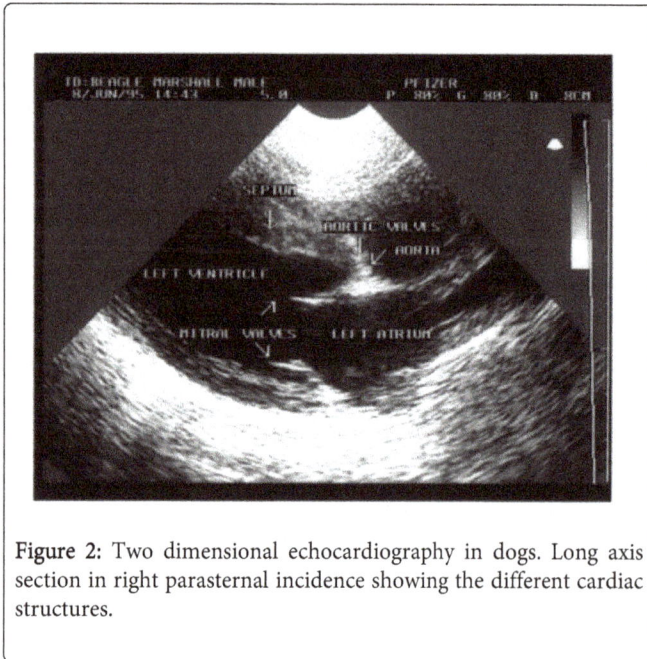

Figure 2: Two dimensional echocardiography in dogs. Long axis section in right parasternal incidence showing the different cardiac structures.

This section is used for the examination of the septum, free wall and cavity of left ventricle, wall and cavity of the left atrium, mitral valves and aortic root.

A short axis section allows visualization of the heart in successive transverse sections, from the apex to the upper part of the heart. The section at the upper level allows visualization of the aortic and pulmonary artery trunk and measurement of the pulmonary artery diameter (Figure 3).

For apical incidence, the transducer is placed on the left side of the animal at the level of the cardiac apex (Figure 4).

The four cardiac cavities are visualized simultaneously (Figure 5) and their areas can be measured in systole and diastole.

In 2-D EC views, guidance lines for M-mode EC or Doppler EC recording can be placed across cardiac structures.

Two-dimensional EC is thus the method of choice for visualizing the cardiac structures and assessing anatomical abnormalities. An ECG that is recorded simultaneously allows following the cardiac cycle. Images 2-D can then be frozen either in ventricular systole or diastole a number of measurements can be taken. For example the surface of the left ventricle can be measured in diastole and systole and the corresponding volumes of the ventricle can be estimated allowing a theoretical calculation of the stroke volume. However in 2-D EC

changes in cardiac structures cannot be followed over the full cardiac cycle.

Time-motion EC

In time-motion (M-mode), the position and movements of the cardiac structures crossed by the guidance line are displayed for a few cycles. In this way, M-mode EC allows the observer to visualize changes in heart morphology over the full cardiac cycle and to monitor cardiac function. However the time-related changes can only be seen in a single dimension. M-mode EC is recorded from a 2-D view of the heart in either short axis or long-axis section.

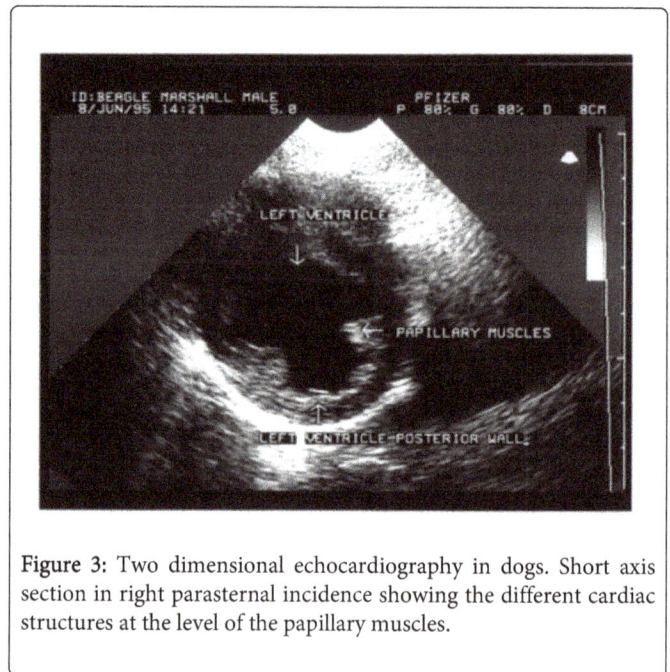

Figure 3: Two dimensional echocardiography in dogs. Short axis section in right parasternal incidence showing the different cardiac structures at the level of the papillary muscles.

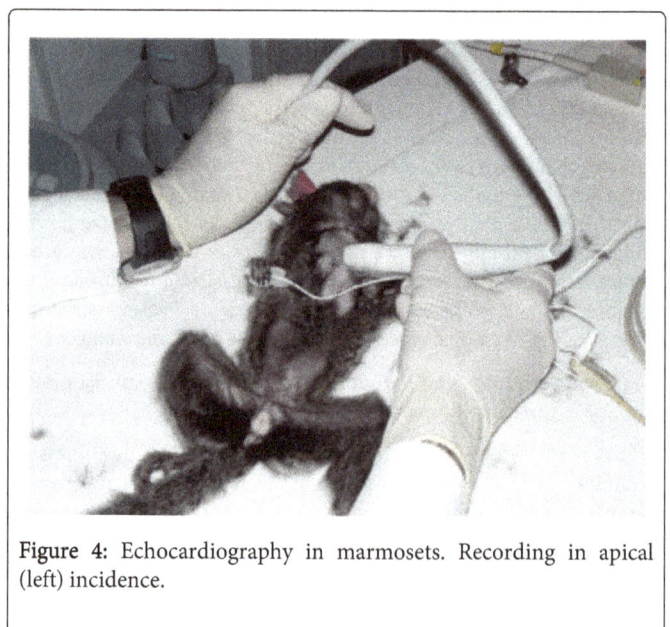

Figure 4: Echocardiography in marmosets. Recording in apical (left) incidence.

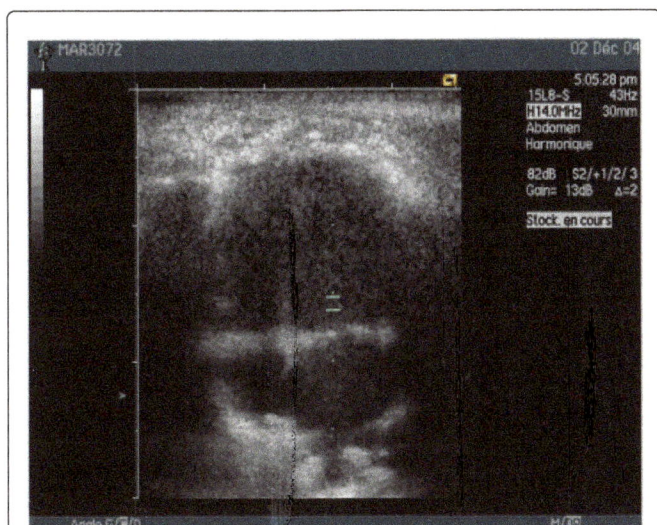

Figure 5: Two dimensional echocardiography in marmoset. Four cavity section in apical incidence showing the different cardiac structures and positioning of the Doppler guidance line for recording mitral flow. LV: Left Ventricle; RV: Right Ventricle; LA: Left Atrium; RA: Right Atrium.

In a short axis section, the upper part of the ventricle is visualized at the level of the papillary muscles close to the chordae tendinae. The guideline is positioned between the papillary muscles and the movements of the cardiac walls and septum are recorded (Figure 6A). Left ventricular end-diastolic (LVDd) and end-systolic (LVDs) diameters are measured at the time of maximum diastolic and minimum systolic dimensions. Thicknesses of the interventricular septum (IVSd and IVSs) and of the left ventricular posterior wall (PWTd and PWTs) are measured in diastole and systole (Figure 6B).

A number of parameters can be calculated

- End diastolic and end systolic volumes (EDV and ESV), calculated with the Teicholz formula: $V = 7D^3/(2.4 + D)$ with D=LVIDd or LVIDs respectively or EDV and ESV.
- Stroke volume: SV= EDV- ESV.
- Cardiac output and cardiac index: CO=SV*HR and CI=CO/body weight.
- Fractional shortening: FS=(LVIDd - LVIDs)/LVIDd.
- Ejection fraction: EF=SV/EDV (EF indicates the fraction of the ventricular diastolic volume that is ejected at each beat and is therefore considered as a key indicator of the ventricular contractile function).
- Percent of septum thickening: PST=(STd - STs)/STd.
- Percent of left ventricle posterior wall thickening: PWT=(LVPWd - LVPWs)/LVPWd.

The mean slope of the systolic wave of the free wall of ventricle is calculated between the onset and the peak of the wave, whereas the maximal slope is measured as a tangent of the wave at its onset. These slopes are further indices of left ventricle contractile function.

In long axis section, an area of the heart giving a clear longitudinal view of the cavities and walls, in particular these of the left heart is selected, and the guidance line is usually placed at two levels. For the evaluation of the ventricular function and morphology, the guidance line is positioned at the tips of the mitral valves and the movements of the cardiac walls and septum are recorded. The same parameters as those measured or calculated from M-mode recordings in short axis section can be obtained from this long axis section.

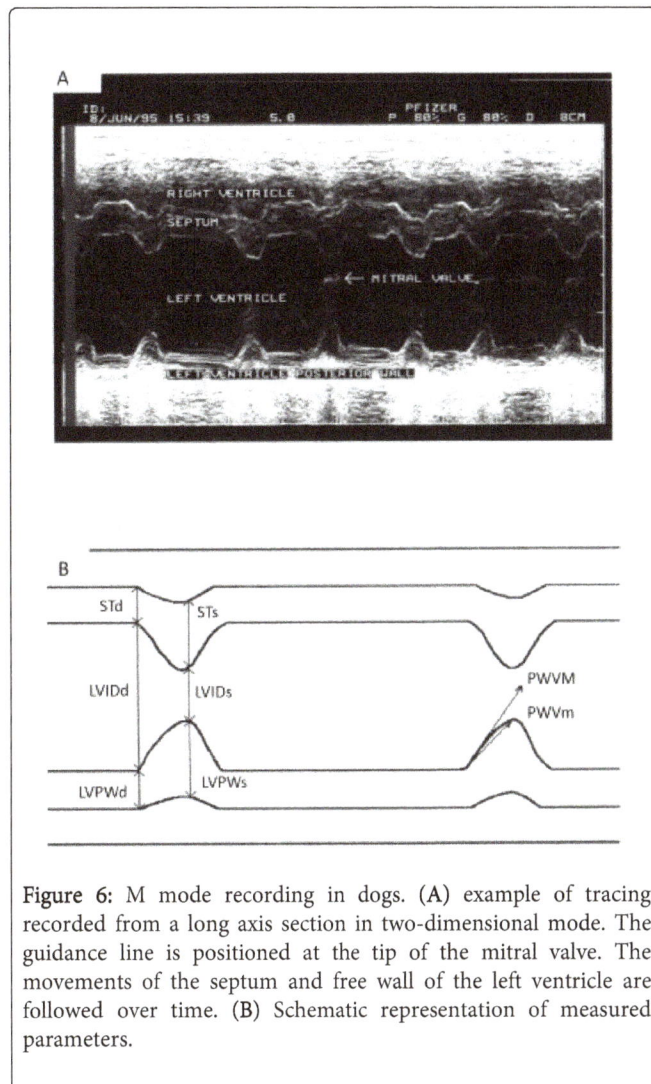

Figure 6: M mode recording in dogs. (**A**) example of tracing recorded from a long axis section in two-dimensional mode. The guidance line is positioned at the tip of the mitral valve. The movements of the septum and free wall of the left ventricle are followed over time. (**B**) Schematic representation of measured parameters.

In addition, the guidance line can be placed in long axis section in the upper part of the heart, across the aortic root and left atrium, for recording of their movements (Figure 7). Aortic diameter of the aorta and left atrium are measured in systole and diastole (ADs and ADd).

M-mode and 2-D EC give no information on intra-cardiac blood flows and only an indirect evaluation of stroke volume based on measurement of ventricle volumes in systole and diastole.

Doppler echocardiography

In pulsed Doppler EC, blood velocity is measured at the level of a window selected in a 2-D section. The spectrum of distribution of the velocities of the red blood cells and their variations over the cardiac cycle are recorded as successive waves produced by the pulsatile flows. The waves appear positive on the screen when the blood is flowing to the transducer and the waves are negative when the blood is flowing in the opposite direction. By measuring the speed of blood motion in vessels and cardiac cavities, pulsed Doppler EC allows the assessment of flows patterns and, consequently, of the systolic and diastolic cardiac function. Physiological and pathological changes in pulmonary, aortic and atrio-ventricular flows can be investigated. Doppler EC is also a reliable method for measurement of stroke volume.

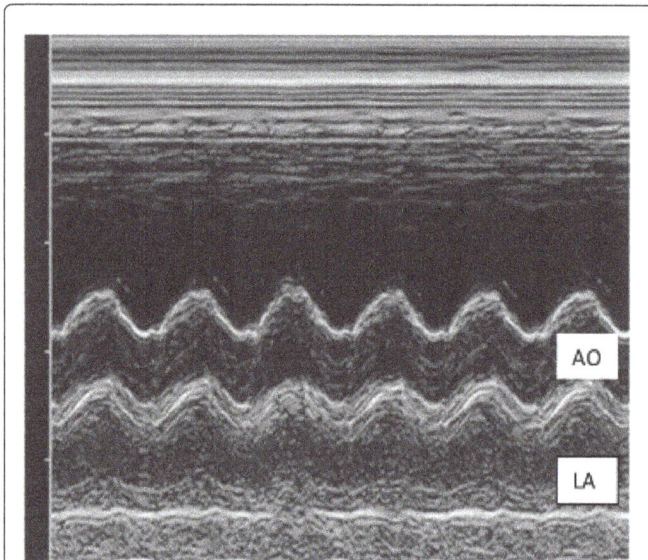

Figure 7: M mode recording at the level of upper part of the heart in marmosets from a long axis section in two-dimensional mode. The guidance line is positioned across the aorta and left atrium. The movements of aorta (AO) and left atrium (LA) are recorded over time.

The atrio-ventricular flows are assessed from a four-cavity section obtained in apical incidence. The Doppler windows are placed downstream of the flows, below the mitral or the tricuspid valves (Figure 5).

The flows are recorded and two positive waves occur at each cardiac beat (Figure 8). The rapid inflow E wave corresponds to the passive filling of the ventricle occurring during its diastole and is recorded during the isoelectric section of the ECG, between T and P waves. The A wave corresponds to the ventricular filling associated with atrial contraction and occurs at the time of the P wave. Peak velocities (V max) of E and A waves, their ratio (E/A), wave acceleration and the integral of velocity over time (VTI) of the two waves together are recorded and serve as indices of ventricle diastolic and/or atrial systolic functions. In particular, E/A gives an indication of the relative contribution of ventricle diastole and atrial systole to the ventricular filling.

Measurements

- Pre-ejection time from the Q wave of the ECG (a) to the onset of the Doppler velocity spectrum(b),
- Acceleration time from the onset to the peak of the velocity spectrum (c) and
- Ejection time from the onset to the end of the velocity spectrum (d).

The stroke volume (SV) is calculated for the pulmonary (SVPul) or aortic flows (SVAo) with VTI of the corresponding flow and the diameter (D) of the artery measured from a two-dimensional section.

$$SV_{Pul} = VTI_{Pul} * \pi * 1/4\ D_{Pul}^2$$

$$SV_{Ao} = VTI_{Ao} * \pi * 1/4\ D_{Ao}^2$$

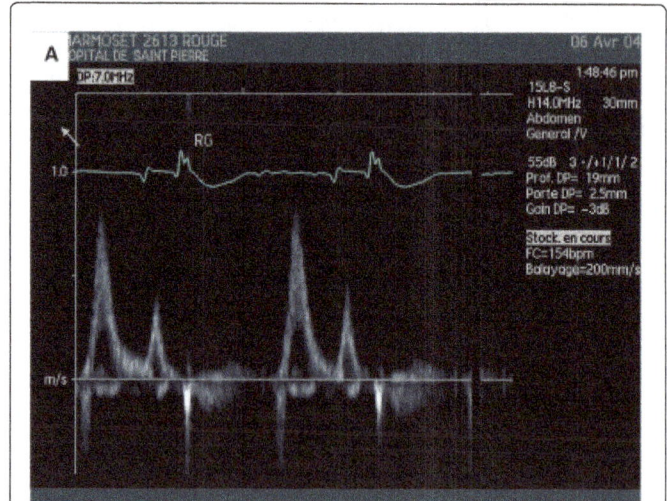

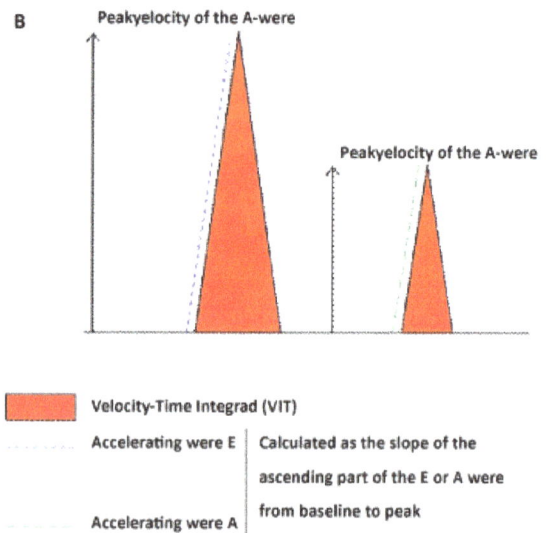

Figure 8: Doppler recording of mitral flow in marmosets. (A) example of tracing recorded from an apical section in two-dimensional mode. (B) Schematic representation of measured parameters.

In color Doppler EC, the flows in the cavities and large vessels are visualized in real time from a two-dimensional section, based on a color code. On a four-cavity apical view of the heart, the atrio-ventricular flows during ventricular diastole and atrial systole and the arterial flows during ventricular systole are observed at each cardiac beat. The flow appears in blue when the blood is flowing toward the transducer or in red when blood is flowing in the opposite direction. The brightness of blue or red color indicates the velocity of the blood.

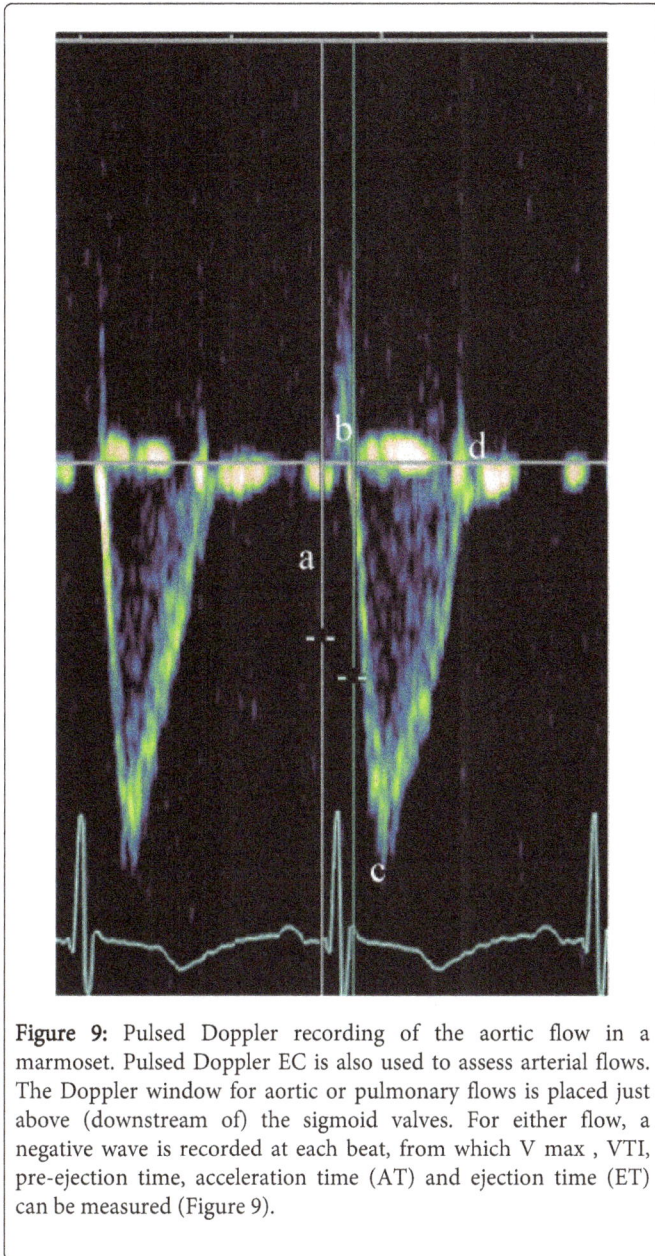

Figure 9: Pulsed Doppler recording of the aortic flow in a marmoset. Pulsed Doppler EC is also used to assess arterial flows. The Doppler window for aortic or pulmonary flows is placed just above (downstream of) the sigmoid valves. For either flow, a negative wave is recorded at each beat, from which V max , VTI, pre-ejection time, acceleration time (AT) and ejection time (ET) can be measured (Figure 9).

Color Doppler EC shows a number of qualitative blood flow changes, for example, laminar versus turbulent flows or abnormal timing and location of blood flows. Color Doppler is therefore a useful tool for the assessment of disturbed flow patterns associated with valve insufficiency or stenosis.

Doppler EC gives thus the information on intra-cardiac blood flows and the direct evaluation of stroke volume, which are missing when only 2-D and M-mode EC is recorded. Therefore Doppler is a key complement of the other EC modes but cannot be substituted to them, since it gives no information on cardiac morphology.

Usefullness of Echocardiography in Preclinical Toxicology

EC has been widely used in humans to investigate cardiac physiology and pathology and to evaluate the pharmacological effects of drugs.

EC has a number of applications in laboratory animals, in particular in dogs and nonhuman primates, but also in rodents and rabbit.

In dogs, the method of EC recording is well established and has been described in a number of papers, together with values in normal subjects [1-4]. In canine or feline veterinary practice, EC is routinely used and can assist in the diagnosis of cardiac morphological alterations or dysfunction.

EC is frequently used to assess toxicity of drugs in humans and in particular, Doppler EC is the gold method to assess the functional consequences of anthracycline's cardiotoxic effects [5-7]. In contrast, this technique is not routinely used for the preclinical toxicological evaluation of drugs despite its potential interest, mainly in dogs and non-human primates [8,9].

Using 2-D EC, it is possible to visualize and evaluate morphological changes induced by drug treatment, such as myocardium hypertrophy or cardiac chamber dilation.

Furthermore, the functional consequences of treatment induced arrhythmia or cardiac lesions in laboratory animals can be assessed by M-mode or Doppler EC. Changes in hemodynamic parameters (SV and flows patterns) and indicators of cardiac contraction (ejection fraction, fractional shortening and velocities of cardiac structures movements) would allow evaluation of the degree of cardiac function impairment.

EC is also of prime interest in assessing the cause of cardiac lesions. Toxic effects of cardiovascular drugs on the heart or blood vessels are often due to exaggerated pharmacological effects [10,11], resulting in marked changes in the cardiovascular function. M-mode and Doppler EC can quantify drug-induced changes in the patterns of cardiac contraction, flows, SV and cardiac output and in this way help to clarify the pathogenesis of cardiac or arterial lesions [12].

Value of echocardiography as a method of refinement

In contrast to most methods presently used in animal experimentation to investigate cardiac or vascular function, EC is non-invasive and does not necessitate surgery. It requires only a gentle restraint and, in some species, sedation or light anesthesia. EC does not induce any pain and no or minimal stress. It does not alter the cardiovascular function that it seeks to measure. Similarly, EC has no or little interference with the measurement of other parameters recorded in toxicity or pharmacology studies and has no effect on the health status of the animal. EC measurements are easily repeatable and therefore allow subsequent follow-up in the same animal.

Limitations of echocardiography

For obtaining accurate data from echocardiographic investigations, recordings should be done by highly trained people using a well standardized method. Even when it is the case, a full EC examination using the 3 modes is rather time consuming. Moreover measurements of changes in cardiac function are usually less accurate than for invasive methods. EC should therefore be limited to toxicological investigations or in some occasions pharmacological investigations, when major changes in cardiac function are expected.

Example of application of echocardiography for assessment of the pathogenesis of cardiac lesions

EC is routinely used in the clinic and there are a number of publications describing the application of echocardiography for evaluating the functional consequences of drug-induced cardiac toxicity, in particular for monitoring patients treated with chemotherapeutic agents [13-16]. The consequences of cardiac lesions produced by doxorubicin in dogs have been assessed by EC [17]. Thus EC is occasionally used in preclinical toxicology but is not apply to the assessment of the cause of cardiac lesions [18]. Therefore we used echocardiography to assess the pathogenesis of cardiac lesions associated with minoxidil treatment in dogs. This compound is a potent vasodilator and produces necrotic lesions in the myocardium of the left ventricle when given at suprapharmacological doses. These adverse effects are considered to be due to marked changes in ventricular function and hemodynamics. The aim of the study was to confirm that these changes can be investigated by echocardiography. Details on these experiments can be found in previous publications [19,20].

Groups of three beagles received a single administration of minoxidil at doses of 0.5 or 2 mg/kg or the vehicle alone (controls). M-mode and Doppler echocardiography was performed under two-dimensional echocardiography guidance on three occasions the day before treatment, immediately before dosing and 1, 3 and 24 h after dosing. Lead I ECG was recorded by the echographic equipment and heart rate (HR) was calculated. From M-mode recording, the following parameters were measured or calculated: end diastolic, end systolic, and stroke volumes (EDV, ESV and SV), fractional shortening (FS), ejection fraction (EF), the percentage of thickening of the septum and of the left ventricle posterior wall (PST and PWT). Doppler was used for recording aortic flows and calculating the corresponding Vmax, VTI, ejection time (ET) and stroked volume. Cardiac output was calculated at SV*HR.

Minoxidil produced a marked tachycardia. The treatment was associated with a decrease in ESV and with marked increases in FS, EF, PST and PWT, in comparison with data from controls (Table 1), (Figures 10 and 11).

	PST	PWT	EDV	ESV	EF	HR
Control	-14	-17	-7	-10	2	2
0.5 mg/kg	72	25	-21	-62	28	59
2 mg/kg	51	25	-21	-74	34	111

PST: Percent of septum thickening; PWT: Percent of left ventricle posterior wall thickening; EDV, ESV: End diastolic, End systolic volumes; EF: Ejection fraction; HR: Heart rate

Table 1: Minoxidil effects on parameters of left ventricle function in dogs, measured by M-mode echocardiography. Change (%) in mean values recorded 1 hour after treatment (time of maximal amplitude of changes) compared to values recorded the day before treatment.

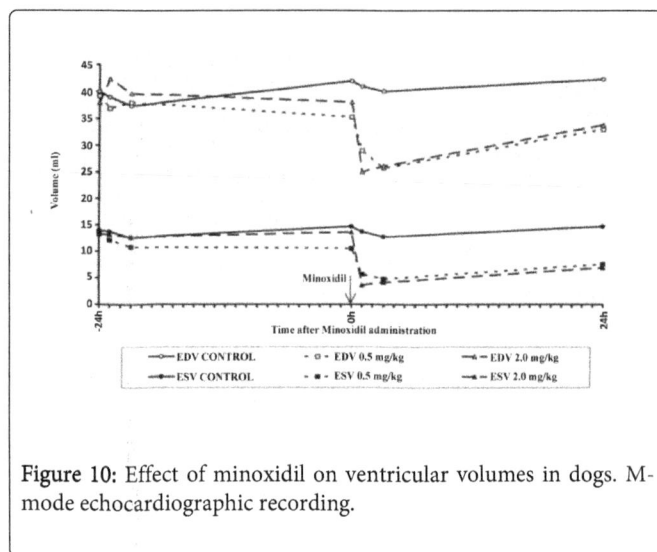

Figure 10: Effect of minoxidil on ventricular volumes in dogs. M-mode echocardiographic recording.

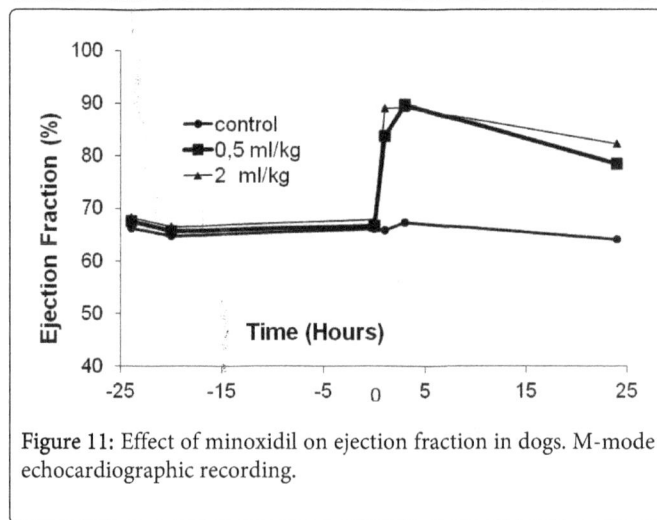

Figure 11: Effect of minoxidil on ejection fraction in dogs. M-mode echocardiographic recording.

	Vmax	VTI	ET	SV	CO
Control	16	14	-2	8	10
0.5 mg/kg	29	18	-17	22	93
2 mg/kg	53	25	-18	33	181

Table 2: Minoxidil effects on aortic flow in dogs, measured by Doppler echocardiography. Change (%) in mean values recorded 1 hour after treatment (time of maximal amplitude of changes) compared to values recorded the day before treatment.

Vmax: Maximum velocity of the wave; VTI: Velocity time integral; ET: Ejection time; SV: Stroke volume; CO: Cardiac output.

These changes are indicative of an increase in the amplitude of cardiac contraction. Minoxidil also produced a decrease in EDV, which indicates a decrease in left ventricle filling probably due to the tachycardia and consequent decrease in inter systolic time. Doppler measurements in table 2 showed an increase in the velocity of the aortic flow, which confirmed the increase in cardiac contractility. A decrease in ET is consistent with an increase in heart rate and a faster ventricular contraction. There was also a mild increase in stroke volume, which together with the tachycardia resulted in a marked increase in cardiac output. Overall, the effects were dose-related.

The tachycardia and echocardiographic evidence of increased cardiac contractility are consistent with the vasodilatory properties of minoxidil [21,22]. The consequent hypotension provoked a reflex inotropic and chronotropic compensatory reaction on the heart [23]. Furthermore, by decreasing the afterload, the vasodilation also resulted in the increase in velocity and amplitude of ventricle contraction [24,25].

The increase in rate and force of contraction of the myocardium increases its energy expenditure and oxygen requirements [10]. Because of the tachycardia, the ventricular filling is reduced as indicated by a decrease in EDV. In addition, the increase in heart rate decreases the duration of the diastole when most of the coronary perfusion occurs. The compound-induced hypotension further decreases the coronary perfusion [26]. Therefore, the increase in energy requirement coupled with an impaired perfusion resulted in a condition of relative coronary insufficiency, which is the likely cause of the necrotic lesions in the left ventricular myocardium (Figure 12).

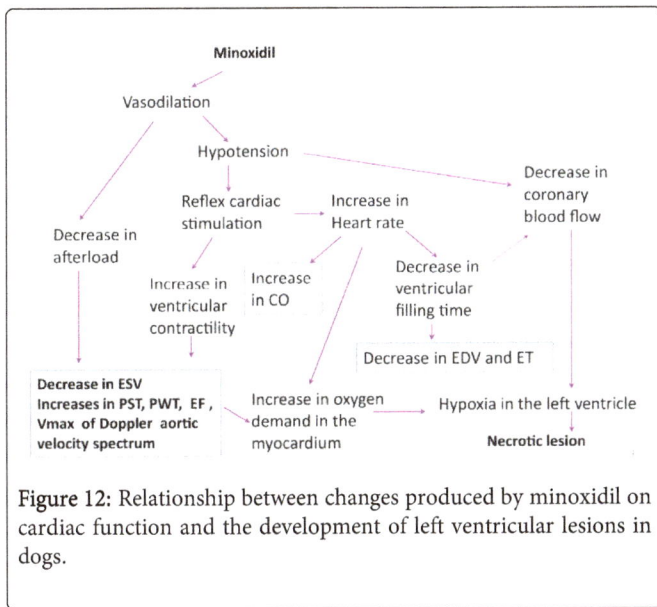

Figure 12: Relationship between changes produced by minoxidil on cardiac function and the development of left ventricular lesions in dogs.

Decrease in end systolic volume (ESV) and increases in percent thickening of the septum and left ventricle wall (PST and PWT), in ejection fraction (EF) and in maximum value of the Doppler aortic velocity spectrum (Vmax), which can be evaluated by echocardiography play a critical role and the development of the left ventricular necrosis. EDV: End diastolic volume; ET: ejection time; CO: cardiac output.

In conclusion, we have shown that echocardiography allows a non-invasive investigation of the changes in cardiac function that are considered to play a key role in the development of cardiac lesions produced by supra-pharmacological doses of a potent vasodilator in dogs.

References

1. Bonagura JD (1983) M-mode echocardiography. Basic principles. Vet Clin North Am Small Anim Pract 13: 299-319.

2. Bonagura JD, O'Grady MR, Herring DS (1985) Echocardiography. Principles of interpretation. Vet Clin North Am Small Anim Pract 15: 1177-1194.

3. Crippa L, Ferro E, Melloni E, Brambilla P, Cavalletti E (1992) Echocardiographic parameters and indices in the normal beagle dog. Lab Anim 26: 190-195.

4. Hanton G, Geffray B, Lodola A (1998) Echocardiography, a non-invasive method for the investigation of heart morphology and function in laboratory dogs: 1. Method and reference values for M-mode parameters. Lab Anim 32: 173-182.

5. Marchandise B, Schroeder E, Bosly A, Doyen C, Weynants P, et al. (1989) Early detection of doxorubicin cardiotoxicity: interest of Doppler echocardiographic analysis of left ventricular filling dynamics. Am Heart J 118: 92-98.

6. Sandor GG, Puterman M, Rogers P, Chan KW, Pritchard S, et al. (1992) Early prediction of anthracycline cardiomyopathy using standard M-mode and digitized echocardiography. Am J Pediatr Hematol Oncol 14: 151-157.

7. Tan TC, Scherrer-Crosbie M (2012) Assessing the Cardiac Toxicity of Chemotherapeutic Agents: Role of Echocardiography. Curr Cardiovasc Imaging Rep 5: 403-409.

8. Hanton G, Baneux PJR (2000) Echocardiography in laboratory dogs: a method of refinement for the assessment of cardiovascular toxicology. Example of minoxidil and quinidine: Progress in the Reduction, Refinement and Replacement of Animal Experimentation Elsevier, Amsterdam 1175 -1186.

9. Hug M-C, Singer T (1996) Echocardiography as a new tool in toxicology. Toxicol Lett 88: 105.

10. Balazs T, Bloom S (1982) Cardiotoxicity of adrenergic bronchodilator and vasodilating anti-hypertensive drugs: Cardiovascular Toxicology. Raven Press, New York, pp 199 -220.

11. Mesfin GM, Piper RC, DuCharme DW, Carlson RG, Humphrey SJ, et al. (1989) Pathogenesis of cardiovascular alterations in dogs treated with minoxidil. Toxicol Pathol 17: 164-181.

12. Hanton G (2007) Preclinical cardiac safety assessment of drugs. Drugs R D 8: 213-228.

13. Florescu M, Magda LS, Enescu OA, Jinga D, Vinereanu D (2014) Early detection of epirubicin-induced cardiotoxicity in patients with breast cancer. J Am Soc Echocardiogr 27: 83-92.

14. Thavendiranathan P, Poulin F, Lim KD, Plana JC, Woo A, et al. (2014) Use of Myocardial Strain Imaging by Echocardiography for the Early Detection of Cardiotoxicity in Patients During and After Cancer Chemotherapy - A Systematic Review. J Am Coll Cardiol .

15. Oreto L, Todaro MC, Umland MM, Kramer C, Qamar R, et al. (2012) Use of echocardiography to evaluate the cardiac effects of therapies used in cancer treatment: what do we know? J Am Soc Echocardiogr 25: 1141-1152.

16. DeCara JM (2012) Early detection of chemotherapy-related left ventricular dysfunction. Curr Cardiol Rep 14: 334-341.

17. Hanai K, Takaba K, Manabe S, Nakano M, Kohda A, et al. (1996) Evaluation of cardiac function by echocardiography in dogs treated with doxorubicin. J Toxicol Sci 21: 1-10.

18. Hanton G, Eder V, Rochefort G, Bonnet P, Hyvelin JM (2008) Echocardiography, a non-invasive method for the assessment of cardiac function and morphology in preclinical drug toxicology and safety pharmacology. Expert Opin Drug Metab Toxicol 4: 681-696.

19. Hanton G, Lodola A (1998) Echocardiography, a non-invasive method for the investigation of heart morphology and function in laboratory dogs: 2. Effects of minoxidil and quinidine on the left ventricle function. Lab Anim 32: 183-190.

20. Hanton G, Gautier M, Bonnet P (2004) Use of M-mode and Doppler echocardiography to investigate the cardiotoxicity of minoxidil in beagle dogs. Arch Toxicol 78: 40-48.

21. DuCharme DW, Freyburger WA, Graham BE, Carlson RG (1973) Pharmacologic properties of minoxidil: a new hypotensive agent. J Pharmacol Exp Ther 184: 662-670.

22. Jett GK, Herman EH, Jones M, Ferrans VJ, Clark RE (1988) Influence of minoxidil on myocardial hemodynamics, regional blood flow, and morphology in beagle dogs. Cardiovasc Drugs Ther 1: 687-694.

23. Humphrey SJ, Zins GR (1984) Whole body and regional hemodynamic effects of minoxidil in the conscious dog. J Cardiovasc Pharmacol 6: 979-988.

24. Kittleson MD, Pipers FS, Knauer KW, Keister DM, Knowlen GG, et al. (1985) Echocardiographic and clinical effects of milrinone in dogs with myocardial failure. Am J Vet Res 46: 1659-1664.

25. Baum T (1990) Fundamental principles governing regulation of circulatory function: Cardiovascular Pharmacology. Raven Press, New York. pp 1-36.

26. Herman EH, Ferrans VJ, Young RS, Balazs T (1989) A comparative study of minoxidil-induced myocardial lesions in beagle dogs and miniature swine. Toxicol Pathol 17: 182-192.

9

Evaluation of Two Different Screening ELISA Assays for Synthetic Cathinones (Mephedrone/Methcathinone and MDPV) with LC-MS Method in Intoxicated Patients

Roda E[1*], Lonati D[1], Buscaglia E[1], Papa P[2], Rocchi L[2], Locatelli CA[1] and Coccini T[1]

[1]Laboratory of Clinical & Experimental Toxicology and Poison Control Centre and National Toxicology Information Centre, Toxicology Unit of the Pavia's Hospital, IRCCS Maugeri Foundation, Pavia, Italy

[2]Laboratory of Analytical Toxicology, Clinical Chemistry Service of Pavia's Hospital, IRCCS Policlinico San Matteo Foundation, Pavia, Italy

*Corresponding author: Dr. Elisa Roda, IRCCS Maugeri Foundation, Medical Institute of Pavia Laboratory of Clinical & Experimental Toxicology and Poison Control Centre and National Toxicology Information Centre, Via Maugeri, 10 - 27100 Pavia, Italy, E-mail: elisa.roda@fsm.it; elisa.roda@unipv.it

Abstract

Context: Synthetic cathinones are a new trend in the recreational drug market and the paucity of human toxicological data combined with their widespread abuse generated great concern in the international scientific community.

Objective: Inside the Italian National Early Warning System (NEWS), clinical urine specimens were collected from patients (n=202) admitted to the Emergency Departments (April 2011-January 2013) for clinically suspected abuse of any kind of unknown new psychoactive substances, to measure synthetic cathinones demonstrating the consistency and reliability of the employed screening assays as useful tools to detect these drugs, with the ultimate objective to advance patients care and management.

Methods: Screening analyses were performed using two specific ELISA assays, targeting Mephedrone/methcathinone and MDPV (LOD 0.40 and 20.0 ng/ml, respectively). Data were then compared to determinations gained by LC-MS (LOD 5 ng/ml).

Results: (i) Mephedrone/methcathinone: 195/202 samples gave values <7 ng/ml by screening ELISA assay and tested negative by LC-MS. Seven specimens showed concentrations >16 ng/ml (above the upper limit of the standard curve) by screening immunoassay, and only 4 of them resulted positive by LC-MS; (ii) MDPV: 162/167 samples gave values ≤ 60 ng/ml by screening ELISA and tested negative by LC-MS. Five samples showed concentration above the upper limit of the standard curve (>850 ng/ml). Among these, 3/5 samples were confirmed positive by LC-MS (2 for butylone and MDPV, 1 for pentedrone and MDPV).

Discussion and conclusion: These results emphasize a good overall match between data obtained by the two analytical methods, showing disagreement in few cases concerning positive results; no false negatives were detected by ELISA screening, suggesting the promising usefulness of this reliable tool as first approach in the emergency setting to rapidly detect synthetic cathinones, allowing the clinician to improve differential diagnosis, aiding real-time patient care and management.

Keywords: Designer drugs; Bath salts; Cross reactivity; Immunoassay; Emergency departments

Introduction

The worldwide drug scenario is incessantly transforming in that common drugs of abuse have been joined by "new psychoactive substances" (NPS) that fall outside international drug control conventions. Many of these substances were synthesized and patented in the early 1970s, but only over the last decades they have rapidly emerged in the market supposedly as "legal" alternatives to internationally controlled drugs, thus posing serious risks to human safety. These novel psychoactive substances are marketed as 'designer drugs', being this term used, and continuously broadened, to identify and include synthetic substances mimicking the effects of illicit drugs, produced by introducing slight modifications to the chemical structure of controlled substances to circumvent drug controls [1].

In 2000s, among NPS, many synthetic cathinones (amphetamine- and cocaine-type stimulants) have received a renewed popularity. These novel compounds, derived from the vegetable cathinone, naturally present in the Khat plant (Catha edulis), are marketed as "bath salts" or "plant food" and labeled "not for human consumption" to circumvent the legislation on drugs of abuse [2-4]. The internet market greatly increased the spread of these NPS, sold in specialized shops known as "head" or "smart shops" as well as in online store, being able to respond quickly to changes in the legal status of recreational drugs offering for sale new legal alternatives, thus becoming a matter of threat to public health [5-10].

These "bath salts" are synthetic cathinone powders, distributed under trade names such as 'Ivory Wave', 'White Lightning' and 'Vanilla Sky', typically taken by inhalation (snorting), ingestion, or intravenous/intramuscular injection [6,11]. As with tablets, mephedrone is the most commonly abuse in Europe, whereas MDPV and methylone are more prominent in US bath salts [1]. Abuse is documented across population from mid-to-late adolescent to older adults [12].

Like amphetamines, synthetic cathinones exert their stimulant effects via (i) increasing synaptic concentration of catecholamines such as dopamine, serotonin and norepinephrine, and (ii) inhibiting monoamine uptake transporters, with a consequent decreased clearance of the neurotransmitters from the synapse. Furthermore, they may cause release of biogenic amines from intracellular stores [2,13].

Since synthetic cathinones are a pandemic trend, the paucity of human toxicological data combined with the numerous cases of abuse, dependence, severe intoxication and drug-related deaths, signalled in several Countries, has generated great concern in the scientific community. Thus, International agencies and national institutions have issued extensive reports to monitor this emerging trend of abuse, as well as to schedule and banned some NPS [1,14-20]. In Italy, as a result of acute intoxications including deaths, mephedrone was placed under the regulatory control in June 2010, as reported in the Presidential Decree 309/90 (as amended) on the "regulation of narcotic drugs and psychotropic substances, prevention, treatment and rehabilitation of drug addiction". Subsequently, new decrees entered into force placing under control synthetic cathinone 3,4-methylendioxypyrovalerone (MDPV) and structure analogues, derived from 2-amino-1-phenyl-1-propanone, for one or more substitutions on the aromatic ring and/or on the nitrogen and/or on the terminal carbon [18,21].

Currently, the information available about the human pharmacokinetics and pharmacodynamics of cathinone derivatives as well as the short and long-term toxicological effects of these NPS are very limited, thus their potential consequences are not well defined and generally poorly known.

In Italy the dimension of this problem is still indefinite; ambiguous signs/symptoms often characterize the clinical presentation of the patients admitted to the National Emergency Departments (EDs), contributing to underestimate or misjudge this phenomenon, potentially reverberating on the patient management. The identification of intoxication cases consistently related to synthetic cathinones abuse on the Italian EDs may allow the national regulatory agencies to engage actions designed to prevent and control this growing misuse.

So far, even though a number of national and international bans have been enacted, [15,16,18,19,22] the abuse of these designer drugs still continues and exponentially grows. For this reason it is difficult to validate and maintain comprehensive analytical methods for accurate detection of these compounds in biological specimens. Commonly, screening methods, such as immunoassay, are employed by toxicology laboratories for the first, presumptive identification of drugs of abuse, followed by confirmatory analysis, such as gas chromatography (GC) or liquid chromatography (LC) coupled with mass spectrometry (MS). As a consequence, in recent years, a critical need emerged in the field of toxicology to (i) study the activities of these NPS in screening assays, as well as to (ii) identify and validate reliable screening tests for multiple designer drugs, to be successfully applied other than classical analytical methods in human specimens.

With this purpose, inside the Italian National Early Warning System (NEWS) Project - Department for Antidrug Policies-Presidency of the Italian Council of Ministers (Rome), in which the Pavia Poison Control Centre (IRCCS Salvatore Maugeri Foundation) is the National Coordinating Centre for clinico-toxicological aspects, our Laboratory of Clinical Toxicology (IRCCS Salvatore Maugeri Foundation) performed screening analysis in urine samples of poisoned patients, admitted to EDs for a clinically suspected abuse of any kind of unknown NPS, followed by confirmatory analyses carried out by the Laboratory of Analytical Toxicology of the IRCCS Foundation Policlinico San Matteo. The investigation aimed at measuring synthetic cathinones to demonstrate the consistency and reliability of the employed screening assays as useful tools to rapidly detect these NPS, with the final goal to improve patient care and management.

Materials and Methods

Human urine specimens

The present study design was reviewed and approved by the Ethic Committee of our Hospital (1099 CE/2015).

The study was conducted on a total of 202 clinical urine specimens collected from severely intoxicated patients admitted to Italian emergency departments (EDs) inside the NEWS Project, from April 2011 to January 2013, for a clinically suspected abuse of a broad range of unknown NPS. Patients were informed of their biological specimens use for this research project and signed the consent forms, following the regulation established by Department for Antidrug Policies-Presidency of the Italian Council of Ministers (Rome). The urine samples sent to our lab were collected in plastic containers (not adsorbing drugs), divided into two aliquots (one for the first-step screening ELISA analysis and the other one for the following confirmatory determination, respectively) and immediately stored at -20°C until examinations.

In addition, twenty-five healthy, non-smoker, non-drug abusers volunteers were recruited and their urines underwent contextual screening analysis to determine synthetic cathinones (i.e. both Mephedrone/Methcathinone and MDPV) background levels.

Reagents and consumables

Mephedrone/Methcathinone (Bath Salt I) and MDPV (Bath Salt II) determination was achieved using two specific enzyme-linked immunosorbent (ELISA) commercial kits, purchased from RANDOX Laboratories Ltd (Crumlin, Co. Antrim, UK).

For confirmatory analyses, all chemical reagents were obtained from Sigma Aldrich (Sigma, Milan, Italia), and the certified reference standards from LGC (LGC Standards, Teddington, Middlesex, UK).

Immunoassay screening procedure

The ELISA assays allow to semi-quantitatively measure, with high specificity, the level of several Mephedrone/Methcathinone and MDPV parent compounds and derivates (see Table 1). Standard curves for Mephedrone/Methcathinone and MDPV kits ranged between 0 to 0.16 ng/ml and 0 to 850 ng/ml, respectively. LOD: 0.40 and 20.0 ng/ml for Mephedrone/methcathinone (Bath Salt I) and MDPV (Bath Salt II), respectively.

According to the manufacturer's instructions, urines were centrifuged at 13000 rpm for 60 sec and then diluted 1:4 with sample diluent. Subsequently, 25 microL of standard solution or urine samples and 100 microL of conjugate diluent were added to each appropriate well. All calibrators and samples were performed in duplicate. After incubation at room temperature for 1 h in the dark, the plates were washed six times with diluted wash buffer.

Compound	% Cross Reactivity
Mephedrone/Methcathinone (Bath Salt I) kit	
Mephedrone HCl (4-MMC)	100
Methylone	63
Flephedrone HCl (4-FMC)	45
R(+)-Methcathinone HCl	44
Methcathinone	43
3-FluoroMethcathinone (3-FMC)	16
4-Methylethcathinone (4-MEC)	10
Ethylone HCl	7
N-ethylcathinone HCl	4
Buphedrone HCl	<1
S(-)-Methcathinone	<1
S(-)-cathinone	<1
R(+)-cathinone	<1
Bupropion HCl	<1
Beta-ethyl Methcathinone	<1
MDPV (Bath Salt II) kit	
3,4-Methylenedioxypyrovalerone (MDPV) HCl	100
3'-4'-Methylenedioxy-alpha-pyrrolidinobutiophenone (MDPBP) HCl	96
Naphyrone HCl	27
Pyrovalerone HCl	17
4'- Methyl-alpha-pyrrolidinohexaphenone (4'-Me-a-PHP) HCl	15
4' Methyl-alpha-pyrrolidinobutiophenone (MPBP) HCl	13
Pentylone HCl	9
3',4'-Methylenedioxy-alpha-pyrrolidinopropiophenone (MDPPP) HCl	4
Butylone HCl	4
Desmetyl pyrovalerone (alpha-PVP) HCl salt	2
Pentedrone HCl	<1

Table 1: Summarized specificity of the ELISA kits employed for the screening analyses, based on the manufacturer's indications.

Next, 125 microL of one shot substrate solution was added and the plates were placed in the dark at room temperature for 20 min. The reaction was stopped by adding 100 microL of stop solution and the absorbance was read at 450 nm, also using a reference 630 nm filter. Finally, to interpret the results and to calculate the urine concentrations, a 4 parameter curve fit method was used to generate a standard log10 curve; the mean absorbance of controls and samples was calculated and then plotted against the standard curve.

Confirmatory urine samples study: Liquid chromatography-tandem mass spectrometry (LC/MS) analysis

Presumptive positive and negative urine specimens, based on the values obtained by screening assay, were confirmed with a liquid chromatography-tandem mass spectrometry (LC-MS) method, modified from Chimalakonda et al. and Dresen et al. [23,24]. Specifically, for the LC-MS analysis, urine samples (1 ml) were additivated with 100 ng of dosulepin as internal standard, 100 microL of NaOH 1N (pH 14) and extracted with a mixture of exane:ethylacetate (3:1 v/v) by vortex mixing for 2 min. The organic layer was transferred to a new glass tube and evaporated to dryness under nitrogen stream.

The samples were then reconstituted in 10 microL of methanol and 100 microL of mobile phase A. 20 microL of the reconstituted sample was injected into a Waters LC-MS apparatus, constituted by an Alliance liquid chromatographic system coupled with a Waters Quattro Micro triple quadrupole equipped with a Z-spray electrospray source. The chromatographic separation was performed using a Waters Xbridge C18 column operating in gradient mode at 30°C. The mobile phases were: (A) 5 mM ammonium formate in water, pH 3 with formic acid, (B) 0.1% formic acid in acetonitrile. The gradient started from 95% A, 5% B, got up to 20% A, 80% B in 12 min and returned to the original condition in 6 min. Flow rate was 0.2 ml/min. Mass spectrometer analysis was performed in positive ionization (ESI) and the acquisition was made in Multiple Reaction Monitoring mode (MRM) with two transitions for each analyte.

Results

Presumptive negative and positive urine specimens, based on ELISA screening determinations, were analysed with a LC-MS confirmatory method for 15 parent cathinones and derivates. Limits of detection (LOD) was 5 ng/ml for all the screened cathinones, based on the availability of certified reference standards.

Specifically, the followings were determined: Mephedrone or 4-methylmethcathinone (4-MMC), 3,4-Dimethylmethcathinone (3,4-DMMC), Flephedrone or 4-FluoroMethcathinone (4-FMC), 4-Methylethcathinone (4-MEC), Ethylone (βk-MDEA), Buphedrone or α-methylamino-butyrophenone (MABP), 3,4-Methylenedioxypyrovalerone (MDPV), Naphyrone or naphthylpyrovalerone (O-2482), Pentylone (βk-MBDP), Butylone (βk-MBDB), Pentedrone or α-methylamino-valerophenone, N,N-DimethylCathinone or metamfepramone, Ethcathinone or ethylpropion (ETH-CAT), Methedrone or 4-methoxymethcathinone (βk-PMMA), Methylone or 3,4-methylenedioxy-N-methylcathinone (MDMC or bk-MDMA).

We identified the analyzed urine samples as following: (i) true positive specimens, those screened and confirmed positive, (ii) true negative specimens, those negative in both assays, (iii) false (i.e. mismatching) positive specimens, those screened positive, but not confirmed by LC-MS for synthetic cathinones; (iv) false negatives, sample screened negative but confirmed positive for one or more synthetic cathinones.

Table 2 details which drug of abuse screened by ELISA assay, as specified by the manufacturer, was determined by LC-MS, based on certified reference standards supply.

Confirmatory LC-MS analyses	Screening Analyses % Cross Reactivity	ELISA kits
Mephedrone (4-MMC)	100	(Mephedrone/Methcathinone)
Methylone	63	(Mephedrone/Methcathinone)
4-FluoroMethcathinone (4-FMC)	45	(Mephedrone/Methcathinone)
4-Methylethcathinone (4-MEC)	10	(Mephedrone/Methcathinone)
Ethylone (βk-MDEA)	7	(Mephedrone/Methcathinone)
Buphedrone (MABP)	1	(Mephedrone/Methcathinone)
MDPV	100	(MDPV)
Naphyrone (O-2482)	27	(MDPV)
Pentylone (βk-MBDP)	9	(MDPV)
Butylone (βk-MBDB)	4	(MDPV)
Pentedrone	1	(MDPV)
N,N-DimethylCathinone	not detected	---
3,4-Dimethylmethcathinone (3,4-DMMC)	not detected	---
Ethcathinone (ETH-CAT)	not detected	---
Methedrone (βk-PMMA)	not detected	---

Table 2: Drug of abuse screened by ELISA, as reported in given manufacturer's indications, was determined by LC-MS, based on certified reference standards supply.

Regarding the n=25 samples from healthy volunteers (considered as controls), tested to determine the cathinones background levels, screening analysis measured urinary values ranging from 0.0 to 0.8 ng/ml and 0.0 to 57.2 ng/ml, for Mephedrone/Methcathinones (Bath Salt I) and MDPV (Bath Salt II), respectively.

Mephedrone/methcathinone (Bath Salt I) determination: on a total of 202 biological specimens, 195 samples gave values <7 ng/ml by screening ELISA assay, thus being considering as presumptive negatives; the same samples subsequently were tested as negative by LC-MS analysis, with value <5 ng/ml, thus demonstrating that all 195 samples were true negatives.

Seven urine samples showed concentrations >16 ng/ml (above the upper limit of the standard curve) by screening immunoassay, and only 4 of them resulted true positive when dosed by LC-MS (Table 3A). Regarding the n=3 false (i.e. mismatching) positive specimens (Table 3A), it has to be pointed out that 2 samples belonged to subjects screened and confirmed as polydrug abusers; specifically, one urine

was positives for delta-9-tetrahydrocannabinol (Δ-9-THC), Amphetamine (AMP) and 3,4-methylenedioxy-methamphetamine (MDMA) and the second sample for benzoylecgonine (i.e. cocaine) (COC) and MDMA, respectively, while the remaining one was tested positive for Methoxetamine (MXE) by LC-MS. Notably, no false negatives were detected.

MDPV (Bath Salt II) determination: On a total of 167 specimens analyzed, 162 samples gave values ≤ 60 ng/ml by screening ELISA assay and considered as presumptive negatives. When tested by LC-MS, the same samples were confirmed as true negatives. 5 urine samples were screened as presumptive positive; among these, 3 specimens, showing concentrations above the upper limit of the standard curve (>850 ng/ml) in screening, were confirmed as true positive by LC-MS analysis (Table 3B). Concerning the false (i.e. mismatching) positive specimens (n=2) not confirmed by LC-MS (Table 3B), n=1 urine was screened positive for COC and the other sample for Ketamine (KET), as further confirmed by the following LC-MS analyses. Importantly, once more, no false negatives were determined.

A: Mephedrone/Methcathinones				
Total biological samples	True Confirmed Negatives	False negatives	True Confirmed positives	FALSE (i.e. mismatching) positives
n=202	n=195	0	n=4	n=3 (*)
	<7 ng/ml (Screening analyses)		>16 ng/ml (Screening analyses)	
	<5 ng/ml (LC-MS analyses)		>5 ng/ml (LC-MS analyses)	
B: MDPV				
Total biological samples	True Confirmed Negatives	False negatives	True Confirmed positives	FALSE (i.e. mismatching) positives
n=167	n=162	0	n=3	n=2 (*)
	≤ 60 ng/ml (Screening analyses)		>850 ng/ml (Screening analyses)	
	<5 ng/ml (LC-MS analyses)		>5 ng/ml (LC-MS analyses)	

Table 3: Comparison between screening results (ELISA assay) and LC-MS data. (*) Discrepancy between ELISA results for Mephedrone/Methcathinones and MDPV (>16 ng/ml and >850 ng/ml, respectively) and LC-MS data (negative).

Notably, Table 4 details the true positives samples, n=4. The urine specimens screened as presumptive positive for both Mephedrone/methcathinone and MDPV, were the same, except for one sample screened as presumptive negative for MDPV only.

Among the four urines screened positives for Mephedrone/methcathinone (Bath Salt I), n=1 specimen was positive for 4-MEC and n=1 for mephedrone, fully matching with the declared specificity of the ELISA assay package insert (see Table 1, Bath Salt I).

Regarding the other two presumptive positives in screening, they were both LC-MS confirmed positive for butylone, which is known to crossreact (about 50%) with Bath Salt I, targeting Mephedrone/methcathinone, although butylone is exclusively included in the specificity stated by the manufacturer for MDPV kit (Bath Salt II) [25].

Concerning the n=3 samples screened as positives for MDPV, LC-MS confirmatory analyses demonstrated n=2 sample were positive for

both butylone and MDPV, and the other one for pentedrone and MDPV, accordingly to the specificities enumerated in the MDPV ELISA kit package insert (see Table 1, Bath Salt II).

| Sample ID | ELISA Screening | | LC-MS analyses | | | | | |
	Mephedrone/ Methcathinone	MDPV	Mephedrone	Butylone	Other Cathinones	4-MEC	Pentedrone	MDPV
1	+	+	–	+	–	–	–	+
2	+					+		
3	+	+		+				+
4	+	+	+				+	+

Table 4: True positive samples. +: positive; −: negative. Full colours (i.e. green and yellow) indicate accordance between LC-MS results and screening data obtained with the specific ELISA kit. Merged colours (green+yellow in LC-MS analyses) indicate accordance between LC-MS results (specifically for butylone) and screening data obtained with both ELISA kit. Weak yellow is just to indicate the specimen screened and confirmed as true negative by both methods.

Moreover, the LC-MS analyses showed that the only specimen determined as presumptive negative for MDPV (but also presumptive positive for Mephedrone/methcathinone) in screening, tested as true negative for Butylone, Pentedrone and MDPV, resulting as true positive for the 4-MEC only, which is included among the compounds detected by the Mephedrone/methcathinones kit (Bath Salt I).

| | LC-MS determination | ELISA Screening analyses | |
	MXE	Mephedrone/Methcathinone (*)	MDPV (*)
Sample ID	+	0.1	2.4
#1	+	0.2	5.7
#2	+	0	3.1
#3	+	0	7.5
#4	+	0.4	14.7
#5	+	0.7	8.8
#6	+	0.2	2.6
#7	+	0.3	15.9

Table 5: Comparison between urinary specimens screened and confirmed negative for both Mephedrone/Methcathinones and MDPV,

and confirmed positive for MXE by LC-MS. (*) Urinary values determined by both ELISA assays fell within the background range levels (0.0-0.8 ng/ml for Mephedrone/Methcathinones and 0.0-57.2 ng/ml for MDPV).

Based on the clinical history and health conditions at admission to EDs, n=7 subjects were evaluated for suspected MXE assumption, and confirmed positive by LC-MS. The same patients were screened with both Mephedrone/Methcathinone (Bath Salt I) and MDPV (Bath Salt II) assays resulting negatives, as further confirmed by LC-MS (Table 5).

Discussion

Even though (i) several confirmatory LC-MS/MS and GC-MS methods have been previously published for the determination of synthetic cathinones in biological samples, [26-33] and (ii) an increasing number of labs are using MS-based technology, regrettably rather few hospital-based clinical laboratories possess the capability to perform these tests and to give a robust clinical toxicological consultation. Thus, screening methods such as ELISA immunoassays continue to be widely employed in hospital-based laboratories, representing a rapid and cost-efficient approach to gain basic information about the drug content of a biological specimen [34-36].

Few specific immunoassays are available for new designer drugs, including the newest compounds such as the synthetic cathinones and their derivatives [25,26,27]. Noteworthy, it has to be remarked that the recently developed ELISA assays, presently applied in our study, were specifically designed to detect synthetic cathinones.

Altogether, our results highlighted a good global correspondence between results obtained with the Mephedrone/Methcathinone and MDPV kits and data gained by LC-MS, employed to confirm cathinones (and their derivatives) presence, showing the complete absence of false negative data, and evidencing a mismatch only in very few cases related to positive results. Thus, the total lack of false negatives further support the reliability of the screening test approach.

Specifically, with regard to Mephedrone/Methcathinone (Bath Salt I), in accordance to our results, previous literature data demonstrated that the Randox Mephedrone/Methcathinone kit was specific for several cathinone derivatives (i.e. mephedrone, methcathinone, methylone, 4-MEC, and 4-FMC) [36]. The same authors also reported that the Mephedrone/Methcathinone kit did neither demonstrate cross-reactivity towards MDPV (indicating the possibility that the nitrogen-containing ring system on MDPV hindered the antibodies activity) nor towards other phenethylamines. Regarding the n=3 false (i.e. mismatching) positive specimens, not confirmed by LC-MS, it has to be reported that two samples belonged to subjects screened and confirmed as polydrug abusers, positives for Δ-9-THC, AMP, MDMA and for COC and MDMA, respectively, while the remaining one was tested positive for MXE by LC-MS. We can exclude the occurrence of potential interference/crossreactivities of these substances with the antibodies/enzyme employed for the ELISA assay, based on (i) the manufacturer's indications, clearly reporting that even urinary concentrations as high as 7 - 10 microg/ml of Δ-9-THC, AMP, MDMA, and COC elicited a negative response when tested with Mephedrone/Methcathinone kit, (ii) our lab experience testing THC-, AMP-, MDMA- and COC-true positive specimens (other than those included in these study), demonstrating the lack of any reactivity using Mephedrone/Methcathinone assay (data not shown), as well as (iii) recent experimental literature data from Swortwood et al., [36] assessing the crossreactivities of designer drugs, e.g. cathinones, with several types of immunoassay. Moreover, it has to be mentioned that Ellefsen et al. [25] using Randox Drugs of Abuse (DOA-V) biochip array technology assay, assessed crossreactivities of some cathinones, included in those determined by MDPV (Bath Salt II) kit, with Bath Salt I targeting Mephedrone/Methcathinone. In particular, crossreactivities of about 50% and 1% were reported for methedrone/butylone and for 4-MPBP/MDPPP, respectively.

Concerning the MDPV analysis, accordingly to our data, previous experimental investigation demonstrated that the Randox MDPV kit was extremely selective, particularly for butylone [36]. With respect to the false (i.e. mismatching) positives (n=2), not confirmed by LC-MS, these two urine specimens were screened and confirmed positive for different substances (i.e. COC and KET), belonging to subjects recognized as polydrug abusers. Similarly to what previously hypothesised for Mephedrone/Methcathinone test, once more, for MDPV kit, we can rule out the occurrence of non-specific crossreactivities of the two mentioned substances (i.e. COC and KET) based on our previous lab dosages showing that COC- and KET-true positive samples resulted negative when tested with MDPV assay (data not shown), in accordance to the manufacturer's data (MDPV-negative response even at COC and KET urinary concentrations as high as 10 microg/ml).

Otherwise, it has to be considered for the mismatching data obtained from either screening ELISA assay that these not confirmed positive specimens were tested by LC-MS only for certified reference standards available in our labs (see Materials and Methods section and Table 2 for details). Therefore, the discrepancy between screening and confirmatory data could be ascribable to the presence of substance/metabolites not yet included in LC-MS analyses, but still identified by ELISA assay. In fact, further recent literature data seem to support this hypothesis demonstrating that even 4-MPBP and MDPPP cross-react with Bath Salt II (targeting MDPV/MDPBP) [25].

Moreover, even though the patient samples were collected within 12 hours from the admission to EDs, and properly stored at -20°C until the analyses, we cannot exclude that the instability of synthetic cathinones in urines (over the interval between screening and confirmatory determination) could have also contributed to the false positive screening rate [30].

Approaching another issue, grounding on previous literature demonstrating that some cathinones, including MDPV and butylone, produced false positive results in Phencyclidine (PCP) immunoassays, [8,38-40] we reason about the possibility that an inverse mechanism may occur.

Thus, with the aim to clarify this hypothesis, we evaluated the potential cross-reactivity of NPS, structural analogues of KET and PCP, i.e. MXE, [41-44] with the employed ELISA screening assays. These data plainly demonstrated that no interferences/crossreactivities occur when testing MXE-positive urine specimens for cathinones presence with the two ELISA kits.

Current literature data on the metabolism of the available bath salts are still limited, and predicting their half life time as well as detection window is complex.

Furthermore the required "effective" dose for these synthetic stimulants is much lower than their cocaine/ecstasy/amphetamine counterparts (usual dose of about 100 mg), thus resulting in lower excreted metabolite levels, even though accompanied by higher psychoactive potency. To date, MDPV is known to produce psychoactive effects with intake doses as low as 3 to 5 mg, depending on its route of administration, with reported average dose of approximately 5-20 mg, [45] while mephedrone has typical doses ranging between 25 and 75 mg, with 90 mg being considered an elevated dose [46].

The pharmacokinetics of bath salts (i.e. MDPV) has not yet been rigorously studied; Ross and co-authors [45] produced preliminary data, based on a single case report study, of a rapid clearance from the blood with a half-life of 1.88 hours. A recent epidemiological investigation demonstrated that drug effect timing depends on the route of administration, possibly starting within minutes after with nasal insufflation. Furthermore, the drug's "rush" may peak at 90 minutes, with duration of action of 3-4 hours, subsequently followed by about 1 hour come-down, for a total experience typically in the range of 6-8 hours [47].

Marinetti and Antonides [31] reported the occurrence of desired effects within 30-45 min (after intake), enduring from 1 to 3 hours, with the counterpart undesirable side outcomes lasting from hours to days. Winder et al. [46] provided detailed information on both MDPV and Mephedrone pharmacokinetics, summarizing the available literature data. Specifically, typical intake doses of 5-25 and 25-75 mg were reported for MDPV and Mephedrone, respectively. The drug onset ranged from 60 to 90 minutes for MDPV, with an estimated duration effect of 2.5 hours. Regarding the Mephedrone, the peak effect was expected within 30 minutes, followed by a rapid withdrawal.

Based on (i) the available pharmacokinetic and pharmacodynamic study, and (ii) the comparison with the pharmacokinetic of classical stimulant drugs, a predicted detection window of 48-72 hours can be hypothesised in urine specimens [45,46,48-52].

Regarding to bath salt concentrations detected in biological fluids, despite MDPV and mephedrone have been directly implicated in a number of case reports/series/fatalities relating to individuals presenting to healthcare facilities with acute toxicity, [53-56] there is no unanimous consensus on what constitutes toxic or lethal levels.

Our screening data reporting MDPV and Mephedrone/methcathynone urinary levels of about 850 and 16 ng/ml, respectively, in positive samples, further corroborated by the confirmatory analyses by LC-MS, seem to be in line with the available literature data.

In a retrospective case series of 236 patients reported by two USA poison centres with exposures to bath salts, [57] MDPV was detected in 13 of 17 live patients, with blood serum levels ranging from 24 to 241 ng/ml (mean 58 ng/ml). GC-MS determination in urine samples demonstrated MDPV values ranging between 34 and 1386 ng/ml, with a mean level of 856 ng/ml. Furthermore, quantitative analysis performed on postmortem samples detected MDPV in blood at 170 ng/ml and in urine at 1400 ng/ml.

Thornton and colleagues [34] described a case report of psychosis after reportedly insufflating a "bath salt" product; LC-TOF/MS testing revealed both MDPV and flephedrone. MDPV concentrations in serum and urine were 186 and 136 ng/ml, respectively, while flephedrone levels of 346 and 257 ng/ml were determined in the serum and urine, respectively. Ojanperä et al. [29] evaluating urine specimens from patients with a history of stimulant misuse, reported a range of MDPV of 40 to 3800 ng/ml, with a median value of 160 ng/ml. In a case report documenting hyperthermia and multiorgan failure after abuse of bath salts, patient urine, from the day of admission, tested positive for MDPV showing a concentration of 140 ng/ml by LC/MS [58]. Marinetti and Antonides [31] describing several intoxication cases, reported MDPV blood concentration of 6 - 368 ng/ml, with an average of 100 ng/ml. Moreover, in a recent case of confirmed MDPV related death, the serum and urine concentrations were 82 ng/ml and 670 ng/ml respectively [9,55].

Parally, several cases of fatal poisoning with mephedrone have been reported in the last years, [59-61] as also described by Advisory Council on the Misuse of Drugs from the UK. [22]. Some of these cases involved combined use with other drugs, such as cannabis or heroin, and tested mephedrone levels in blood and urine as high as 500 and 198000 ng/ml, respectively. In a published series of 4 fatalities in Scotland measured mephedrone concentrations in blood ranged from 1200 to 22000 ng/ml.

On the other hand, Lusthof et al. [53] descript a case of extreme agitation and death after the use of mephedrone in The Netherlands; toxicological analyses by GC-MS in post-mortem samples demonstrated mephedrone levels of 5100 and 186000 ng/ml in blood and urine, respectively.

A recent work evaluating clinical features in analytically confirmed cases of 3-Methylmethcathinone (3-MMC, a structural analogue of mephedrone) exposure among patients presenting to hospitals in Sweden, established serum concentrations ranging between 2 to 1490 ng/ml (median 91 ng/ml), while urinary levels were 7-290000 ng/ml (median 3050 ng/ml) [62].

From a clinical point of view, patients coming to medical attention with bath salt intoxication can display agitation, combative behavior, psychosis, tachycardia, and hyperthermia [57,58,63,64]. Health care workers should be cognizant that patients presenting with this constellation of symptoms may have taken bath salts, other than cocaine, ecstasy or amphetamine, thus needing a primarily supportive treatment with benzodiazepines for agitation and excessive sympathetic stimulation, as well as aggressive cooling for severe hyperthermia [2,45,57,65].

In this clinical context, a pivotal support to improve differential diagnosis as well as to aid real-time patient care and management may come from the employment of both Mephedrone/Methcathinone and MDPV screening assay as useful tools in emergency setting to rapidly detect these NPS, also allowing the clinician to address a focused and quick treatment.

Conclusions

In summary, our data highlight a good overall match between results obtained with the two analytical methods, evidencing an incongruity only in very few cases related to positive results.

This discrepancy may be due to: (i) non-specific interference/crossreactivities of substances, other than cathinones, with the ELISA kit, (ii) presence of substance/metabolites not yet included in LC-MS evaluated standards, but still identified by ELISA assay or (iii) instability of synthetic cathinones in urines, over the interval between screening and confirmatory determination.

Importantly, no false negatives were detected by screening analysis, thus suggesting the promising usefulness of this rapid and reliable tool as first approach in the emergency setting, followed by confirmatory LC-MS determination, even though the current availability of reference standards is limited, due to the continuous turnover of new synthetic substances in the drug market.

Acknowledgements

This publication arises from the activities of the Italian National Early Warning System (NEWS) Alert Project from the Department for Antidrug Policies-Presidency of the Italian Council of Ministers, Rome, Italy. We wish to thank our technical staff for the analytical determinations.

References

1. German CL, Fleckenstein AE, Hanson GR (2014) Bath salts and synthetic cathinones: an emerging designer drug phenomenon. Life Sci 97: 2-8.

2. Baumann MH, Partilla JS, Lehner KR (2013) Psychoactive "bath salts": not so soothing. Eur J Pharmacol 698: 1-5.

3. Zawilska JB, Wojcieszak J (2013) Designer cathinones--an emerging class of novel recreational drugs. Forensic Sci Int 231: 42-53.

4. Hill SL, Thomas SH (2011) Clinical toxicology of newer recreational drugs. Clin Toxicol (Phila) 49: 705-719.

5. Davies S, Wood DM, Smith G, Button J, Ramsey J, et al. (2010) Purchasing 'legal highs' on the internet-is there consistency in what you get? QJM 103: 489-493.

6.   Addiction (EMCDDA) (2011) Report on the risk assessment of mephedrone in the framework of the council decision on new psychoactive substances. Luxembourg. The Publications Office of the European Union; 2011193.

7.   Winstock AR, Mitcheson LR, Deluca P, Davey Z, Corazza O, et al. (2011) Mephedrone, new kid for the chop? Addiction 106: 154-161.

8.   Kasick DP, McKnight CA, Klisovic E (2012) "Bath salt" ingestion leading to severe intoxication delirium: two cases and a brief review of the emergence of mephedrone use. Am J Drug Alcohol Abuse 38: 176-180.

9.   Coppola M, Mondola R (2012) Synthetic cathinones: chemistry, pharmacology and toxicology of a new class of designer drugs of abuse marketed as "bath salts" or "plant food". Toxicol Lett 211: 144-149.

10.   DAWN (drug abuse warning network) Report (2013) Highlights of the 2011 Drug Abuse Warning Network (DAWN) Findings on Drug-Related Emergency Department.

11.   Kavanagh P, O'Brien J, Power JD, Talbot B, McDermott SD (2013) 'Smoking' mephedrone: the identification of the pyrolysis products of 4-methylmethcathinone hydrochloride. Drug Test Anal 5: 291-305.

12.   European Monitoring Centre for Drugs and Drug Addiction (EMCDDA) (2012) Drug profiles: synthetic cathinones. EMCDDA, Lisbon, Portugal.

13.   Cozzi NV, Sievert MK, Shulgin AT, Jacob P 3rd, Ruoho AE (1999) Inhibition of plasma membrane monoamine transporters by beta-ketoamphetamines. Eur J Pharmacol 381: 63-69.

14.   Council Decision (2010) Council decision of 2 December 2010 on submitting 4-methylmethcathinone (mephedrone) to control measures (2010/759/EU).

15.   Drug Enforcement Administration (DEA) (2011) Schedules of controlled substances: temporary placement of three synthetic cathinones in Schedule I. Fed Regist 76: 65371-65375.

16.   American Association of Poison Control Centers (AAPCC) (2013) Bath salts data.

17.   EMCDDA-Europol Joint Report (2010) Joint report on a new psychoactive substance: 4-methylmethcathinone (mephedrone).

18.   European Monitoring Centre for Drugs and Drug Addiction (EMCDDA) (2015). New psychoactive substances in Europe. An update from the EU Early Warning System. EMCDDA, Publications Office of the European Union, Luxembourg.

19.   Dargan PI, Sedefov R, Gallegos A, Wood DM (2011) The pharmacology and toxicology of the synthetic cathinone mephedrone (4-methylmethcathinone). Drug Test Anal 3: 454-463.

20.   Schifano F, Albanese A, Fergus S, Stair JL, Deluca P, et al. (2011) Mephedrone (4-methylmethcathinone; 'meow meow'): chemical, pharmacological and clinical issues. Psychopharmacology (Berl) 214: 593-602.

21.   National Early Warning System (NEWS), http://www.en.allertadroga.it

22.   Advisory Council on the Misuse of Drugs (ACMD) (2010). Consideration of the cathinones.

23.   Chimalakonda KC, Hailey C, Black R, Beekman A, Carlisle R, et al. (2010) Development and validation of an LC-MS/MS method for determination of phencyclidine in human serum and its application to human drug abuse cases. Anal Methods 2: 1249-1254.

24.   Dresen S, Kempf J, Weinmann W (2006) Electrospray-ionization MS/MS library of drugs as database for method development and drug identification. Forensic Sci Int 161: 86-91.

25.   Ellefsen KN, Anizan S, Castaneto MS, Desrosiers NA, Martin TM, et al. (2014) Validation of the only commercially available immunoassay for synthetic cathinones in urine: Randox Drugs of Abuse V Biochip Array Technology. Drug Test Anal 6: 728-738.

26.   Meyer MR, Wilhelm J, Peters FT, Maurer HH (2010a) Beta-keto amphetamines: Studies on the metabolism of the designer drug mephedrone and toxicological detection of mephedrone, butylone, and methylone in urine using gas chromatography-mass spectrometry. Anal Bioanal Chem 397: 1225-1233.

27.   Meyer MR, Du P, Schuster F, Maurer HH (2010b) Studies on the metabolism of the a-pyrrolidinophenone designer drug

28.   methylenedioxypyrovalerone (MDPV) in rat and human urine and human liver microsomes using GC-MS and LC-high-resolution MS and its detectability in urine by GC-MS. J Mass Spectrom 45: 1426-1442.

28.   Strano-Rossi S, Cadwallader AB, de la Torre X, Botre F (2010) Toxicological determination and in vitro metabolism of the designer drug methylenedioxypyrovalerone (MDPV) by gas chromatography/mass spectrometry and liquid chromatography/quadrupole time-of-flight mass spectrometry. Rapid Commun Mass Spectrom 24: 2706-2714.

29.   Ojanperä IA, Heikman PK, Rasanen IJ (2011) Urine analysis of 3,4-methylenedioxypyrovalerone in opioid-dependent patients by gas chromatography-mass spectrometry. Ther Drug Monit 33: 257-263.

30.   Concheiro M, Anizan S, Ellefsen K, Huestis MA (2013) Simultaneous quantification of 28 synthetic cathinones and metabolites in urine by liquid chromatography-high resolution mass spectrometry. Anal Bioanal Chem 405: 9437-9448.

31.   Marinetti LJ, Antonides HM (2013) Analysis of synthetic cathinones commonly found in bath salts in human performance and postmortem toxicology: method development, drug distribution and interpretation of results. J Anal Toxicol 37: 135-146.

32.   De Castro A, Lendoiro E, Fernández-Vega H, Steinmeyer S, López-Rivadulla M, et al. (2014) Liquid chromatography tandem mass spectrometry determination of selected synthetic cathinones and two piperazines in oral fluid. Cross reactivity study with an on-site immunoassay device. J Chromatogr A 1374: 93-101.

33.   Namera A, Kawamura M, Nakamoto A, Saito T, Nagao M (2015) Comprehensive review of the detection methods for synthetic cannabinoids and cathinones. Forensic Toxicol 33: 175-194.

34.   Thornton SL, Gerona RR, Tomaszewski CA (2012) Psychosis from a bath salt product containing flephedrone and MDPV with serum, urine, and product quantification. J Med Toxicol 8: 310-313.

35.   Wohlfarth A, Weinmann W, Dresen S (2010) LC-MS/MS screening method for designer amphetamines, tryptamines, and piperazines in serum. Anal Bioanalysis Chem 396: 2403-2414.

36.   Swortwood MJ, Hearn WL, Decaprio AP (2014) Cross-reactivity of designer drugs, including cathinone derivatives, in commercial enzyme-linked immunosorbent assays. Drug Test Anal 6: 716-727.

37.   Petrie M, Lynch KL, Ekins S, Chang JS, Goetz RJ, et al. (2013) Cross-reactivity studies and predictive modelling of " Bath Salts " and other amphetamine-type stimulants with amphetamine screening immunoassays. Clin Toxicol 51: 83-91.

38.   Bell C, George C, Kicman AT, Traynor A (2011) Development of a rapid LC-MS/MS method for direct urinalysis of designer drugs. Drug Test Anal 3: 496-504.

39.   Penders TM, Gestring RE, Vilensky DA (2012) Intoxication delirium following use of synthetic cathinone derivatives. Am J Drug Alcohol Abuse 38: 616-617.

40.   Macher AM, Penders TM (2012) False-positive phencyclidine immunoassay results caused by 3,4-methylenedioxypyrovalerone (MDPV). Drug Test Anal 5: 130-132.

41.   Hofer KE, Grager B, Müller DM, Rauber-Lüthy C, Kupferschmidt H, et al. (2012) Ketamine-like effects after recreational use of methoxetamine. Ann Emerg Med 60: 97-99.

42.   Coppola M, Mondola R (2012) Methoxetamine: from drug of abuse to rapid-acting antidepressant. Med Hypotheses 79: 504-507.

43.   Corazza O, Schifano F, Simonato P, Fergus S, Assi S, et al. (2012) Phenomenon of new drugs on the Internet: the case of ketamine derivative methoxetamine. Hum Psychopharmacol 27: 145-149.

44.   Zawilska JB (2014) Methoxetamine--a novel recreational drug with potent hallucinogenic properties. Toxicol Lett 230: 402-407.

45.   Ross EA, Reisfield GM, Watson MC, Chronister CW, Goldberger BA (2012) Psychoactive "bath salts" intoxication with methylenedioxypyrovalerone. Am J Med 125: 854-858.

46.   Winder GS, Stern N, Hosanagar A (2013) Are "bath salts" the next generation of stimulant abuse? J Subst Abuse Treat 44: 42-45.

47. Psychonaut Webmapping Research Group (2009) MDPV Report. London, UK, Institute of Psychiatry, King's College London.

48. Erowid Vaults (2011) 4-MethylMethcathinone/mephedrone.

49. Erowid Vaults (2011) MDPV.

50. Rosenbaum CD, Carreiro SP, Babu KM (2012) Here Today, Gone Tomorrow...and Back Again? A Review of Herbal Marijuana Alternatives (K2, Spice), Synthetic Cathinones (Bath Salts), Kratom, Salvia divinorum, Methoxetamine, and Piperazines. J Med Toxicol 8: 15-32.

51. Paillet-Loilier M, Cesbron A, Le Boisselier A, Bourgine J, Debruyne D (2014) Emerging drugs of abuse: current perspectives on substituted cathinones. Subst Abuse Rehab 5: 37-52.

52. Katz DP, Bhattacharya D, Bhattacharya S, Deruiter J, Clark CR, et al. (2014) Synthetic cathinones: "a khat and mouse game". Toxicol Lett 229: 349-356.

53. Lusthof KJ, Oosting R, Maes A, Verschraagen M, Dijkhuizen A, et al. (2011) A case of extreme agitation and death after the use of mephedrone in The Netherlands. Forensic Sci Int 206: e93-95.

54. Maskell PD, De Paoli G, Seneviratne C, Pounder DJ (2011) Mephedrone (4-methylmethcathinone)-related deaths. J Anal Toxicol 35: 188-191.

55. Murray BL, Murphy CM, Beuhler MC (2012) Death following recreational use of designer drug "bath salts" containing 3,4-Methylenedioxypyrovalerone (MDPV). J Med Toxicol 8: 69-75.

56. Wood DM, Dargan PI (2012) Mephedrone (4-methylmethcathinone): what is new in our understanding of its use and toxicity. Prog Neuropsychopharmacol Biol Psychiatry 39: 227-233.

57. Spiller HA, Ryan ML, Weston RG, Jansen J (2011) Clinical experience with analytic confirmation of "bath salts" and "legal highs" (synthetic cathinones) in the United States. Clin Toxicol 49: 499-505.

58. Borek HA, Holstege CP (2012) Hyperthermia and multiorgan failure after abuse of "bath salts" containing 3,4-methylenedioxypyrovalerone. Ann Emerg Med 60: 103-105.

59. Gustavsson D, Escher C (2009) Mephedrone-Internet drug which seems to have come and stay. Fatal cases in Sweden have drawn attention to previously unknown substance. Lakartidningen 106: 2769-2771.

60. Torrance H, Cooper G (2010) The detection of mephedrone (4-methylmethcathinone) in 4 fatalities in Scotland. Forensic Sci Int 202: e62-63.

61. Dickson AJ, Vorce SP, Levine B, Past MR (2010) Multiple-drug toxicity caused by the coadministration of 4-methylmethcathinone (mephedrone) and heroin. J Anal Toxicol 34: 162-168.

62. Bäckberg M, Lindeman E, Beck O, Helander A (2015) Characteristics of analytically confirmed 3-MMC-related intoxications from the Swedish STRIDA project. Clin Toxicol (Phila) 53: 46-53.

63. Kyle PB, Iverson RB, Gajagowni RG, Spencer L (2011) Illicit bath salts: not for bathing. J Miss State Med Assoc 52: 375-377.

64. Prosser JM, Nelson LS (2012) The toxicology of bath salts: a review of synthetic cathinones. J Med Toxicol 8: 33-42.

65. Ross EA, Watson M, Goldberger B (2011) "Bath salts" intoxication. N Engl J Med 365: 967-968.

10

Ex vivo Effects of Sorafenib and Regorafenib on Murine Hepatocytes

Ali S. Alfazari[1], **Saeeda Almarzooqi**[3], **Alia Albawardi**[3], **Sami Shaban**[4], **Bayan Al-Dabbagh**[2], **Dhanya Saraswathiamma**[3], **Saeed Tariq**[5] and **Abdul-Kader Souid**[6,*]

[1]*Departments of Internal Medicine, UAE University, Al-Ain, Abu Dhabi, United Arab Emirates*

[2]*Department of Chemistry, College of Science, United Arab Emirates University, Al Ain, United Arab Emirates*

[3]*Pathology, UAE University, Al-Ain, Abu Dhabi, United Arab Emirates*

[4]*Medical Education, Al-Ain, Abu Dhabi, United Arab Emirates*

[5]*Anatomy, UAE University, Al-Ain, Abu Dhabi, United Arab Emirates*

[6]*Pediatrics, UAE University, Al-Ain, Abu Dhabi, United Arab Emirates*

*****Corresponding author:** Abdul-Kader Souid, Departments of Pediatrics, UAE University, Al-Ain, Abu Dhabi, United Arab Emirates,
E-mail: asouid@uaeu.ac.ae

Abstract

Sorafenib and regorafenib are structurally-related small-molecular-weight inhibitors of cellular kinases. Regorafenib has a Boxed Warning stating: "Severe and sometimes fatal hepatotoxicity has been observed in clinical trials", while sorafenib is considered less hepatotoxic. This *ex vivo* study assessed the effects of sorafenib (2.5 and 50 µM) and regorafenib (5.0 and 50 µM) on liver structure, ultrastructure, cellular respiration (mitochondrial O_2 consumption), ATP, caspase activity, urea synthesis, and glutathione. Liver fragments from Taylor Outbred mice were incubated in Krebs-Henseleit buffer (continuously gassed with 95% O_2:5% CO_2) with and without the drugs for 3 to 4 h. The presence of sorafenib or regorafenib had insignificant effects on liver structure, cellular respiration, ATP, caspase-3 activity, urea synthesis, and glutathione. At 3 h, liver histology with and without 2.5 µM sorafenib or 5.0 µM regorafenib was similar. Liver histology with 50 µM sorafenib was slightly worse than untreated tissue at 3 h, showing single hepatocyte necrosis and cellular disintegration. With 50 µM regorafenib, the histology was closely mirroring untreated tissue at 3 h. Similarly, caspase-3, caspase-9, cytochrome c, BAX and annexin A2 immunostains showed no significant drug effects at 4 h (2.5 µM sorafenib or 5.0 µM regorafenib). Electron microscopy revealed a more prominent loss of rough endoplasmic reticulum (rER) integrity with regorafenib treatment compared with sorafenib treatment. Thus, derangements in the rER were more prominent with regorafenib. Otherwise, the studied hepatic surrogate biomarkers did not distinguish between the two compounds.

Keywords: Mitochondria; Respiration; Caspases; Apoptosis; Liver tissue; Murine; Sorafenib; Regorafenib

Abbreviations

ER: Endoplasmic Reticulum; Rer: Rough endoplasmic reticulum; ROS: Reactive O_2 species; GSG: Glutathione; Pd phosphor: Pd(II) complex of *meso*-tetra-(4-sulfonatophenyl)-tetrabenzoporphyrin; mBBr: Monobromobimane; zVAD-fmk: *N*-benzyloxycarbonyl-val-ala-asp(O-methyl)-fluoromethylketone; Ac-DEVD-AMC: *N*-acetyl-asp-glu-val-asp-7-amino-4-methylcoumarin; AMC: Amino-4-methylcoumarin; TFA: Trifluoroacetic Acid; DTNB: 5,5'-dithio-bis(2-nitrobenzoic acid)]; KH buffer: Krebs-Henseleit buffer; EM: Electron Microscopy; MSA: Methanesulfonic Acid

Introduction

The use of medications is often limited by "off target" adverse events that frequently involve the mitochondria [1]. Drug development, thus, requires screening the candidate compounds for potential mitochondrial disturbances. Hepatic failure associated with the nucleoside reverse transcriptase inhibitors, for example, is due to a mitochondrial toxicity, which includes inhibition of mitochondrial DNA polymerases [2]. The "mitochondrial cell death pathway" is another example, which involves leakage of cytochrome c from the mitochondrial intermembrane to the cytosol. In combination with the apoptotic protease activating factor-1, cytochrome c triggers caspase cascades (cysteine, aspartate-specific proteases) [3]. Biomarkers for these events include decreased cellular respiration (mitochondrial O_2 consumption), reduced cellular ATP synthesis, and generation of reactive O_2 species (ROS; commonly associated with depletion of cellular glutathione, GSH) [4,5]. These changes are often associated with altered cellular and mitochondrial structures and ultrastructures.

Sorafenib (a biaryl urea) and regorafenib (fluoro-sorafenib) are novel anticancer drugs. These structurally-related, small molecular weight inhibitors of cellular kinases [e.g., vascular endothelial growth factor receptor 2 (VEGFR-2), platelet-derived growth factor receptor (PDGFR), rapidly accelerated fibrosarcoma (Raf) kinase, and Fms-like tyrosine kinase-3 (FLT3)] are known to induce various levels of liver injuries. Regorafenib has a Boxed Warning, stating: "Severe and sometimes fatal hepatotoxicity has been observed in clinical trials" [6]. The hepatotoxicity of sorafenib, on the other hand, is less pronounced [7]. Sorafenib is an approved treatment for renal cell carcinoma and hepatocellular carcinoma and regorafenib is an approved treatment for colorectal cancer.

The cytotoxicities of sorafenib and regorafenib include alterations in multiple signaling pathways, mitochondrial disturbances, execution of apoptosis (via caspase dependent and independent pathways), induction of endoplasmic reticulum (ER) stress, inhibition of protein synthesis, generation of ROS and depletion of cellular GSH. These mechanisms are mainly studied in malignant cells [8-15]. Thus, it is unclear whether these modes of action are applicable to normal tissue (e.g., the liver). Furthermore, it is unknown whether the fatal hepatotoxicity of regorafenib is mediated through the same mechanisms. This study addressed some of these issues by testing liver fragments from Taylor Outbred mice, using highly-sensitive structural and functional biomarkers [4,5].

An *in vitro* liver preparation based on the work of Berry and others [16] was recently developed to study the effects of various drugs on hepatocyte bioenergetics (the biochemical processes involved in cellular energy metabolism and conversion) [4,5]. Exposure of liver fragments to 8 μM dactinomycin for 60 min was used as a positive control for induction of apoptosis [4], confirming the analytical system could detect hepatotoxicities. The same methodology was employed here to investigate whether regorafenib hepatotoxicity could be identified *in vitro*.

Experimental Section

Reagents

Sorafenib [*m.w.* 464.8; 4[4-({[4-chloro-3-(trifluoromethyl)phenyl]carbamoyl}amino)phenoxy] N-methylpyridine2carboxamide]andregorafenib[*m.w.* 482.8;4[4-({[4chloro3(trifluoromethyl)phenyl]carbamoyl}amino)-3-fluorophenoxy]-N-methylpyridine-2-carboxamide] were purchased from Selleck Chemicals (Houston, TX, USA). Pd(II) complex of meso-tetra-(4-sulfonatophenyl)-tetrabenzoporphyrin (Pd phosphor) was purchased from Porphyrin Products (Logan, UT). Monobromobimane (mBBr, *m.w.*=271.1) was purchased from Molecular Probes (Eugene, Oregon).A lyophilized powder of the pan-caspase inhibitor N-benzyloxycarbonyl-val-ala-asp(O-methyl)-fluoromethylketone (zVAD-fmk, *m.w.*=467.5) was purchased from Calbiochem (La Jolla, CA). The caspase-3 substrate Ac-DEVD-AMC (N-acetyl-asp-glu-val-asp-7-amino-4-methylcoumarin; *m.w.*=675.64) was purchased from Axxora LLC (San Diego, CA).Complete® protease inhibitor cocktail was purchased from Roche Applied Science (Indianapolis, IN).Rabbit anti-cleaved caspase-3 antibody, rabbit anti-BAX antibody (#D2E11) and rabbit anti-annexin antibody (#D11G2) were purchased from Cell Signaling Technology (Boston, MA, USA).Rabbit anti-cytochrome c antibody [(H-104): sc-7159] was purchased from Santa Cruz Biotechnology, Inc. (Texas, USA). Rabbit anti-caspases-9 antibody (ab52299) was purchased from Abcam (Cambridge, MA, USA). Glucose, DTNB [5,5'-dithio-bis(2-nitrobenzoic acid)], GSH (*m.w.*=307.43), HPLC-grade methanol, dichloromethane, trifluoroacetic acid (TFA), methanesulfonic acid (MSA), MTT [3-(4,5-dimethylthiazol-2-yl)-2,5-diphenyltetrazolium bromide] and remaining reagents were purchased from Sigma-Aldrich (St. Louis, MO).

Sorafenib and regorafenib were dissolved in dimethyl sulfoxide (DMSO) and stored at -20oC. GSH was dissolved in dH$_2$O and stored at -80°C; its concentration was measured by Ellman's reagent [17]. GS-bimane derivative, sodium methane sulfonate, mBBr (0.1 M in acetonitrile) and DTNB (10 mM in 100 mM Tri-Cl, pH 8.0) solutions were prepared and stored as described [18]. GSH standard (10 μM) was used to generate a calibration curve, which was linear from 10 to 200 picomoles. zVAD-fmk (2.14 mM), Ac-DEVD-AMC solution (7.4 mM), Pd phosphor solution (2.5 mg/mL=2 mM), NaCN (1.0 M), glucose oxidase (10 mg/mL), and Complete® protease inhibitor cocktail were prepared and stored as described [4,5].

Mice

Taylor Outbred (9-10 weeks old) mice were housed at the animal facility in rooms maintained at 22°C, 60% humidity and 12-h light-dark cycles. The use of Taylor Outbred mice was simply due to availability. The mice had ad libitum access to standard rodent chow and filtered water. The study received approval from the Animal Ethics Committee-United Arab Emirates University - College of Medicine and Health Sciences.

Liver specimens

Mice were anesthetized by sevoflurane inhalation (10 μL/g). Liver specimens (20 to 30 mg each; giving an average radius of ~1.5 mm, sufficiently small to allow penetration of O$_2$ and nutrients throughout the piece) were collected by 4-mm skin biopsy punches (Miltex GmbH, Germany) and *immediately* immersed in ice-cold *modified* Krebs-Henseleit (KH) buffer (115 mMNaCl, 25 mM NaHCO$_3$, 1.23 mM NaH$_2$PO$_4$, 1.2 mM Na$_2$SO$_4$, 5.9 mM KCl, 1.0 mM EDTA, 1.18 mM MgCl$_2$, 10 mM glucose, and 0.5 μL/mL Complete® protease inhibitor cocktail, pH 7.5) gassed with 95% O$_2$: 5% CO$_2$ as previously described [4,5]. The samples were then incubated at 37oC in 50 mL in normal KH buffer (115 mM NaCl, 25 mM NaHCO$_3$, 1.23 mM NaH$_2$PO$_4$, 1.2 mM Na$_2$SO$_4$, 5.9 mMKCl, 1.25 mM CaCl$_2$, 1.18 mM MgCl$_2$, and 10 mM glucose, pH 7.5) supplemented with 0.5 μL/mL Complete® protease inhibitor cocktail and gassed with 95% O$_2$: 5% CO$_2$.

Each drug was tested at its therapeutic concentration and at 50 μM. In humans, the geometric mean peak plasma level (C$_{max}$) of sorafenib is about 2.5 μM and of regorafenib is about 5.2 μM [6,7]. The duration of drug exposure was 3 to 4 h. The drug vehicle dimethyl sulfoxide was added to the control experiments.

Specimens were also processed for histology, electron microscopy, respiration, ATP, caspase activity, and urea synthesis as previously described [4,5,19-22]. A brief description of these analytical methods is given below.

Histology

The tissue was fixed in 10% neutral formalin, dehydrated in increasing concentrations of ethanol, cleared with xylene and embedded in paraffin. Three-micrometer sections were prepared from paraffin blocks, stained with hematoxylin and eosin (H&E), and immunostained for caspase-3, caspase-9, cytochrome c, BAX, and annexin [4,5].

Electron microscopy (EM)

Samples were processed for electron microscopy as previously described [19]. The tissue was immersed at 25°C for 3 h in McDowell and Trump fixative. It was then rinsed with phosphate-buffered saline (PBS) and fixed with 1% osmium tetroxide for 1 h. The sample was washed with dH$_2$O, dehydrated in graded ethanol and propylene oxide. The mixture was infiltrated and embedded in agar-100 epoxy resin. Polymerization was allowed to occur at 65°C for 24 h. Semi-thin (1 μm) and ultra-thin (95 nm) sections were prepared using Reichert–Jung Ultracut Ultramicrotome (Leica Microsystems, Wetzlar, Germany). Semithin sections were stained on glass slides with 1% aqueous toluidine blue. Ultrathin sections were contrasted on 200-mesh copper grids with uranyl acetate; this step was followed by lead citrate double stain. The grids were imaged on CM10 transmission electron microscope (Philips, Amsterdam, Netherlands).

Cellular respiration

The phosphorescence O_2 analyzer was used to monitor O_2 consumption by the liver fragments [4,5]. O_2 detection was performed with the Pd phosphor (absorption maximum=625 nm and phosphorescence maximum=800 nm).Samples were exposed to 600 per min light flashes from a pulsed light-emitting diode array (peak output, 625 nm). Emitted phosphorescent light was detected by the Hamamatsu photomultiplier tube after passing through 800 nm filter.

A program was developed using Microsoft Visual Basic 6, Microsoft Access Database 2007, and Universal Library components (Universal Library for Measurements Computing Devices), which allowed direct reading from the PCI-DAS 4020/12 I/O Board (PCI-DAS 4020/12 I/O Board) [20].

The phosphorescence decay rate $(1/\tau)$ was characterized by a single exponential. The values of 1/ were linear with dissolved O_2: $1/o=1/ + k_q[O_2]$, $1/\tau$=the phosphorescence decay rate in the presence of O2, $1/\tau o$=the phosphorescence decay rate in the absence of O_2, and k_q=the second-order O_2 quenching rate constant in $s^{-1} \cdot \mu M^{-1}$ [21].

In the vials sealed from air, $[O_2]$ decreased linearly with time (zero-order kinetics). The rate of respiration $(k,$ in μM O_2 $min^{-1})$ was the negative of the slope $d[O_2]/dt$. NaCN inhibited respiration, confirming O_2 was consumed in the mitochondrial respiratory chain.

ATP content

Liver fragments were homogenized in ice-cold 2% trichloroacetic acid and neutralized with 100 mM Tris-acetate, 2 mM ethylenediaminetetraacetic acid (pH 7.75). The supernatants were stored at -20°C until analysis. ATP was measured using the Enliten ATP Assay System (Bioluminescence Detection Kit, Promega, Madison, WI). The luminescence reaction contained 2.5 µL of the acid-soluble supernatant and 25 µL of the luciferin/luciferase reagent. The luminescence intensity was measured at 25°C using the Glomax Luminometer (Promega, Madison, WI) [4,5].

Intracellular caspase activity

Liver specimens were incubated at 37°C in oxygenated KH buffer containing 37 µM Ac-DEVD-AMC with and without 32 µM zVAD-fmk (final volume, 0.5 mL). The tissue was disrupted by vigorous homogenization. The supernatants were centrifuged (16,300g for 90 min) through a Microcentrifuge Filter (m.w. limit=10,000 Dalton, Sigma©), separated on HPLC, and analyzed for the free fluorogenic AMC moiety [4,5].

Urea synthesis

Liver specimens were incubated at 37°C in 50 ml KH buffer (gassed with 95% O_2: 5% CO_2) for 3 h. Specimens were placed in 1.0 mL KH buffer supplemented with 10 mM NH_4Cl and 2.5 mM ornithine. The reactions were continued at 37°C for 50 min. The solutions were analyzed for urea as previously described [22].

Cellular GSH

Cellular GSH was labeled with mBBr in a 0.5 mL reaction containing the liver specimen, 10 mMTris-MSA (pH 8.0) and 1.0 mM mBBr. The mixture was incubated at 25°C in the dark for 15 min. The labeling was quenched with 100 µL of 70% perchloric acid. The solution was diluted with 10 mM Tris-MSA and the tissue was disrupted by homogenization. The supernatant was collected by centrifugation (13,000xg at 4°C for 10 min) and stored at -20°C until HPLC analysis [18].

HPLC

Reversed-phase HPLC system (Waters, Milford, MA, U.S.A.) was used. Ultrasphere IP column, 4.6×250 mm (Beckman, Fullerton, CA, U.S.A.) was operated at 25°C at 1.0 mL/min. For GSH detection, the analysis was performed as previously described [18]. Solvent A was 0.1% (v/v) TFA/water and solvent B was HPLC-grade methanol. The gradient was: 0 min, 10% B; 5 min 10% B; 13 min, 100% B; 15 min, 10% B; 20 min, re-inject. The excitation and emission wavelengths were 390 nm and 480 nm, respectively. Injection volume was 50 µL.

For AMC (amino-4-methylcoumarin) detection, the excitation wavelength was 380 nm and the emission wavelength 460 nm. Solvents A and B were HPLC-grade methanol:dH_2O 1:1 (isocratic). The run time was 15 min [4,5].

Statistical analysis

Data were analyzed on SPSS statistical package (version 19), using the nonparametric (2 independent samples) Mann-Whitney test.

Results

Histology

Figure 1A shows representative H&E assessments of liver fragments incubated with and without 2.5 µM sorafenib and 5.0 µM regorafenib for 3 h. Histology was similar in the three specimens, revealing mild cellular disintegrations in the forms of cytoplasmic ballooning, vacuolar degeneration and micro-steatosis (Figure 1A). Another experiment (Figure 1B) shows representative H&E images with and without 50 µM sorafenib or 50 µM regorafenib at 0 h and at 3 h. Cytoplasmic vacuolization (processing artifact) and early cytoplasmic ballooning were noted at 0 h; otherwise, the nuclear details, cell membrane integrity and hepatic architecture were preserved. Inflammation, apoptosis, necrosis and cholestasis were absent. At 3 h (untreated), hepatic architecture was relatively preserved. Hepatocyte ballooning, vacuolar degeneration, cell membrane disintegration, early nuclear disintegration and spotty necrosis were more evident. Thus, there were structural changes associated with *in vitro* incubations without addition of drugs.

With sorafenib, the histology was slightly worse than untreated tissue at 3 h, showing more single hepatocyte necrosis and cellular disintegration. The hepatic architecture, however, was preserved and inflammation and cholestasis were absent. With regorafenib, the histology was closely mirroring untreated tissue at 3 h (Figure 1B). Histological changes, thus, were not clearly noticeable at 3 h.

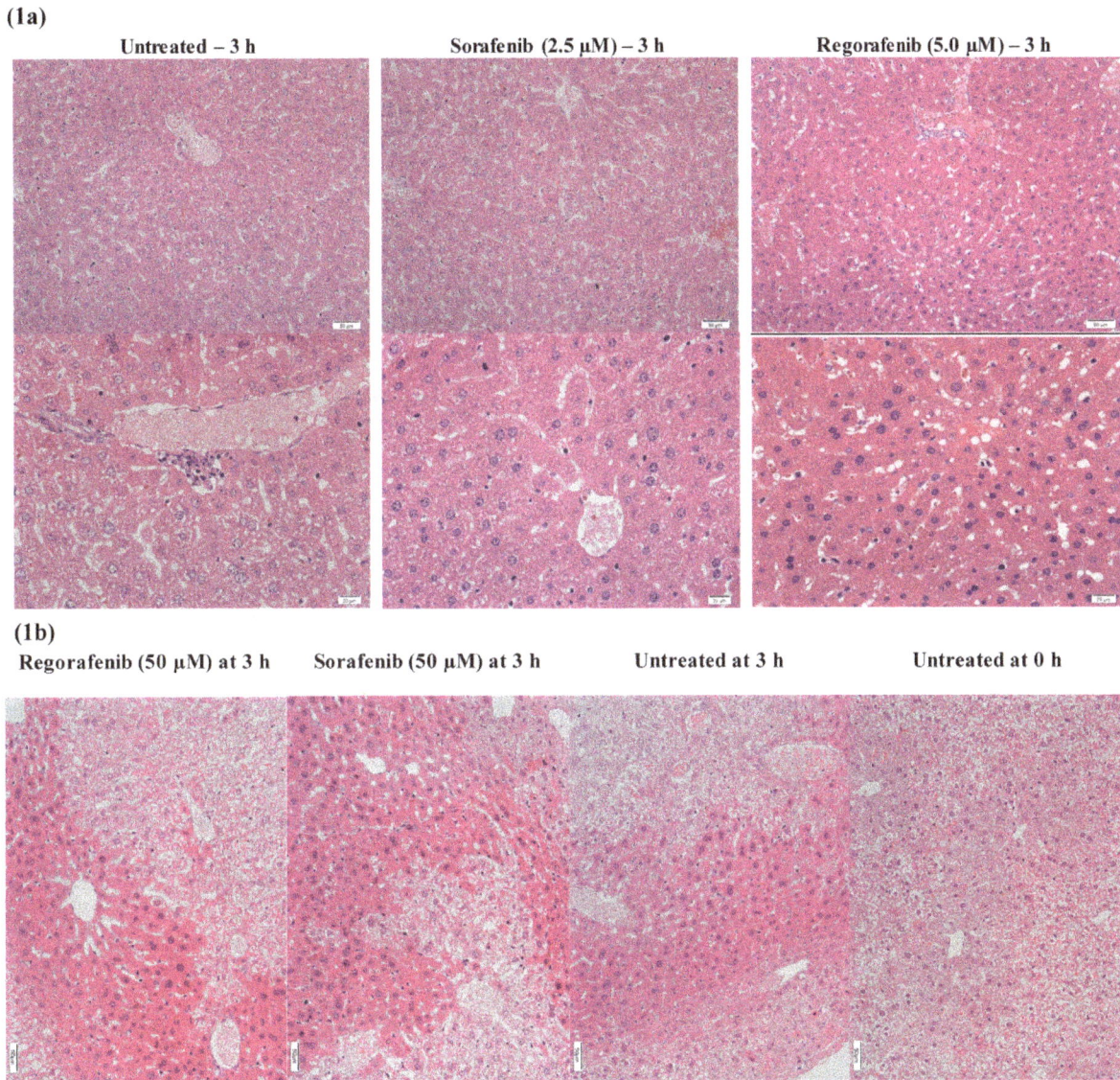

Figure 1: Liver histology. Panel A (H&E staining, 20x and 40x): Untreated at 3 h, 2.5 µM sorafenibat 3 h and 5.0 µM regorafenib at 3 h. Panel B (H&E staining, 20x): Untreated at 0 h, untreated at 3 h, 50 µM sorafenib at 3 h and 50 µM regorafenib at 3 h.

Liver fragments were incubated at 37oC in 50 mL KH buffer (continuously gassed with 95% O2: 5% CO2) with and without 2.5 µM sorafenib or 5.0 µM regorafenib for 4 h. The specimens were then processed for immunostaining with several apoptosis biomarkers. At 0 h (untreated liver fragment), the caspase-3 stain was negative. At 4 h, the caspase-3 stain in both untreated and treated specimens was 1%, mostly localized to Kupffer cells (Figure 1S, Supplementary Material). Cytoplasmic cytochrome c stain of the untreated liver fragment at 0 h was negative; at 4 h, the cytoplasmic staining was more intense than the treated tissue. Sorafenib treatment demonstrated a slightly more intense cytoplasmic positivity than regorafenib treatment (Figure 2S, Supplementary Material). BAX immunostain of the untreated liver fragment at 0 h was undetectable. BAX expression increased at 4 h in untreated and treated liver fragments (Figure 3S, Supplementary Material). Annexin A2 immunostain of the untreated liver fragment at

0 h was undetectable. The expression of annexin A2 increased at 4 h in untreated more than treated liver fragments (Figure 4S, Supplementary Material). The intensity of caspase-9 immunostain of untreated liver fragment at 0 h and 4 h and treated liver fragments at 4 h was zero (Figure 5S, Supplementary Material).

Electron microscopy

Since histological findings were not prominent at 3 h, EM studies were performed at 4 h. Representative images of liver fragments at 0 h and at 4 h with and without 2.5 µM sorafenib or 5.0 µM regorafenib are shown in Figure 2A. The hepatocyte architecture was preserved at 0 h. For untreated tissue at 4 h, the hepatocyte showed minimal distension of the mitochondria and minimal disintegration of the rER. For tissue treated with sorafenib, the mitochondrial swelling and the rER disintegration were slightly more than in untreated tissue at 4 h. For tissue treated with regorafenib, the rER changes were evidently more prominent (Figure 2A). Thus, derangements in the rER were more prominent with a therapeutic dosing of regorafenib.

Figure 2B shows representative images of liver fragments at 0 h and at 3 h with and without 50 μM sorafenib or 50 μM regorafenib. For untreated tissue at 0 h, the hepatocyte showed intact mitochondria and rER. For untreated tissue at 3 h, the hepatocytes demonstrated minimal mitochondrial swelling and relatively preserved rER with attached ribosomes. For tissue treated with sorafenib, the hepatocyte showed mild swelling of the mitochondria and relatively preserved rER. The focal minimal detachment of ribosomes from the rER was similar to untreated tissue at 3 h. For tissue treated with regorafenib, the hepatocyte showed mild swelling (distension) of the mitochondria and disruption of the rER with focal detachments of ribosomes. Thus, exposure to high-dose regorafenib produces more noticeable rER derangements.

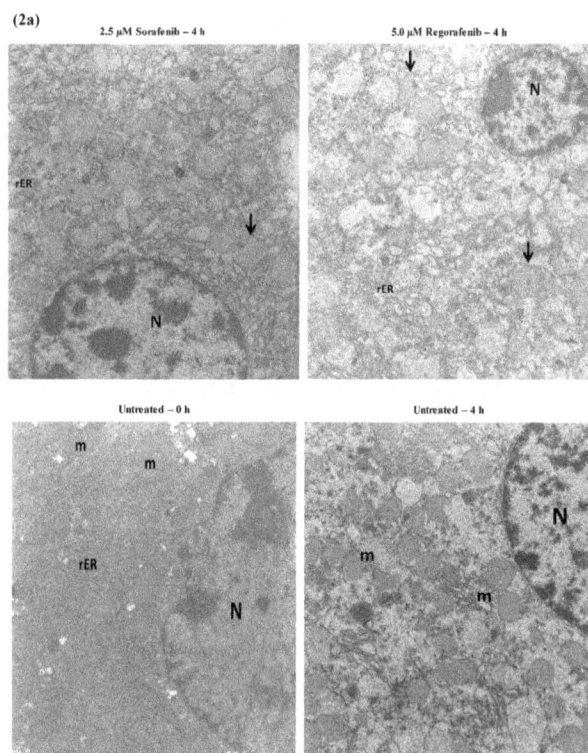

Figure 2: Hepatocyte ultrastructure. Panel A: Untreated tissue at 0 h, showing a hepatocyte with preserved architecture. Note hepatocyte nucleus (N), numerous intact mitochondria (m) and rER; magnification =98,000. Untreated tissue at 4 h, showing a hepatocyte with minimal distension of the mitochondria (m) and minimal disintegration of the rER; magnification =7,000. Tissue treated with 2.5 μM sorafenibat 4 h, showing a hepatocyte with mild distension of the mitochondria (arrow) with amorphous densities. Early loss of integrity of rER was also noted; magnification =7,000. Tissue treated with 5.0 μM regorafenib at 4 h, showing a hepatocyte with mild distension of the mitochondria (arrows) with amorphous densities. The rER changes were more evident; magnification =7,000.

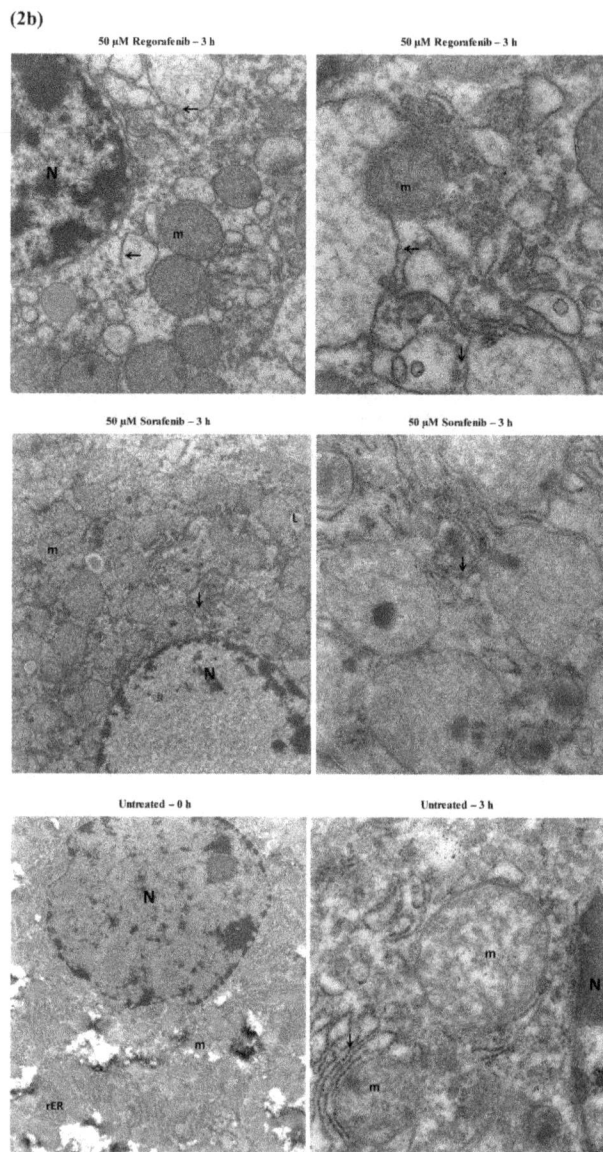

Figure 2B: Untreated tissue at 0 h, showing a hepatocyte with preserved architecture; magnification =7,000. The white areas represented an artifact from specimen collection or preparation. Untreated tissue at 3 h, showing a hepatocyte with relatively preserved cellular architecture. Note hepatocyte nucleus (N), mitochondria (m) with minimal swelling, relatively preserved rER (arrow) with attached ribosomes; magnification =27,500. Tissue treated with 50 μM sorafenib at 3 h, showing a hepatocyte with swollen mitochondria and relatively preserved rER. The focal minimal detachment of ribosomes (arrows) from rER was similar to untreated liver at 3 h; magnification =27,500.Tissue treated with 50 μM regorafenib at 3 h,showing a hepatocyte with mildly distended mitochondria (m), significant disruption of the rER and focal detachments of the ribosomes (arrows); magnification =14,000.

Cellular respiration

Five separate experiments, each involving five mice, were performed in KH buffer for each compound. Representative O2 runs are shown in Figure 3, and a summary of all results is shown in Table 1. The rate of respiration (mean ± SD, in μM O_2 min^{-1} mg^{-1}) without addition was 0.21 ± 0.05, with the addition of 2.5 or 50 μM sorafenib was 0.19 ± 0.01 (p=0.797), and with the addition of 5.0 or 50 μM regorafenib was 0.19 ± 0.02 (p=0.606).Thus, the drugs had no noticeable effects on hepatocyte respiration.

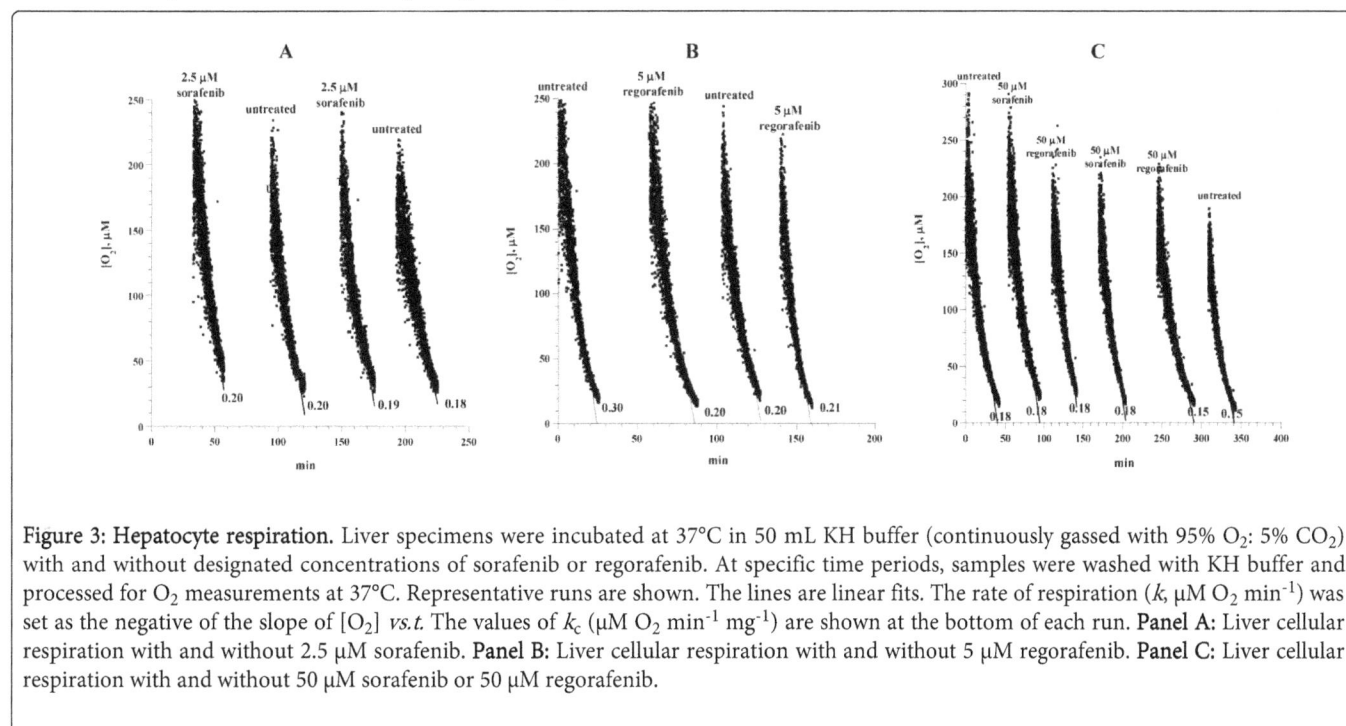

Figure 3: Hepatocyte respiration. Liver specimens were incubated at 37°C in 50 mL KH buffer (continuously gassed with 95% O_2: 5% CO_2) with and without designated concentrations of sorafenib or regorafenib. At specific time periods, samples were washed with KH buffer and processed for O_2 measurements at 37°C. Representative runs are shown. The lines are linear fits. The rate of respiration (k, μM O_2 min^{-1}) was set as the negative of the slope of $[O_2]$ $vs.t$. The values of k_c (μM O_2 min^{-1} mg^{-1}) are shown at the bottom of each run. **Panel A:** Liver cellular respiration with and without 2.5 μM sorafenib. **Panel B:** Liver cellular respiration with and without 5 μM regorafenib. **Panel C:** Liver cellular respiration with and without 50 μM sorafenib or 50 μM regorafenib.

The same experiments were repeated in RPMI medium. The conditions were no addition, 2.5 and 5.0 μM sorafenib and 5.0 and 50 μM regorafenib. The incubation time was 0 to 300 min. The results are in Supplementary Material (Figure 6S). For t=0 min, the values of k_c were 0.41 ± 0.08 (n=4). For the sorafenib experiments and $0 < t \leq 300$ min, the values of k_c for untreated specimens were 0.25 ± 0.05 (n=8) and for treated specimens 0.29 ± 0.05 (n=8), p=0.130. For the regorafenib experiments and $0 < t \leq 300$ min, the values of k_c for untreated specimens were 0.25 ± 0.09 (n=8) and for treated specimens 0.24 ± 0.08 (n=8), p=0.867. Thus, the rate of respiration was slightly higher in RPMI medium than in KH buffer (Table 1).

Cellular ATP

Four separate experiments, each involving four mice, were performed. Hepatocyte ATP ($pmol^{-1}mg^{-1}$) without addition was 56 ± 23 (n=5), with 2.5 or 50 μM sorafenib was 47 ± 42 (n=4, p=0.556) and with of 5.0 or 50 μM regorafenib was 41 ± 22 (p=0.556), Table 1. Thus, the drugs had no noticeable effects on hepatocyte ATP.

Intracellular caspase activity

The caspase-3 substrate analogue Ac-DEVD-AMC was used to measure hepatocyte caspase activity. Three separate experiments each involving three mice were performed. Representative HPLC runs are shown in Figure 4A-4D, and a summary of all of the results is shown in Table 1. Briefly, liver specimens were incubated with and without 50 μM sorafenib or regorafenib. At t=3 h, the specimens were transferred to the Ac-DEVD-AMC cleavage reaction in the presence and absence of zVAD-fmk. The tissue was then vigorously disrupted and the

supernatants were separated on HPLC and analyzed for the released AMC moiety (retention time=4.6 min). zVAD-fmk inhibited the release of AMC, confirming Ac-DEVD-AMC was mainly cleaved by intracellular caspases (Figure 4). The AMC peak area (arbitrary unit mg^{-1} ÷ 10^3) in untreated sample at t=0 h was 72, and at t=3 h was 145. The AMC peak area in the sample treated with sorafenib was 81 and with regorafenib was 70 (Figure 4). In another experiment, the AMC peak area at t=3 h without treatment was 66, with 2.5 μM sorafenib was 65 and with 5.0 μM regorafenib was 30. Thus, the drugs had no noticeable effects on hepatocyte caspase activity. Consistently, the drugs had no significant effects on casaspe-3, cytochrome c, BAX, caspase-9 and annexin A2 immunostains (Figure 1S-5S, Supplementary Material) and MTT assay (Table 1S, Supplementary Material).

Urea synthesis

Liver specimens were incubated as above with and without sorafenib (2.5 or 50 μM) or regorafenib (5.0 or 50 μM). At t=3 h, specimens were rinsed and incubated in 1.0 mL KH buffer supplemented with 10 mM NH_4Cl and 2.5 mM ornithine for 50 min. The solutions were then analyzed for urea. Four individual experiments involving four mice were performed for sorafenib and five individual experiments involving five mice were performed for regorafenib. The concentration of urea (mg/dL mg^{-1}) without addition was 0.16 ± 0.03, with sorafenib was 0.17 ± 0.03 (p=0.610), and with regorafenib was 0.17 ± 0.06 (p=0.429). The concentration of urea in specimens that were immediately placed $KH-NH_4Cl$-ornithine solution (t=0 h) was 0.25 ± 0.01 mg/dL mg^{-1} (Table 1). Thus, the drugs had no noticeable effects on hepatocyte urea synthesis.

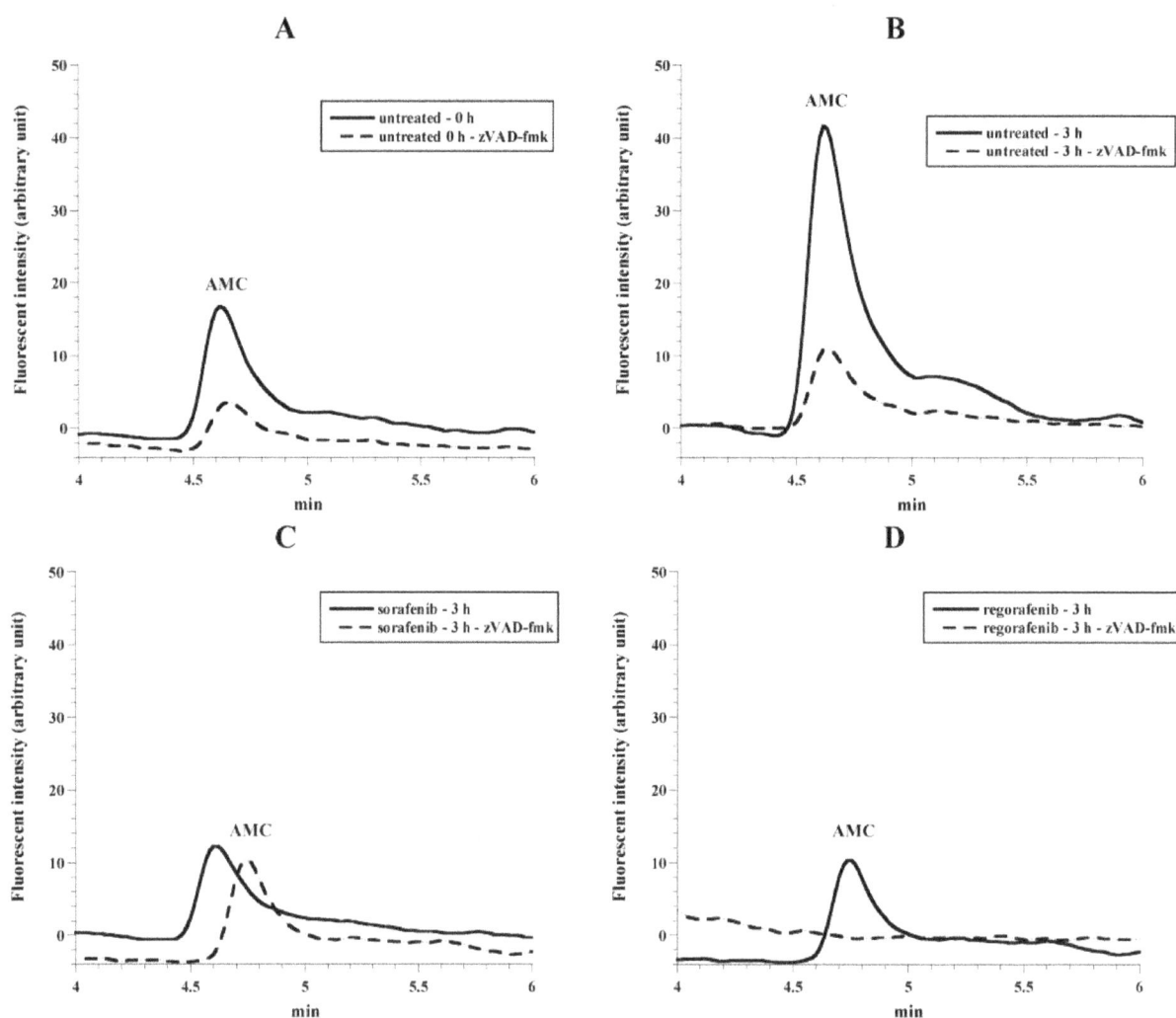

Figure 4: Hepatocyte caspase activity. Representative HPLC runs of liver tissue extracts showing intracellular caspase activity. Specimens were incubated at 37°C in 50 mL KH buffer (continuously gassed with 95% O_2: 5% CO_2) without additions or with the addition of 50 μM sorafenib or 50 μM regorafenib. At t=3 h, the specimens were transferred to the Ac-DEVD-AMC (caspase-3 substrate) reaction in the presence and absence of zVAD-fmk (pancaspase inhibitor). Tissues were then vigorously disrupted and the supernatants were separated on HPLC and analyzed for the AMC moiety (AMC retention time =4.6 min). **Panel A:** Intracellular caspase activity with and without zVAD-fmk at 0 h. **Panel B:** Intracellular caspase activity with and without zVAD-fmk at 3 h. **Panel C:** Intracellular caspase activity at 3 h in the presence of 50 μM sorafenib with and without zVAD-fmk. **Panel D:** Intracellular caspase activity at 3 h in the presence of 50 μM regorafenib with and without zVAD-fmk.

Cellular GSH

Liver specimens were incubated as above with and without sorafenib (50 μM) or regorafenib (50 μM). At t=180 min, the specimens were rinsed and transferred to the mBBr labeling reaction. Cellular GS-bimane was determined on HPLC as shown in Figure 5.Two individual experiments involving two mice were done. Cellular GSH (pmol mg^{-1}) without addition was 279 ± 9, with the addition of sorafenib was 384 ± 76, and with the addition of regorafenib was 312 ± 45. GSH content in specimens that were immediately placed in the mBBr reaction at t=0 min was 685 ± 129 pmol mg^{-1} (Table 1). Thus, the drugs had no noticeable effects on hepatocyte GSH.

Discussion

The Food and Drug Administration (FDA) approved the kinase inhibitor sorafenib for treatment of advanced renal cell (2005) and hepatocellular carcinomas (2007). Regorafenib, as approved in 2012 for colorectal cancer. Although these two compounds are closely related, their clinical adverse events differ. For example, regorafenib may produce fatal hepatotoxicity, a complication that has not been linked to sorafenib [6,7].

This study employed structural (hepatocyte histology and EM) and functional (hepatocyte respiration, ATP, caspase activity, and urea synthesis) surrogate biomarkers to investigate the toxic effects of sorafenib and regorafenib *in vitro*. The measured functional biomarkers were similar in treated and untreated liver specimens (Table 1). The ultrastructural changes, most notably loss of rER integrity and detachment of ribosomes, were more evident with regorafenib than sorafenib (Figures 2A and B). At 0 h, the untreated liver specimen showed well preserved hepatocyte architecture. At 4 h, the hepatocytes demonstrated only *minimal* mitochondrial distension and rER disintegration. Sorafenib treatment (2.5 μM for 4 h) produced *mild* mitochondrial distension and rER disintegration. The rER changes were more noticeable with regorafenib treatment (2.5 μM for 4 h), Figure 2A. Higher sorafenib dose (50 μM for 3 h) showed only mitochondrial distension with relatively preserved rER. Significant disruption of the rER and focal detachments of the ribosomes were evident in the tissue treated with 50 μM regorafenib at 3 h (Figure 2B).

Biologic activities of sorafenib and regorafenib can be demonstrated *in vitro* within a few hours of exposure to 0.1-10 μM of the drugs [8-13]. The cytotoxicity is cell specific and includes alterations in multiple signaling pathways, execution of apoptosis, induction of ER stress, and inhibition of protein synthesis. At 5 to 50 μM, for example, sorafenib inhibited the proliferation of hepatocellular carcinoma cell lines; the degree of inhibition was dependent on pERK expression [10]. Exposure of human leukemia cells to 10 μM sorafenib produced

cytotoxicity that involved inducing ER stress and generation of ROS [12]. At 3 to 20 μM, sorafenib induced apoptosis in melanoma cells in 4 h, mainly by nuclear translocation of the apoptosis-inducing factor [14]. In cell lines, apoptosis is induced via caspase dependent (e.g., caspase-2 and caspase-4 processing) and independent (e.g., nuclear translocation of the apoptosis-inducing factor) pathways.Regorafenib also inhibited the proliferation of human hepatocellular carcinoma cell lines, but the cells regrew after drug removal [13,15].

In contrast to these malignant cells, the findings here show high doses of sorafenib and regorafenib (50 μM) do not alter normal liver caspase-3 activity (Figure 4) or GSH content (Figure 5). The results also show hepatocyte bioenergetics (respiration and ATP content) following *in vitro* exposure to sorafenib or regorafenib for several hours is similar to that of untreated tissue (Figure 3 and Table 1). Consistently, hepatocyte urea synthesis is similar with and without the drugs (Table 1). By contrast, both compounds produce subtle derangements in hepatocyte ultrastructure (Figure 2). The rER changes, however, are more prominent with regorafenib, perhaps accounting for its potential hepatotoxicity (Figures 2A and 2B). Of note, the mitochondrial swelling is relatively similar in samples treated with sorafenib or regorafenib (Figures 2A and 2B).

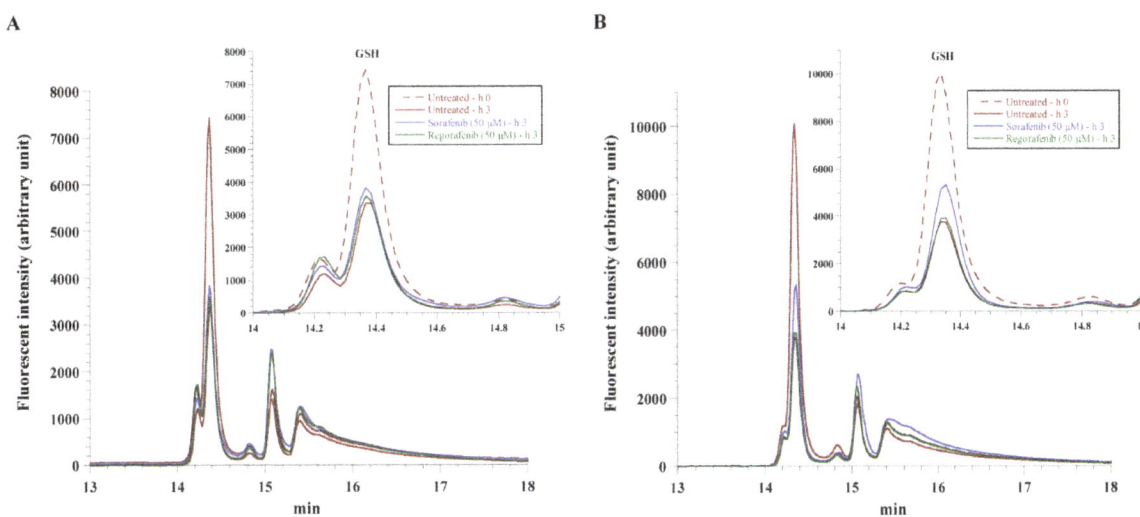

Figure 5: Hepatocyte GSH. HPLC runs of liver acid-soluble supernatants, showing the GS-bimane peaks with a retention time of 14.3 min. Specimens were incubated at 37°C without addition with 50 μM sorafenib or 50 μM regorafenib. At *t*=3 h, the specimens were transferred to the mBBr labeling reaction and processed and analyzed as described in Methods.

Sorafenib and regorafenib are tested at their therapeutic concentrations (2.5 and 5 μM, respectively [6,7] and at a 10- to 20-fold higher than the therapeutic concentration (50 μM). The first objective of using 50 μM was to investigate potential concentration-dependent hepatotoxicity. Of note, a few of the fatal regorafenib-associated hepatotoxicity were in patients with dehydration, a complication that increased serum drug concentration. The second aim was to compensate for the relatively short drug exposure (3-4 h).

In contrast to previous toxicology studies that were performed on isolated hepatocytes [23], this study utilized viable liver fragments. Advantages of our approach include minimum tissue handling and avoiding extensive collagenase digestion required for single cell preparations. Successful liver fragment collection, however, requires

rapid sampling of thin (<0.2 mm) slices, preferably <20 mg, while the liver is still perfused [24].The specimens should be immediately immersed in appropriate buffer supplemented with protease inhibitors.

Important limitation of this study is deterioration of the measured biomarkers with time in KH buffer (Table 1) and RPMI medium (Figure 6S, Supplementary Material). The biomarker values at *t*=0 (immediately after tissue collection) corresponded to the best possible results (Table 1). At $180 \leq t \leq 240$ min, hepatocyte respiration decreased by 30%, ATP decreased by 66%, caspase-3 activity increased by 47%, urea synthesis decreased by 36%, and GSH decreased by 59% (Table 1). This limitation prevented extending the incubation beyond 4.5 h.

	t=0 min	$180 \leq t \leq 240$ min		
	No addition	No addition	Sorafenib	Regorafenib
k_c [a] (μM O_2 min^{-1} mg^{-1})	0.30 ± 0.08 (n=4)	0.21 ± 0.05 (n=9)	0.19 ± 0.01 (n=5)	0.19 ± 0.02 (n=5)
ATP [b] (pmol mg^{-1})	167	56 ± 23 (n=6)	47 ± 40 (n=4)	41 ± 22 (n=4)
AMC peak area [c] (arbitrary unit mg^{-1} + 10^3)	71	104 ± 41 (n=4)	96 ± 41 (n=3)	47 ± 21 (n=3)
Urea synthesis [d] (mg/dL mg^{-1})	0.25 ± 0.01 (n=6)	0.16 ± 0.03 (n=6)	0.17 ± 0.03 (n=4)	0.17 ± 0.06 (n=5)

[a]Five individual experiments involving five mice were done for each compound. The concentration of sorafenib was 2.5 μM in three experiments and 50 μM in two experiments. The concentration of regorafenib was 5 μM in three experiments and 50 μM in two experiments. The in vitro incubation with the drugs was up to 6 h. There was no statistical significance between the untreated and treated pairs.

[b]Four individual experiments involving four mice were done for each compound. The concentration of sorafenib was 2.5 μM in three experiments and 50 μM in one experiment. The concentration of regorafenib was 5 μM in three experiments and 50 μM in one experiment. The in vitro incubation with the drugs was 180 to 240 min. There was no statistical significance between the untreated and treated pairs (p>0.556).

[c]Three individual experiments involving three mice were done for each compound. The concentration of sorafenib was 2.5 μM in two experiments and 50 μM in one experiment (Figure 4). The concentration of regorafenib was 5 μM in two experiments and 50 μM in one experiment (Figure 4). The in vitro incubation with the drugs was 180 to 240 min. There was no statistical significance between the untreated and treated pairs (p>0.114).

[d]For sorafenib, four individual experiments involving four mice were done. The concentration of sorafenib was 2.5 μM in two experiments and 50 μM in two experiments. For regorafenib, five individual experiments involving five mice were done. The concentration of regorafenib was 5 μM in three experiments and 50 μM in two experiments. The in vitro incubation with the drugs was 180 min. There was no statistical significance between the untreated and treated pairs (p>0.429).

Values are mean ± SD

Table 1: Effects of sorafenib and regorafenib on liver tissue respiration, ATP content, caspase activity, and urea synthesis.

Intracellular caspase activity is measured on viable liver fragments, using Ac-DEVD-AMC. This substrate is cleaved by several caspases, including caspase-3 (k_{cat}/K_m=218,000 s^{-1}), caspase-7 (k_{cat}/K_m=37,000 s^{-1}), caspase-1/interleukin-1 converting enzyme (k_{cat}/K_m=30,000 s^{-1}), caspase-6 (k_{cat}/K_m=2,000 s^{-1}), and caspase-4 (k_{cat}/K_m=1,800 s^{-1}) [25]. Of note, ER stress triggers a specific cascade involving caspase-12, -9, and -3 in a cytochrome c-independent manner [26]. Consistently, caspase-3 labeling at 4 h was similar in treated and untreated specimens; the few caspase-3 positive cells were mostly localized to Kupffer cells (Figure 1S, Supplementary Material). Similarly, compared with untreated specimens, cytochrome c, BAX, caspase-9 and annexin A2 labeling showed no significant drug effects at 4 h (Figure 2S – 5S, Supplementary Material).

The concentrations used in this study were therapeutics and 10 to 20-fold higher than therapeutics. These drug levels produced structural and ultrastructural changes in the liver (Figures 1 and 2). It is unclear, however, whether the observed adverse effects were due to

multikinase inhibition (e.g., VEGFR-2, PDGFR, Raf kinase, FLT3, Ret, and cKit) or "off" target effects. Further studies are needed to address this important issue.

In conclusion, this *in vitro* study shows murine hepatocyte bioenergetics, caspase-3 activity, urea synthesis and GSH are not significantly affected by sorafenib or regorafenib. Altered hepatocyte rER is more noticeable with regorafenib. Thus, these data demonstrate ultrastructural changes with regorafenib treatment, justifying its Boxed Warning of hepatotoxicity. The findings call for novel methods that allow early detection of regorafenib and sorafenib hepatotoxicities.

Author Contributions

The manuscript was written through contributions of all authors. All authors have given approval to the final version of the manuscript.

Funding Sources

This research was supported by a grant from the United Arab Emirates University - NRF (31M096).

References

1. Dykens JA, Will Y (2007) The significance of mitochondrial toxicity testing in drug development. Drug Discov Today 12: 777-785.

2. Lewis W, Day BJ, Copeland WC (2003) Mitochondrial toxicity of NRTI antiviral drugs: an integrated cellular perspective. Nat Rev Drug Discov 2: 812-822.

3. Green DR, Kroemer G (2004) The pathophysiology of mitochondrial cell death. Science 305: 626-629.

4. Alfazari AS, Al-Dabbagh B, Almarzooqi S, Albawardi A, Souid AK (2013) A preparation of murine liver fragments for in vitro studies: liver preparation for toxicological studies. BMC Res Notes 6: 70.

5. Alfazari AS, Al-Dabbagh B, Almarzooqi S, Albawardi A, Souid AK (2013) Bioenergetic study of murine hepatic tissue treated in vitro with atorvastatin. BMC PharmacolToxicol 14: 15.

6. Centers for Disease Control and Prevention (2013) Provisional CDC guidelines for the use and safety monitoring of bedaquilinefumarate (Sirturo) for the treatment of multidrug-resistant tuberculosis. MMWR Recomm Rep 62: 1-12.

7. http://www.accessdata.fda.gov/drugsatfda_docs/label/2011/021923s011lbl.pdf

8. Carr BI, D'Alessandro R, Refolo MG, Iacovazzi PA, Lippolis C, et al. (2013) Effects of low concentrations of regorafenib and sorafenib on human HCC cell AFP, migration, invasion, and growth in vitro. J Cell Physiol 228: 1344-1350.

9. Ramakrishnan V, Timm M, Haug JL, Kimlinger TK, Halling T, et al. (2012) Sorafenib, a multikinase inhibitor, is effective in vitro against non-Hodgkin lymphoma and synergizes with the mTOR inhibitor rapamycin. Am J Hematol 87: 277-283.

10. Zhang Z, Zhou X, Shen H, Wang D, Wang Y (2009) Phosphorylated ERK is a potential predictor of sensitivity to sorafenib when treating hepatocellular carcinoma: evidence from an in vitro study. BMC Med 7: 41.

11. Rahmani M, Davis EM, Bauer C, Dent P, Grant S (2005) Apoptosis induced by the kinase inhibitor BAY 43-9006 in human leukemia cells involves down-regulation of Mcl-1 through inhibition of translation. J Biol Chem 280: 35217-35227.

12. Rahmani M, Davis EM, Crabtree TR, Habibi JR, Nguyen TK et al (2007). The kinase inhibitor sorafenib induces cell death through a process

involving induction of endoplasmic reticulum stress. Mol Cell Biol 27: 5499-5513.

13. Carr BI, Cavallini A, Lippolis C, D'Alessandro R, Messa C, et al. (2013) Fluoro-Sorafenib (Regorafenib) effects on hepatoma cells: growth inhibition, quiescence, and recovery. J Cell Physiol 228: 292-297.

14. Panka DJ, Wang W, Atkins MB, Mier JW (2006) The Raf inhibitor BAY 43-9006 (Sorafenib) induces caspase-independent apoptosis in melanoma cells. Cancer Res 66: 1611-1619.

15. Wilhelm SM, Dumas J, Adnane L, Lynch M, Carter CA, et al. (2011) Regorafenib (BAY 73-4506): a new oral multikinase inhibitor of angiogenic, stromal and oncogenic receptor tyrosine kinases with potent preclinical antitumor activity. Int J Cancer 129: 245-255.

16. Berry MN (1962) Metabolic properties of cells isolated from adult mouse liver. J Cell Biology 15: 1-8.

17. Jocelyn PC (1987) Spectrophotometric assay of thiols. Methods Enzymol 143: 44-67.

18. Souid AK, Fahey RC, Aktas MK, Sayin OA, Karjoo S, et al. (2001) Blood thiols following amifostine and mesna infusions, a pediatric oncology group study. Drug MetabDispos 29: 1460-1466.

19. McDowell EM, Trump BF (1976) Histologic fixatives suitable for diagnostic light and electron microscopy. Arch Pathol Lab Med 100: 405-414.

20. Shaban S, Marzouqi F, Al Mansouri A, Penefsky HS, Souid AK (2010) Oxygen measurements via phosphorescence. Comput Methods Programs Biomed 100: 265-268.

21. Lo LW, Koch CJ, Wilson DF (1996) Calibration of oxygen-dependent quenching of the phosphorescence of Pd-meso-tetra (4-carboxyphenyl) porphine: A phosphor with general application for measuring oxygen concentration in biological systems. Anal Biochem. 236:153-160.

22. Saheki T, Katunuma N (1975) Analysis of regulatory factors for urea synthesis by isolated perfused rat liver. I. Urea synthesis with ammonia and glutamine as nitrogen sources. J Biochem 77: 659-669.

23. Ferrigno A, Richelmi P, Vairetti M (2013) Troubleshooting and improving the mouse and rat isolated perfused liver preparation. J PharmacolToxicol Methods 67: 107-114.

24. Al Samri MT, Al Shamsi M, Al-Salam S, Marzouqi F, Al Mansouri A, et al. (2011) Measurement of oxygen consumption by murine tissues in vitro. J PharmacolToxicol Methods 63: 196-204.

25. Talanian RV, Quinlan C, Trautz S, Hackett MC, Mankovich JA, et al. (1997) Substrate specificities of caspase family proteases. J Biol Chem 272: 9677-9682.

26. Nobuhiro M, Nakanishi K, Takenouchi H, Shibata T, Yasuhiko Y (2002) An endoplasmic reticulum stress-specific caspase cascade in apoptosis: cytochrome c-independent activation of caspase-9 by caspase-12. J Biol Chem 277: 34287-34294.

11

Fresh Red Blood Transfusion as a Successful Erythrocyte Cholinesterase Supplement in Organophosphate Poisoning

Ying Wang[1,2], Zhi-hui Huang[2,3], Bin-yu Chen[1,2#] and Xiang-min Tong[1,2#*]

[1]Research Center of Blood Transfusion Medicine, Key Laboratory of Laboratory Medicine (Wenzhou Medical University), Ministry of Education, Zhejiang Provincial People's Hospital, Hangzhou, 310014, China

[2]Clinical Research Institute, Zhejiang Provincial People's Hospital, Hangzhou, 310014, China

[3]School of Basic Medicine, Wenzhou Medical University, Wenzhou, 325035, China

[#]These authors contributed equally to this work.

*Corresponding author: Xiangmin Tong, Research Center of Blood Transfusion Medicine, Key Laboratory of Laboratory Medicine (Wenzhou Medical University), Ministry of Education, Zhejiang Provincial People's Hospital, Hangzhou, 310014, China, E-mail: tongxiangmin11@163.com

Abstract

Despite improvements to standard treatments (atropine, oxime) and intensive care management, the mortality associated with organophosphate (OP) poisoning has not substantially decreased. In this study, we evaluated the role of packed red blood cells (RBCs) transfusion in acute OP poisoning. Patients diagnosed with OP poisoning were included in this prospective study, and then were transfused with packed RBCs stored less than 10 days or 10 to 35 days. Cholinesterase (ChE) level in blood, atropine usage and durations were recorded. We found both shorter- and longer-storage RBCs (200~400 ml) significantly increased AChE level in blood, improved ChE recovery, and reduced the usage and shortened the duration of atropine and followed clinical recovery. Shorter-storage RBCs had better effect than longer-storage (longer storage) ones. Due to erythrocyte cholinesterase supplement, packed RBCs might be used as an alternative approach in patients with OP poisoning, especially at the early stages.

Keywords: Organophosphate; Acetylcholinesterase; Butyrylcholinesterase; Atropine; Oximes

Introduction

Organophosphorus (OP) compounds are chemical substances that come up with a significant toxicological threat. Several pesticides, fungicides, rodenticides were made of OPs, such as parathion, malathion, dimethoate, trichlorfon, dichlorvos, that were commonly used in Asia. In acute and chronic forms, OPs poisoning prevail in industry and agriculture [1]. Due to the availability and toxicity, OPs poisoning happen regularly in accidental intoxication and suicides. Actually acute self-poisoning with organophosphate (OP) pesticides is common in rural Asia, and causes hundreds of thousands of deaths each year [2,3].

OP penetrates via the respiratory tract, alimentary tract and dermal integuments. OPs inhibit cholinesterase, and lead to the increase and accumulation of endogenous acetylcholine concentration, which then affect muscarinic ACh receptors functions mostly in central nervous system, heart muscle, bronchi, alimentary tract and nicotinic ACh receptors in muscular lamina. Thus they exert direct toxic influence on the central nervous system, even could cause death due to pulmonary edema, cerebral edema, respiratory paralysis [4]. OPs affect cholinesterase of all types irreversibly, including acetylcholinesterase (AChE), and pseudocholinesterase (PChE, or butyrylcholinesterase, BChE) [5]. Patients with severe acute poisoning may also lead to delayed sudden death. Some types of organic phosphorus poisoning can occur in 8 to 14 days after the poisoning of delayed neuropathy. Standard therapy includes resuscitation, antidote administration, gastric lavage and/or activated charcoal and supportive care [6].

Despite the use of antidote and intensive care, the high mortality with OPs poisoning still calls for new alternative treatments [7]. Red blood cells (RBCs) transfusion as a mail supply of AChE has been posed as an alternative therapy, but few studies have investigated it, and need to be clarified. Recently we found RBCs transfusion, especially the shorter-storage ones as a supplement of active AChE, could promote ChE restoration, help to improve clinical symptoms.

Materials and Methods

Patients who were diagnosed as OP intoxication in our emergency medicine clinic between Jan 1st, 2014 and Jan 1st, 2016, were included in this study. A standard patient data, demographic information, ChE levels, were recorded.

Diagnosis of OP poisoning was based on information taken either from the patient or their family about the agent involved in the exposure. We confirmed the diagnosis of OP poisoning by measuring plasma cholinesterase (ChE) levels [8]. ChE levels were determined using an Olympus U2700 spectrophotometric chemistry analyzer (Beckman Coulter, Tokyo, Japan). The inclusion criteria contains (1) OP intoxication (exposure history/information), and (2) serum ChE activity less than 2000 KU/L (normal 4000~11000 KU/L).

Standard toxication treatment protocol was applied to all patients. As details, gastric lavage was performed with 2000 ml of 0.9% saline; 0.9% saline and 5% dextrose infusion was started at 2000 ml/m^2 per day. Intravenous (IV) atropine was administered with started at 1 mg/kg per day; 2 g IV single dose pralidoxime was administered. The patients were admitted to the ICU based on the severity of the clinical signs and symptoms.

As to the RBCs transfusion group, 200 ml~400 ml packed RBCs were transfused during the 3 hours after toxication; 200 ml~400 ml packed RBCs were transfused at 10 hours after toxication if still not atropinization or with still low ChE. All the packed RBCs were administrated during 72 hrs. As for the shorter-storage RBCs refers to storage less than 10 days (including 10 days), while the longer-storage RBCs refers to storage more than 10 days, but less than 35 days (absolutely qualified RBCs).

Level of statistical significance was taken as P<0.05 for all tests.

Results

To evaluate the role of packed red blood cells (RBCs) transfusion in acute OP poisoning, 60 patients with acute OP poisoning were included in this study. Shorter-storage RBCs (less than 10 days) transfusion were applied to 20 patients, longer-storage RBCs (more than 10 days, but less than 35 days) transfusion were applied to 17 patients, and 23 patients did not received transfusion. All the patients had orally OP intake history either for accident or suicide. 28 patients were poisoned with dimethoate, 12 with methamidophos, 9 with parathion, 6 with malathion, 3 with trichlorfon, and 2 with dichlorvos.

Since OPs main toxicity is ChE inhibition, the duration of ChE recover to normal level is critical of the therapeutic effect. As shown in Table 1, the duration time for patient's blood ChE recovery to 70% (2, 800 KU/L) and 90% of normal level (3, 600 KU/L) were compared, both shorter-storage and longer-storage RBCs transfusion had a significant reduction, while shorter-storage RBCs had even better effects (Table 1).

	n	Time for ChE recover to 2800 KU/L (hr, x ± s)	Time for ChE recover to 3600 KU/L (hr, x ± s)
Shorter storage RBCs transfusion	20	46.8 ± 15.6*	103.4 ± 7.8*
Longer storage RBCs transfusion	17	53.4 ± 12.2#	112.5 ± 8.8#
No RBCs transfusion	23	67.2 ± 14.9	132.3 ± 10.9

Table 1: Effect of RBCs transfusion on duration of ChE recovery. *P<0.01, #P<0.05.

Shorter-storage RBCs transfusion and longer-storage RBCs transfusion shorten the time for ChE recover to 2, 800 KU/L from 67.2 ± 14.9 hours to 46.8 ± 15.6 hours and 53.4 ± 12.2 hours respectively. Shorter-storage RBCs transfusion and longer-storage RBCs transfusion shorten the time for ChE recover to 3, 600 KU/L from 132.3 ± 10.9 hours to 103.4 ± 7.8 hours and 112.5 ± 8.8 hours respectively.

In order to follow AChE elevation effects by RBCs transfusion, the blood AChE levels before and after RBCs transfusion 6 hours were detected. In the shorter-storage RBCs transfusion group, the level of blood AChE after transfusion was significantly increased (Figure 1). This significant increase was due to the fresh RBCs transfusion. However, in the longer-storage RBCs transfusion group, the level of blood AChE was not increased significantly (Figure 2), might due to the reduction of AChE during storage. These results suggest that fresh RBCs transfusion significantly improve ChE recovery.

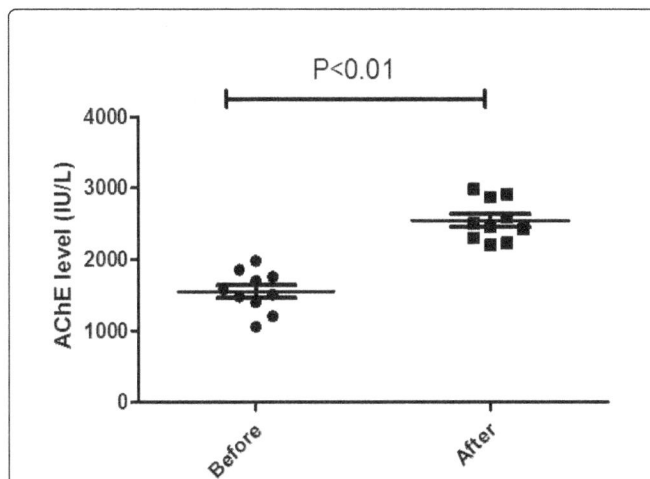

Figure 1: AChE levels of the patients before and after shorter-storage RBCs transfusion. Blood AChE level was detected before and 6 hours after shorter-storage RBCs transfusion respectively. Results were plotted and performed by student t test.

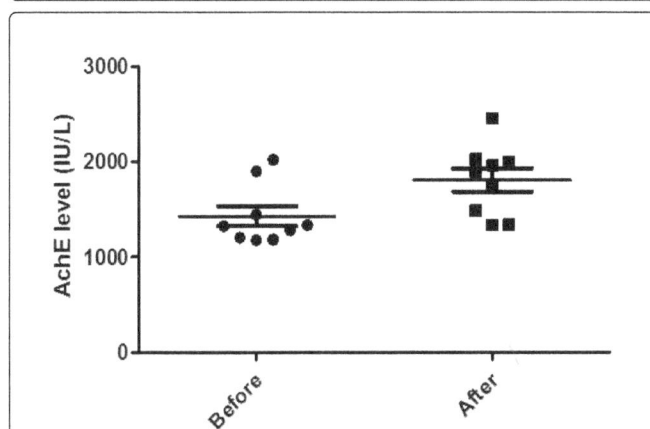

Figure 2: AChE levels of the patients before and after longer-storage RBCs transfusion. Blood AChE level was detected before and 6 hours after longer -storage RBCs transfusion respectively. Results were plotted and performed by student t test.

Atropine usage and durations reflect the severity and progression of the poisoning. We next examined whether RBCs transfusion also reduced the amount and duration of atropine usage. As shown in Table 2, shorter-storage and longer-storage RBCs transfusion significantly reduced the total amount of atropine usage from 685.4 ± 68.4 mg to 423.8 ± 52.8 and 498.2 ± 55.4 mg respectively. Shorter-storage and longer-storage RBCs transfusion also reduced the duration of atropine from 7.2 ± 0.57 days to 6.3 ± 0.48 days and 6.6 ± 0.63 days respectively. These results suggest that RBCs transfusion significantly reduces the amount and duration of atropine usage in OP patients.

	n	Amount of atropine requirement (mg)	Duration of atropine requirement (days)
Shorter storage RBCs transfusion	20	423.8 ± 52.8#	6.3 ± 0.48#

| Longer storage RBCs transfusion | 17 | 498.2 ± 55.4[#] | 6.6 ± 0.63 |
| No RBCs transfusion | 23 | 685.4 ± 68.4 | 7.2 ± 0.57 |

Table 2: Effect of RBCs transfusion on total usage and duration of atropine requirement. [#]$P<0.05$.

Discussion

In the present study, we found that RBCs transfusion significantly improved ChE recovery and reduced the amount and duration of atropine usage. OP intoxications are potentially fatal poisonings which result from both accidental and purposeful intake. These poisoning could be acute or chronic, with high risk of remote consequences [9]. OP compounds are very strong inhibitors for carboxylic ester hydrolases. As a result of ChE inhibition, acetylcholine accumulates, leads to paralysis of acetylcholine receptors due to continuous stimulation, then, muscarnic, nicotinc, and central nervous system symptoms occur [10].

The two types of cholinesterase are AChE and BChE. Among the whole blood ChE activity, AChE from erythrocytes accounts for 60% to 80%, and BChE from plasma accounts for 20% to 40%. AChE is primarily concentrated in the blood on red blood cell membranes, neuromuscular junctions, and other neural synapses. BChE is produced in the liver and found primarily in blood plasma. AChE has a higher specificity to Ach than BChE. After combined by free OPs in the circulation, ChEs both the AChE and BChE will be metabolized, so as to prevent severe damage to central nervous system. In severe poisoning, it needs about four weeks for enzyme recovery. If the low enzyme activity status lasts long, could cause 'rebound' or uintermediate syndrome', and might lead to paralysis of respiratory muscle, that increase the mortality rate.

In present study, we found shorter-storage RBCs transfusion (200~400 ml) on the basis of standard therapy could increase cholinesterase activity, reduce the usage and shortened the duration of atropine significantly, the longer-storage RBCs transfusion had similar but lower improvement effect. These results suggest that RBCs transfusion could improve clinical therapeutic effects on OPs intoxication patients. Red blood transfusion may deliver additional erythrocyte cholinesterase, which could be the potential target substrate for OP. Increasing the activity of AChE over 30% leads to normal neuromuscular transmission and better wearing conditions, and then could improve the overall outcome [11]. In addition, transfusion of red blood cell could not only substitute circulating cholnesterases, but could also bind with OP compounds to prevent them enter central nervous system and muscle. These results help to present additional therapeutic options in the early stage of intoxication in patients with reduced cholinesterase, especially when atropine or specific antidote treatments were ineffective.

It has been reported that RBCs AChE activity remains constant before day 7, and showed significant reduction at day 45 [12]. Although the storage methods have slight different, such we keep 35 days in China, the constant AchE activity during storage was observed [13]. Here we found shorter-storage packed RBCs transfusion improved blood cholinesterase activity and clinical symptoms in OP toxication patients, however longer-storage packed RBCs showed lower effects. These results suggest that in the emergency, both shorter-

storage and longer-storage qualified RBCs could be used to supply AchE, leading to improvement.

Previous studies have reported whole blood transfusion [9] or fresh frozen plasma transfusion [14] could restore the enzymatic function by its biscavenging effect. However, packed RBCs transfusion has advantages over whole blood transfusion, since the total volume administrated into patients is less that could avoid risks of overloading and fever or allergy by substances in serum. Some studies tried to use human ChE substitute's administration [15], however, due to the high costs and large quantity needed, these substitutes could not be used in human now.

In this study, we found application of RBCs could substitute cholinesterases in OP poisoning, help to restoration of enzymatic function and bind with OP compounds. RBC-AChE could function as a natural bioscavenger that binds OP compounds stoichiometrically and inactivates them effectively. Therefore red blood cell transfusion both shorter-storage and longer-storage could be a good alternative approach.

Conclusions

Based on our results, early blood transfusion can effectively reduce the extent of toxic symptoms and prevent further progression, especially when oximes are not available. However, further evaluation needs to be examined.

References

1. Catano HC, Carranza E, Huamani C, Hernandez AF (2008) Plasma cholinesterase levels and health symptoms in peruvian farm workers exposed to organophosphate pesticides. Arch Environ Contam Toxicol 55: 153-159.

2. Eddleston M (2000) Patterns and problems of deliberate self-poisoning in the developing world. QJM 93: 715-731.

3. Li Y, Tse ML, Gawarammana I, Buckley N, Eddleston M (2009) Systematic review of controlled clinical trials of gastric lavage in acute organophosphorus pesticide poisoning. Clin Toxicol (Phila) 47: 179-192.

4. Rickett DL, Glenn JF, Beers ET (1986) Central respiratory effects versus neuromuscular actions of nerve agents. Neurotoxicology 7: 225-236.

5. Eddleston M, Buckley NA, Eyer P, Dawson AH (2008) Management of acute organophosphorus pesticide poisoning. Lancet 371: 597-607.

6. Lotti M (2010) Chapter 72 - Clinical Toxicology of Anticholinesterase Agents in Humans; Krieger R, editor: Acdemic Press p 1543-1589.

7. Rahimi R, Nikfar S, Abdollahi M (2006) Increased morbidity and mortality in acute human organophosphate-poisoned patients treated by oximes: a meta-analysis of clinical trials. Hum Exp Toxicol 25: 157-162.

8. Coskun R, Gundogan K, Sezgin GC, Topaloglu US, Hebbar G, et al. (2015) Retrospective review of intensive care management of organophosphate insecticide poisoning: Single center experience. Niger J Clin Pract 18: 644-650.

9. Ryniak S, Harbut P, Goydzik W, Sokolowski J, Paciorek P, et al. (2011) Whole blood transfusion in the treatment of an acute organophosphorus poisoning--a case report. Med Sci Monit 17: CS109-111.

10. Kwong TC (2002) Organophosphate pesticides: biochemistry and clinical toxicology. Ther Drug Monit 24: 144-149.

11. Thiermann H, Szinicz L, Eyer P, Zilker T, Worek F (2005) Correlation between red blood cell acetylcholinesterase activity and neuromuscular transmission in organophosphate poisoning. Chem Biol Interact 157-158: 345-7.

12. Karon BS, Van Buskirk CM, Jaben EA, Hoyer JD, Thomas DD (2012) Temporal sequence of major biochemical events during blood bank storage of packed red blood cells. Blood Transfus 10: 453-461.

13. Yi Luo, Y-XC, Zhang B (2009) The change of erythrocyte true cholinesterase activity and its clinical value. Lab Med Clin 6: 2.

14. Vucinic S, Zlatkovic M, Antonijevic B, Curcic M, Boskovic B (2013) Fresh frozen plasma as a successful antidotal supplement in acute organophosphate poisoning. Arh Hig Rada Toksikol 64: 87-91.

15. Aurbek N, Thiermann H, Eyer F, Eyer P, Worek F (2009) Suitability of human butyrylcholinesterase as therapeutic marker and pseudo catalytic scavenger in organophosphate poisoning: a kinetic analysis. Toxicology 259: 133-139.

12

GC-MS Analysis and Evaluation of Mutagenic and Antimutagenic Activity of Ethyl Acetate Extract of *Ajuga bracteosa* Wall ex. Benth: An Endemic Medicinal Plant of Kashmir Himalaya, India

Hilal Ahmad Ganaie[1,2], **Md. Niamat Ali**[1*], **Bashir A Ganai**[2], **Jasbir Kaur**[1] and **Mudasar Ahmad**[2]

[1]*Cytogenetic and Molecular Biology Research Laboratory, Centre of Research for Development (CORD), University of Kashmir, Srinagar-190 006, J & K, India*

[2]*Phytochemistry Research Laboratory, Centre of Research for Development (CORD), University of Kashmir, Srinagar-190 006, J & K, India*

[*]**Corresponding author:** Md. Niamat Ali, Cytogenetic and Molecular Biology Research Laboratory, Centre of Research for Development (CORD), University of Kashmir, Srinagar-190 006, J & K, India, E-mail: mdniamat@hotmail.com

Abstract

Herbal medicines as the major remedy in traditional system of medicine have been used in medical practices since antiquity. The natural products remain an important source of new drugs, new drug leads and new chemical entities. The ethyl acetate extract of *Ajuga bracteosa* was evaluated for mutagenic and antimutagenic assay against mice pre-treated with 1/4th LD50 (117.5 mg/kg bw) of ethyl methane sulphonate by micronucleus and chromosomal aberration assay. Mice were treated with ethyl acetate extract of *Ajuga bracteosa* (Ab-EAE) (100, 200 300 & 400 mg/kg bw) for 30 days. Without the doses of EMS, no mutagenic effects were observed in blood and bone marrow samples of the mice. But Ab-EAE showed antimutagenic effects on EMS induced mutagenicity in mice. It was observed that high doses of Ab-EAE showed protective effects. The reduction profiles in the EMS induction MN at concentration of ethyl acetate extract of *Ajuga bracteosa* (100, 200, 300 and 400 mg/kg bw) were estimated as 2%, 4.9%, 16.4% and 20.7% respectively. It can be concluded from the study that ethyl acetate extract of *Ajuga bracteosa* exhibited no mutagenic effects but only possessing antimutagenic effects. This antimutagenic activity is an induction of medicinal relevance.

Keywords: Ajuga; Antimutagenicity; EMS; Micronucleus; GC-MS

Introduction

Traditional herbal medicine practitioners have described the therapeutic effectiveness of many indigenous plants [1]. The plants are the source of synthetic and traditional herbal medicine and hence are useful for healing and curing of human diseases because of the presence of phytochemical constituents [2-4]. These phytochemicals are naturally present in all parts of medicinal plants viz., leaves, vegetables and roots. The Phytochemicals are synthesized by a plant itself as primary and secondary metabolites. Chlorophyll, proteins and common sugars are included in primary constituents while as terpenoids, alkaloids and phenolic compounds come under secondary compounds [5]. Terpenoids and phenols exhibit various important pharmacological activities viz., anti-inflammatory, anticancer, anti-malarial, anti-viral, anti-bacterial activities and inhibition of cholesterol synthesis [6]. Alkaloids are known to possess anesthetic properties [7,8].

The pharmacological and therapeutic properties of traditionally used medicinal plants are attributed to various chemical constituents isolated from their crude extracts [9-11]. It is very common among the people who live in upper reaches of Kashmir Himalaya to use herbs for curing of various diseases [12]. Although the diversity of plant species in Kashmiri Himalayas is a potential source of biologically active compounds, the effects on human health and genetic material are often unknown. Interest in such popular usage has recently gained strength, through recent knowledge that chemicals, such as proteases and antioxidants may prevent or reduce the development of cancer by blocking genetic damage [13-15].

Ajuga bracteosa Wall ex. Benth of family Lamiaceae is commonly known as 'Bungle' in English and 'Jan-i-adam' in Kashmiri. It is a perennial erect, ascending hairy herb, often prostrates with oblanceolate or sub-spathulate leaves and grows up to 5-50 cm tall. It is found along roadsides, open slopes, and rock cervices [16,17]. Its distribution extends from temperate regions of Western Himalayas viz., Kashmir, Pakistan, Afghanistan and China to Bhutan in Eastern Himalayas; Indian subtropical regions [18] viz., plains of Punjab and upper Gangetic plains at an altitude of 1300 m [19] and in tropical regions of Malaysia. In Pakistan, it is found in northern hilly areas, where in local Hindi/Punjabi language it is called kori booti (means bitter herb) owing to its bitter taste. The plant is effectively used for the treatment of gout, rheumatism, palsy, jaundice, hypertension, sore throat and as a blood purifier. Locally, the leaves are used to cure headache, pimples, measles, stomach acidity, burns and boils.

Materials and Methods

Collection and air drying of plant material

Aerial parts of *Ajuga bracteosa* were collected from Sinthan Top area of District Anantnag (Kashmir) in the month July, 2013. The plant was identified at the Centre of Biodiversity and Plant Taxonomy, Department of Botany, University of Kashmir, Srinagar, J & K and a voucher specimen (JKASH/CBT/226 Dated 08. 08. 2014) was deposited there. The parts were allowed to dry under shade (30°C) for 8-10 days.

Preparation of extracts

After shade drying, the aerial parts were macerated to fine powder, 1 kg of leaves were extracted successively with hexane for defatenning and methanol for 16 h using Soxhlet apparatus. The extracts were filtered through a Buchner funnel using Whatman No.1 filter paper, and all the extracts were concentrated to dryness under vacuum using a Heidolph rotary evaporator, yielding hexane, ethyl acetate, methanol and aqueous crude extracts of 65, 52, 46 and 36 g respectively. All the extracts were stored at 4°C in air tight glass bottles before use.

Phytochemical screening

Chemical tests were carried out on the extracts using standard procedures to identify various constituents like Tannin, saponin, flavonoids, steroids, terpenoids, glucosides, alkaloids, carbohydrates, phytosterols, phenol, proteins and amino acids [20-23].

GC-MS analysis

GC-MS analysis was carried out with GCMS-QP2010 Plus, Shimadzu, Japan fitted with programmable head space auto sampler and auto injector. The capillary column used was DB-1/RTX-MS (30 metre) with helium as a carrier gas, at a flow rate of 3 mL/min with 1 µL injection volume. Samples were analysed with the column held initially at 100°C for 2 min after injection, then increased to 170°C with 10°C/min heating ramp without hold and increased to 215°C with 5°C/min heating ramp for 8 min. Then the final temperature was increased to 240°C with 10°C/min heating ramp for 15 min. The injections were performed in split mode (30:1) at 250°C. Detector and injector temperatures were 260°C and 250°C, respectively. Pressure was established as 76.2 kPa and the sample was run for 70 min. Temperature and nominal initial flow for flameionization detector (FID) were set as 230°C and 3.1 mL/min, correspondingly. MS parameters were as follows: scan range (m/z): 40-650 atomic mass units (AMU) under the electron impact (EI) ionization (70 eV). The constituent compounds were determined by comparing their retention times and mass weights with those of authentic samples obtained by GC and as well as the mass spectra from the Wiley libraries and National Institute of Standards and Technology (NIST) database.

Animals and treatments

Both sex of albino mice, Balb/c strain useful for research in cancer and immunology, weighing 25-35 g were obtained from the Indian Institute of Integrative Medicine (IIM), Canal Road Jammu, kept in plastic cages in an experimental room under controlled conditions of temperature ($22 \pm 2°C$), humidity ($55 \pm 10\%$), 12 h light/dark cycles and access to food and water. They were randomized at the beginning of the experiment. The study design was approved by the Institutional Animal Ethical Committee, and the experiments undertaken in accordance with the ethical principles of the CPCSEA norms. The mice were divided into 8 groups, with 5 animals per group (Table 1). Ethyl methane sulfonate (EMS, Sigma Aldrich) was used to induce mutations and chromosomal aberrations for antimutagenic evaluation of ethyl acetate extract of *Ajuga bracteosa*.

Group	Dose	Purpose of group	Duration
Group 1	Distilled water	Negative control	15 days
Group 2	1/4th LD50 EMS	Positive control EMS	24 h
Group 3	Ab-EAE 100 mg/kg bw	Positive control *Ajuga bracteosa*	24 h
Group 4	Ab-EAE 400 mg/kg bw	Positive control *Ajuga bracteosa*	24 h
Group 5	Ab-EAE 100 mg/kg bw + EMS	Treated Group	30 days
Group 6	Ab-EAE 200 mg/kg bw + EMS	Treated Group	30 days
Group 7	Ab-EAE 300 mg/kg bw + EMS	Treated Group	30 days
Group 8	Ab-EAE 400 mg/kg bw + EMS	Treated Group	30 days

Table 1: Grouping, dose (distilled water, EMS and Ab-ME in concentrations of 100, 200, 300 and 400 mg/kg bw) and duration of experiment. Ab-EAE=Ethyl acetate extract of *Ajuga bracteosa*.

The micronucleus test

The method of MacGregor et al. was used for micronucleus test. Mice were injected intraperitoneal with 0. 5 ml of 0.06% colchicine and two hours later, mice were sacrificed by cervical dislocation. Slides were prepared with blood collected from the jugular vein. The slides were air-dried, fixed in absolute methanol, stained in 10% Giemsa and then coded for blind analysis. One thousand polychromatic erythrocytes (PCE) were analysed per mouse. The proportion of PCE and normochromatic erythrocytes (NCE) in 200 erythrocytes/animal was calculated, to detect possible cytotoxic effects. The slides were scored blindly, using a light microscope with a 65x objectives,

Chromosomal aberration

Both the femurs were fleshed out from the muscles and kept in HBSS (Hank's balanced salt solution). The femurs were then rinsed with 3 ml 0.056% KCl solution in a centrifuge tube. The tube was then incubated at 37°C for 20 minutes. After incubation, centrifugation at 800 rpm for 4 minutes was carried out. Supernatant was discarded and fresh Carnoy's fixative was added (3:1methanol: acetic acid). The process of centrifugation was repeated three times. Then slides were prepared, stained with 4% Giemsa, air dried and studied under compound microscope.

Results

Phytochemical screening

Therapeutic values of medicinal and aromatic plants (MAPs) are due to the presence of major bioactive constituents like alkaloids, phenolics, flavonoids, tannins, cardiac glycosides, terpenes, saponins, steroids etc. The phytochemical investigation of *Ajuga bracteosa* extracts in the present study revealed presence of different active ingredients (secondary plant metabolites) like flavonoids, phenolics, alkaloids, tannins, cardiac glycosides, terpenes, saponins, steroids, carbohydrates, amino acids and proteins as shown in Table 2. It supports the resourcefulness of the plant extract.

Phytoconstituents	Test	Result
Alkaloids	Wagner's test	+ +
Phenolics	phenol test	+ +
Tannins	Ferric chloride test	+ +
Cardiac glycosides	Keller-Killani test	+ +
Terpenes	Salkwaski's test	+
Flavonoids	Shinoda's test	+ +
Saponins	Frothing test	+
Steroids	Libermann-Buchard's test	+
Carbohydrates	Molish test	+ +
Proteins	Biuret test	+
Polysterols	Salkowski's Test	+
Amino acids	Ninhydrin Test	+

Table 2: Qualitative phytochemical screening of *Ajuga bracteosa*. (++) = strong presence, (+) = moderate presence

GC-MS analysis

In order to find out the phytocomponents responsible for antimutagenic activity, ethyl acetate fraction of *Ajuga bracteosa* was subjected to GC-MS analysis. The active principals present in the ethyl acetate fraction of *Ajuga bracteosa* along with their retention time (RT), molecular formula, molecular weight (MW) and peak area (%) are presented in Table 3. The chromatogram of Ab-ME showed six major peaks (Figure 1): 1, 2, 3-Propanetriol (18.15%), 1, 2, 3-Propanetriol, 1-acetate (11.35%), Stigmast-5-en-3-ol (11.35%), 2, 6, 10-Trimethyl, 14-ethylene-14-pentadecane (8.51%), 2-Hexadecene-1-ol, 3, 7, 11, 15-tetramethyl-, [R-[R (5.76%) and 1-(+)-Ascorbic acid 2, 6-dihexadecanoate (4.75%) comprising 59.87% of total peak area.

S. No.	Compound	Retention time	% Area	Molecular formula	Molecular weight
1	1, 2, 3-propanetriol	5.7	18.15	$C_3H_8O_3$	92
2	1,2,3-Propanetriol, 1-acetate	7.47	11.35	$C_5H_{10}O_4$	134
3	1,2,3-Propanetriol, 1-acetate	8.5	0.77	$C_5H_{10}O_4$	134
4	1,2,3-Propanetriol, 1-acetate	11.12	0.94	$C_5H_{10}O_4$	144
5	2,3-Dihydroxypropyl acetate	11.23	0.45	$C_5H_{10}O_4$	134
6	1,2,3-Propanetriol, 1-acetate	14.42	0.59	$C_5H_{10}O_4$	134
7	2(4H)-Benzofuranone, 5,6,7,7A-tetrahydro-6-H	24.04	0.83	$C_{11}H_{16}O_3$	196
8	(2E)-3, 7, 11, 15- Tetramethyl-2-Hexadecane	25. 08	0.24	$C_{20}H_{40}$	280
9	2, 6, 10- Trimethyl, 14- Ethylene-14-Pentadecne	25.19	8.51	$C_{20}H_{38}$	278
10	Acetic acid, 3, 7, 11, 15- Tetramethyl-hexadecyl ester	25.32	0.8	$C_{22}H_{44}O_2$	340
11	2-Hexadecen-1-ol, 3,7,11,15-tetramethyl-, [R-[R	25.7	2.82	$C_{20}H_{40}O$	296

12	2-Hexadecen-1-ol, 3,7,11,15-tetramethyl-, [R-[R	26.07	4.37	$C_{20}H_{40}O$	296
13	Hexadecanoic acid, methyl ester	26.89	0.42	$C_{17}H_{34}O_2$	270
14	1-Hexadecne-3-ol, 3, 5, 11, 15-Tetramethyl	27.29	0.24	$C_{20}H_{40}O$	296
15	l- (+)- Ascorbic acid 2, 6-dihexadecanoate	27.69	4.75	$C_{38}H_{68}O_8$	652
16	Hexadecanoic acid, ethyl ester	28.01	0.78	$C_{18}H_{36}O_2$	284
17	9, 12-Octadecenoic acid (Z, Z)-, methyl ester	29.44	0.23	$C_{19}H_{34}O_2$	294
18	9, 12, 15-Octadecenoic acid, methyl ester, (Z, Z, Z)-,	29.53	0.78	$C_{19}H_{32}O_2$	292
19	2-Hexadecen-1-ol, 3,7,11,15-tetramethyl-, [R-[R	29.7	5.76	$C_{20}H_{40}O$	296
20	9,12, 15-Octadecatrienoic acid, (Z,Z,Z)-	30.19	1.55	$C_{18}H_{30}O_2$	278
21	Ethyl (9Z, 12Z)-9, 12-Octadecadienoate	30.35	1.05	$C_{20}H_{36}O_2$	308
22	Octadecanamide	30.6	0.15	$C_{18}H_{37}NO$	283
23	Phytol, acetate	30.9	0.88	$C_{22}H_{42}O_2$	338
24	1-Chloroheptacosane	31.72	0.48	$C_{27}H_{55}Cl$	414
25	9-Hexadecanoic acid, 9-Octadecenyl Ester, (Z)	31.88	0.19	$C_{34}H_{64}O_2$	504
26	13-Octadecenal, (Z)	31.97	0.73	$C_{18}H_{34}O$	266
27	Cyclohexane, Decyl-	32.19	0.43	$C_{16}H_{32}$	224
28	1-Heptacosanol	32.43	0.27	$C_{27}H_{56}O$	396
29	1-Henicosanol	32.64	0.36	$C_{21}H_{44}O$	312
30	1, 3, 5- Trisilacyclohexane	33.42	0.26	$C_3H_{12}Si_3$	132
31	Octadecanal	33.87	0.5	$C_{18}H_{36}O$	268
32	1, 2-Benzenedicarboxylic acid	34.06	0.62	$C_{24}H_{38}O_4$	390
33	Eicosanoic acid, 2-(acetyloxy)-1-[(acetyloxy)methyl] ethyl ester	34.6	0.9	$C_{27}H_{50}O_6$	470
34	1,3-Dioxolane, 4-[(2-Methoxy-4-Hexadecenyl)	34.95	0.14	$C_{23}H_{44}O_4$	384
35	Heneicosane	35.31	0.16	$C_{21}H_{44}$	296
36	14-Beta-H-Pregna	35.74	0.19	$C_{21}H_{36}$	288
37	1-(3,4-dimethoxybenzyl)-6,7-Dimethoxy-2-Meth	35.95	0.44	$C_{21}H_{27}NO_4$	357
38	E, Z-1, 3, 12-Nonadecatriene	36.39	0.62	$C_{19}H_{34}$	262
39	Methyl (Z)-5, 11, 14, 17-Eicosatetraenoate	36.51	0.62	$C_{21}H_{34}O_2$	318
40	Tetracontane	37.61	2.12	$C_{40}H_{82}$	562
41	2-Pentatriacontanone	39.66	1.3	$C_{35}H_{70}O$	506
42	Protopine	40.29	0.59	$C_{20}H_{19}NO_5$	353
43	1, 54- Dibromo tetrapentacontane	41.1	1.35	$C_{54}H_{108}Br_2$	914
44	Stigmast-5-en-3-ol, (3.beta.)-	41.48	0.57	$C_{29}H_{50}O$	414
45	Vitamin E	42.05	0.61	$C_{29}H_{50}O_2$	430
46	Octacosyl acetate	43.54	0.48	$C_{30}H_{60}O_2$	452
47	Ergosta-5, 24-dien-3-ol, (3 beta)	44.39	0.22	$C_{28}H_{46}O$	398

48	Ergost-5-en-3-ol, (3 beta)	44.59	1.32	$C_{28}H_{46}O$	400
49	Octadecanoic acid, octadecyl ester	45.88	0.31	$C_{36}H_{72}O_2$	536
50	Stigmast-5-en-3-ol, (3.beta.)-	47.18	11.35	$C_{29}H_{50}O$	414
51	Cholest-5-en-3-ol, 24-propylidene-, (3 beta)	47.69	1.27	$C_{30}H_{50}O$	426
52	9, 19-Cyclocholeatan-3-ol, 14-methyl- (3 beta)	48.34	0.91	$C_{28}H_{48}O$	400
53	9, 19-Cyclolanost-24-en-3-ol (3 beta)	49.6	0.52	$C_{30}H_{50}O$	426
54	Stigmast-5-en-3-ol, oleate	51.71	3.01	$C_{47}H_{82}O_2$	678
55	2, 6, 10- Trimethyl, 14-Ethylene-14-Pentadecne	56.47	0.74	$C_{20}H_{38}$	278

Table 3: Phytocomponents identified in the ethyl acetate fraction of *Ajuga bracteosa* (Ab-EAE) by GC-MS.

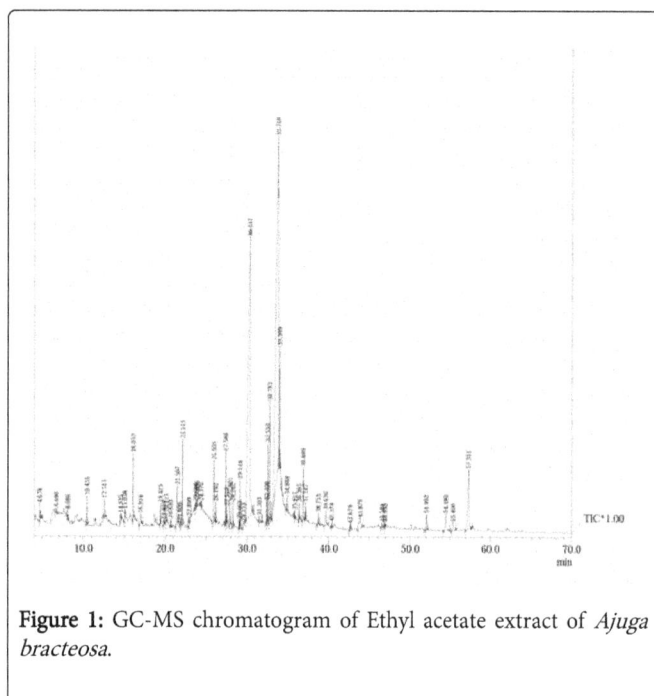

Figure 1: GC-MS chromatogram of Ethyl acetate extract of *Ajuga bracteosa*.

Group 2	Positive control (EMS)	1000	7.23 ± 0.89			0.05*
Group 3	Ab- EAE 100 mg/kg bw	1000	2.32 ± 0.08			
Group 4	Ab- EAE 400 mg/kg bw	1020	2.30 ± 0.05			
Group 5	Ab- EAE 100 mg/kg + EMS	1000	7.09 ± 0.76	98	2	
Group 6	Ab-EAE 200 mg/kg + EMS	1000	6.88 ± 0.54	95.1	4.9	0.05*
Group 7	Ab-EAE 300 mg/kg + EMS	1000	6.05 ± 0.45	83.6	16.4	0.05*
Group 8	Ab-EAE 400 mg/kg + EMS	1000	5.74 ± 0.35	79.3	20.7	0.05*

Micronucleus test

According to MN testing of mouse blood cells the low frequencies of micronucleated cells presumes the meagre effects of ethyl acetate extract of *Ajuga bracteosa* (Ab-EAE) 100 and 400 mg/kg (Table 4), there by indicating the virtual absence of mutagenic effect. In other words, nonstatistically significant difference in the frequency of MN polychromatic erythrocytes (PCE) or the ratio of PCE to normochromatic erythrocytes (NCE), between the negative control and thegroups that ingested extracts could be detected.

Table 4: Effects of Ethyl Acetate Extract of *Ajuga bracteosa* on MNPCE frequencies (mean ± SD) in mice, induced with ethyl methane sulfonate (EMS) 117.5 mg/kg bw (1/4th LD50). Ab-EAE = Ethyl Acetate extract of *Ajuga bracteosa*.

When evaluating antimutagenicity in Ab-EAE, a significant decrease in the frequency of EMS-induced MN PCE was observed only in mice that had received 100, 200, 300 and 400 mg/kg of Ab-EAE (p=0.05). In the present study, the ethyl acetate extract of *A. bracteosa* showed antimutagenic activities by reducing the % age of micronuclei with increase in the dose of the extract (Table 4 and Figure 2). The number of cells with micronuclei also decreased with increase in the dose of the extract i.e., from 100 mg/kgbw to 400 mg/kgbw (Figure 3).

	Treatment	Total No. of cells analysed per mice	No. of cells with micronuclei	% age of MN	% Reduction	P value
Group 1	Negative Control (Distilled water)	1000	2.35 ± 0.12			

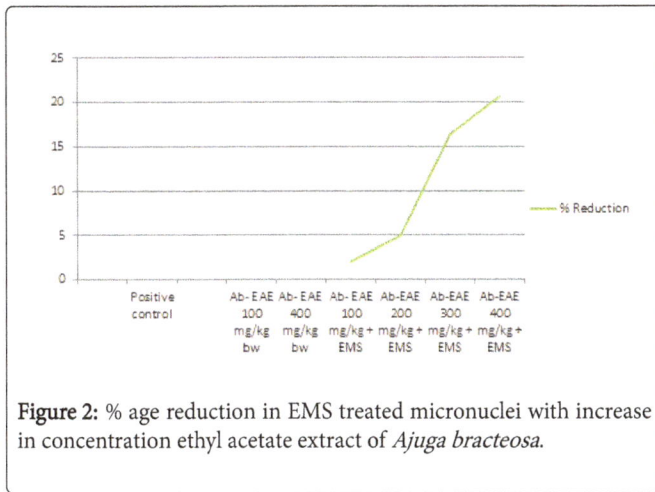

Figure 2: % age reduction in EMS treated micronuclei with increase in concentration ethyl acetate extract of *Ajuga bracteosa.*

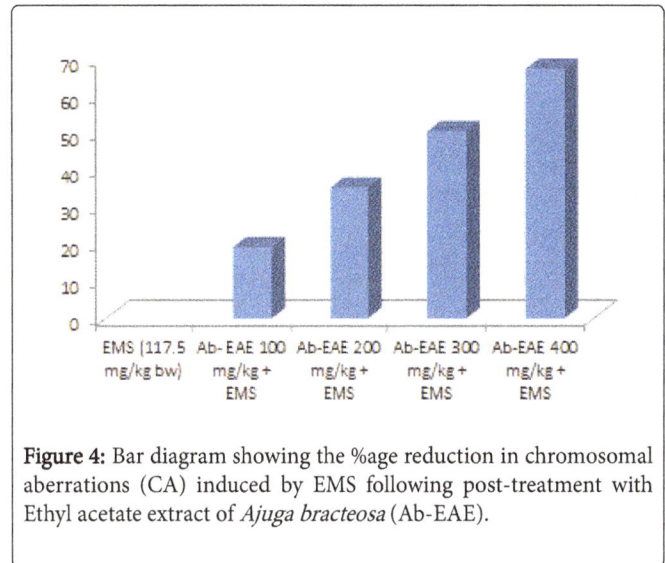

Figure 4: Bar diagram showing the %age reduction in chromosomal aberrations (CA) induced by EMS following post-treatment with Ethyl acetate extract of *Ajuga bracteosa* (Ab-EAE).

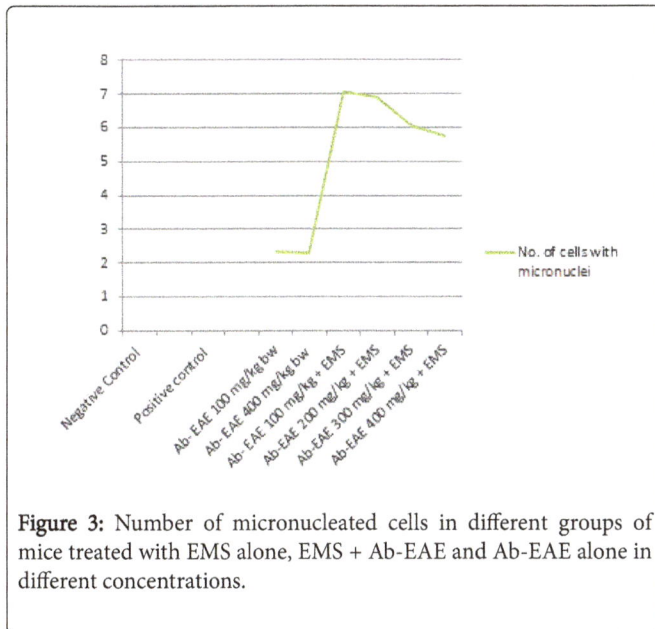

Figure 3: Number of micronucleated cells in different groups of mice treated with EMS alone, EMS + Ab-EAE and Ab-EAE alone in different concentrations.

Chromosomal aberration

Chromosomal aberration frequencies observed after various treatment schedules with EMS and different doses of Ab-EAE is shown in Table 5. The chromosomal aberrations decreased from 25.09% in EMS induced cells to 20.59%, 16.50%, 12.63% and 8.27% at 100, 200, 300 and 400 mg/kg bw of the ethyl acetate extract of *Ajuga bracteosa* (Figure 4). EMS produced predominantly breaks, gaps, fragments and exchanges.

Discussion

From ancient times, medicinal plants are being used as remedies for various diseases in humans. In today's industrialized society, the use of medicinal plants has been traced to the extraction and development of several drugs as they were used traditionally in folk medicine [24]. Medicinal plants have potent phytoconstituents which are important source of antibiotic compounds and are responsible for the therapeutic properties [25-32]. These phytoconstituents bestow them with medicinal properties [33,34]. The antioxidant properties, in many plants, are attributed to the presence of phenolic compounds. These phenolic compounds are known to possess various biological properties such as anti-apoptosis, anti-aging, anti-carcinogen, anti-inflammation, anti-atherosclerosis, cardiovascular protection and improvement of endothelial function, as well as inhibition of angiogenesis and cell proliferation activities [35]. Flavonoids are hydroxylated phenolic substances known to be synthesized by plants in response to microbial infection and they have been found to be antimicrobial substances against wide array of microorganisms *in vitro*. Their activity is probably due to their ability to complex with extracellular and soluble proteins and to complex with bacterial cell wall [36]. They are also effective antioxidants and show strong anticancer activities [37]. Tannins bind to proline rich protein and interfere with protein synthesis. Besides, most of the phytochemicals are known to have therapeutic properties such as insecticidals [38], antibacterial, antifungal [39] and anticonstipative [40] activities etc.

Treatments		Chromosomal Aberrations							
Concentration (mg/kgbw)	No. of cells	Rings	Fragments	Exchange	Breaks	Dicentrics	Gaps	Total Aberrations	%age of Aberrations
Distilled water	1004	2	6	-	15	-	-	23	2.29
EMS 117.5 mg/kg bw	1020	8	35	28	123	-	62	256	25.09
Ab-EAE Alone 100 mg/kg bw	1000	3	4	-	14	-	-	21	2.1

Ab-EAE Alone 400 mg/kg bw	1000	2	6	-	12	-	-	20	2
Ab-EAE 100 mg/kg bw + EMS	1005	8	32	24	102	3	38	207	20.59
Ab-EAE 200 mg/kg bw + EMS	1000	6	28	20	86	-	26	166	16.5
Ab-EAE 300 mg/kg bw+ EMS	1005	4	24	18	62	1	18	127	12.63
Ab-EAE 400 mg/kg bw + EMS	1015	2	18	14	38	-	12	84	8.27

Table 5: Frequency of Chromosomal aberrations observed after post-treatment with Ethyl Acetate extract of *Ajuga bracteosa* in EMS treated mouse bone marrow cells. Ab-EAE=Ethyl Acetate extract of *Ajuga bracteosa*.

The phytochemical screening of *Ajuga bracteosa* showed that their aerial parts were rich in saponins, alkaloids, phenol, tannins and Steroids. The presence of these phytochemicals in the tested plant indicates that this plant may be a good source for production of new drugs for various ailments. Saponins are known to produce inhibitory effect on inflammation [41]. They also have the property of precipitating and coagulating red blood cells. Some of the characteristics of saponins include formation of foams in aqueous solutions, hemolytic activity and cholesterol binding properties [42]. Steroids have been reported to possess antibacterial properties [43] and they are very important compounds especially due to their relationship with compounds such as sex hormones [44,45]. It has been reported that alkaloids possess analgesic [46], antispasmodic and antibacterial [47,48] properties. According to many reports, glycosides are known to show blood pressure lowering property [49]. Thus from the present study, it could be suggested that the identified phytoconstituents from *Ajuga bracteosa* make the plant valuable for bioactive compounds of sustainable medicine.

Important sources of new bioactive agents are the natural products. These natural products are obtained from medicinal herbs which are not only being used world-wide for the treatment of various diseases but also have a great potential for providing novel drug leads with novel mechanism of action [50]. The majority of higher plants contain a number of agents or phytoconstituents that are capable of causing mitigating effects to a number of mutagens [51]. The phytoconstituents from Terminalia arjuna suppressed the mutagenic effect of the aromatic amine, i.e., 2-aminofluorene (2-AF). The observed activity caused the inhibition of the metabolic activation of pro-mutagens [52]. It was also found that the extracts of Acanthopanax divaricatus were able to rapidly eliminate the mutagenic compounds from the cells before they induce the DNA damage [53]. In a similar study, it was observed that the methanol extracts of the lichens have antimutagenic effects against sodium azide [54]. The antimutagenic properties of plant extracts was also demonstrated against cyclophosphamide induced mutagenicity in mice [55]. The different extracts of Dioscorea pentaphylla were found to significantly inhibit the effects of methyl methanesulphonate (MMS) induced mutagenicity [56]. An edible wild plant, Tragopogon longirostis was also evaluated for antioxidant, mutagenic and antimutagenic properties and it was found that the ethanolic extract of its leaves exhibited antimutagenic properties at 2.5, 0.25, and 0.025 mg/plate concentrations [57]. The ethanolic extract of Origanum vulgare also reduced the frequency of MN PCR from 10.52

± 1.07 for CP to 2.17 ± 0.6 for the synergic test of CP and the ethanolic extract [58].

Conclusion

The medicinal plants are the source of the secondary metabolites i.e., alkaloids, flavonoids, terpenoids, phlobatannins and reducing sugars. Medicinal plants play a vital role in preventing various diseases. The presence of secondary metabolites in *Ajuga bracteosa* bestow it with different biological properties like antidiuretic, anti-inflammatory, antianalgesic, anticancer, anti-viral, antimalarial, antibacterial and anti-fungal. Thus, *Ajuga bracteosa* can be used for discovering and screening of the phytochemical constituents which are very helpful for the manufacturing of new drugs. Thus we hope that the important phytochemical properties identified in this study in the local plant of Kashmir Himalaya will be helpful in copping different diseases of this particular region.

Acknowledgements

The authors are highly thankful to the Director, Centre of Research for Development, University of Kashmir for providing the necessary facilities for the smooth research and also to Curator, Centre of Biodiversity and Plant Taxonomy, Department of Botany, University of Kashmir, Srinagar, J & K in proper identification of the plant. The authors are also thankful to Dr Ajai Kumar, Incharge GC-MS Facility, Advanced Instrumentation Research Facility (AIRF), Jawaharlal Nehru University, New Delhi for GC-MS analysis.

References

1. Bharat G, Parabia MH (2010) Pharmacognostic Evaluation of Bark and Seeds of Mimusops elengi. International Journal of Pharmacy and Pharmaceutical Sciences 2:110-113.

2. Nostro A, Germano MP, Dangelo V, Marino A, Cannatelli MA (2000) Extraction methods and bioautography for evaluation of medicinal plant antimicrobial activity. Lett Appl Microbiol 30: 379-384.

3. Rao ML, Savithramma N (2012) Quantification of primary and secondary metabolites of Svensonia hyderobadensis-A rare medicinal plant. International Journal of Pharmacy and Pharmaceutical Sciences 4: 519-521.

4. Choudhary S, Singh B, Vijayvergia TR, Singh T (2013) Preliminary phytochemical screening and primary metabolites of Melothria maderaspatana (Linn.) cong. International Journal of Biological and Pharmaceutical Research 4: 168-171.

5. Krishnaiah D, Sarbatly R, Bono A (2007) Phytochemical antioxidants for health and medicine: A move towards nature. Biotechnology and Molecular Biology Reviews 1: 97-104.

6. Mahato SB, Sen S (1997) Advances in triterpenoid research, 1990-1994. Phytochemistry 44: 1185-1236.

7. Hérouart D, Sangwan RS, Fliniaux MA, Sangwan-Norreel BS (1988) Variations in the Leaf Alkaloid Content of Androgenic Diploid Plants of Datura innoxia. Planta Med 54: 14-17.

8. Kumbhar RR, Godghate AG (2015) Physicochemical and quantitative phytochemical analysis of some medicinal plants in and around Gadhinglaj. International Journal of Science Environment and Technology 4: 172-177.

9. Pereira RP, Fachineto R, Prestes AS, Puntel RL, Boschetti TK, et al. (2009) Antioxidant effects of different extracts from Melissa officinalis, Matricaria recutita and Cymbopogon citratus. Neurochem Res 34: 973-983.

10. Kwak Y, Ju J (2015) Inhibitory activities of Perilla frutescens britton leaf extract against the growth, migration, and adhesion of human cancer cells. Nutr Res Pract 9: 11-16.

11. Liu HX, He MT, Tan HB, Gu W, Yang SX, et al. (2015) Xanthine oxidase inhibitors isolated from Piper nudibaccatum. Phytochemistry Letters 12: 133-137.

12. Dutt HC, Bhagat N, Pandita S (2015) Oral traditional knowledge on medicinal plants in jeopardy among Gaddi shepherds in hills of northwestern Himalaya, J&K, India. J Ethnopharmacol 168: 337-348.

13. Berhow MA, Wagner ED, Vaughn SF, Plewa MJ (2000) Characterization and antimutagenic activity of soybean saponins. Mutat Res 448: 11-22.

14. Hernandez-Ceruelos A, Madrigal-Bujaidadar E, De La Cruz C (2002) Inhibitory affect of chamomile essential oil on the sister chromatid exchanges by daunorubicin and methyl methanesulfonate in mouse bone marrow. Toxicol Lett 135: 103-110.

15. de Sousa AC, Alviano DS, Blank AF, Alves PB, Alviano CS, et al. (2004) Melissa officinalis L. essential oil: antitumoral and antioxidant activities. J Pharm Pharmacol 56: 677-681.

16. Chauhan NS (1999) Medicinal and aromatic plants of Himachal Pradesh Indus publishing company New Delhi 500.

17. Upadhyay SU, Patel VB, Patel AA, Upadhyay UL, Patel NM (2011) Ajuga bracteosa- A promising herb. Pharma science monitor - An international Journal of Pharmaceutical Sciences 2080-2088.

18. Khare CP (2007) Indian Medicinal Plants - An Illustrated Dictionary. 1st Indian Reprint Springer (India) Pvt. Ltd., New Delhi 28.

19. Chandel S, Bagai U (2010) Antiplasmodial activity of Ajuga bracteosa against Plasmodium berghei infected BALB/c mice. Indian J Med Res 131: 440-444.

20. Sofowora AE (1993) Medicinal Plants and Traditional Medicines in Africa. 2nd edition. Spectrum Books, Ibadan, Nigeria. p. 289.

21. Trease GE, Evans WC (1989) Trease and Evans' Pharmacognosy. 13th Edn., Bailliere Tindall, London, UK., ISBN-13: 9780702013577, Pages: 832.

22. Harborne JB (1973) Phytochemical Methods. Chapman and Hall Ltd., London, UK. pp: 49-188.

23. Okwu DE (2004) Phytochemicals and vitamin content of indigenous species of southeastern Nigeria. Journal of Sustainable Agriculture and the Environment 6: 30-37.

24. Shrikumar S, Ravi TK (2007) Approaches towards development and promotion of herbal drugs. Pharmacognosy 1: 180-184.

25. Jeeva S, Johnson M, Aparna JS, Irudayaraj V (2011) Preliminary phytochemical and antibacterial studies on flowers of selected medicinal plants. Int J Med Arom Plants 1: 107-114.

26. Jeeva S, Johnson M (2012) Antibacterial and phytochemical studies on Begonia flaccifera Bedd. flower. Asian Pacific Journal of Tropical Biomedicine 1: 151-154.

27. Florence AR, Joselin J, Jeeva (2012) Intraspecific variation of bioactive principles in select members of the genus Clerodendrum L. Journal of Chemical and Pharmaceutical Research 11. 4908- 4914.

28. Florence AR, Joselin J, Brintha TSS, Sukumaran S, Jeeva S (2014) Preliminary phytochemical studies of select members of the family Annonaceae for bioactive constituents. Bioscience discovery 5: 85-96.

29. Joselin J, Brintha TSS, Florence AR, Jeeva S (2012) Screening of select ornamental flowers of the family Apocyanaceae for phytochemical constituents. Asian Pacific Journal of Tropical Disease 2: 260-264.

30. Joselin J, Brintha TSS, Florence AR, Jeeva S (2013) Phytochemical evaluation of Bignoniaceae flowers. Journal of Chemical and Pharmaceutical Research 5: 106-111.

31. Sainkhediya J, Ray S (2012) Preliminary study of flowering plant diversity of Nimar region. Bioscience Discovery 3: 70-72.

32. Sumathi BM, Uthayakumari F (2014) GC MS analysis of Leaves of Jatropha maheswarii Subram & Nayar. Science Research Reporter 4: 24-30.

33. Brown JE, Rice-Evans CA (1998) Luteolin-rich artichoke extract protects low density lipoprotein from oxidation in vitro. Free Radic Res 29: 247-255.

34. Krings U, Berger RG (2001) Antioxidant activity of roasted foods. Food Chemistry 72: 223-229.

35. Han X, Shen T, Lou H (2007) Dietry polyphenols and their biological significance. Int J Mol Sci 8: 950-988.

36. Marjorie C (1999) Plant products as antimicrobial agents. Clin Microbiol Rev 12: 564-582.

37. Del-Rio A, Obdululio BG, Casfillo J, Main FG, Ortuno A (1997) Uses and properties of citrus flavonoids. Journal of Agriculture and Food Chemistry 45: 4505-4515.

38. Kambu K, Di Phenzu N, Coune C, Wauter JN, Angenot L (1982) Plants Medicine ET. Phytotherapie 34.

39. Lemos TLG, Matos FJA, Alencar JW, Crareiro AA, Clark AM, et al. (1990) Antimicrobial activity of essential oils of Brazilian plants. Phytotherapy Research 4: 82-84.

40. Ferdous AJ, Islam SM, Ahsan M, Hassan CM, Ahmad ZV (1992) In vitro antibacterial activity of the volatile oil of Nigella sativa seeds against multiple drugresistant isolates of Shigella spp. and isolates of Vibrio cholerae and Escherichia coli. Phytotherapy Research 6: 137-140.

41. Just MJ, Recio MC, Giner RM, Cuéllar MJ, Máñez S, et al. (1998) Anti-inflammatory activity of unusual lupane saponins from Bupleurum fruticescens. Planta Med 64: 404-407.

42. Sodipo OA, Akiniyi JA, Ogunbamosu JU (2000) Studies on certain on certain characteristics of extracts of bark of Pansinystalia macruceras (K schemp) picrre Exbeille. Global Journal of Pure and Applied Sciences 6: 83-87.

43. Epand RF, Savage PB, Epand RM (2007) Bacterial lipid composition and the antimicrobial efficacy of cationic steroid compounds (Ceragenins). Biochim Biophys Acta 1768: 2500-2509.

44. Okwu DE (2001) Evaluation of chemical composition of medicinal plants belonging to Euphorbiaceae. Pakistan Veterinary Journal 14: 160-162.

45. Nobori T, Miura K, Wu DJ, Lois A, Takabayashi K, et al. (1994) Deletions of the cyclin-dependent kinase-4 inhibitor gene in multiple human cancers. Nature 368: 753-756.

46. Antherden LM (1969) Textbook Of Pharmaceutical Chemistry. 8th edn., Oxford University Press, London, pp. 813-814.

47. Stray F (1998) The Natural Guide to Medicinal herbs And Plants. Tiger Books International, London, pp. 12-16.

48. Okwu DE, Okwu ME (2004) Chemical composition of Spondias mombin linn. plant parts. Journal of Sustainable Agriculture and the Environment 6: 140-147.

49. Nyarko AA, Addy ME (1990) Effects of aqueous extract of Adenia cissampeloides on blood pressure and serum analyte of hypertensive patients. Phytotherapy Research 4: 25-28.

50. Dar SA, Ganai FA, Yousuf AR, Balkhi MU, Bhat TM, et al. (2013) Pharmacological and toxicological evaluation of Urtica dioica. Pharm Biol 51: 170-180.

51. Mitscher LA, Telikepalli H, McGhee F, Shankel DM (1996) Natural antimutagenic agents. Mutat Res 350: 143-152.

52. Kaur S, Kumar S, Kaur P, Chandel M (2010) Study of antimutagenic potential of phytoconstituents isolated from Terminalia arjuna in the Salmonella/microsome assay. Am J Biomed Sci 2: 164-177.

53. Hong CE, Cho MC, Jang HA, Lyu SY (2011) Mutagenicity and anti-mutagenicity of Acanthopanax divaricatus var. albeofructus. J Toxicol Sci 36: 661-668.

54. Nardemir G, Yanmis D, Alpsoy L, Gulluce M, Agar G, et al. (2013) Genotoxic, antigenotoxic and antioxidant properties of methanol extracts obtained from Peltigera horizontalis and Peltigera praetextata. Toxicol Ind Health 31: 602-613.

55. Durnova NA, Kurchatova MN (2015) [THE EFFECT OF PLANT EXTRACTS ON THE CYCLOPHOSPHAMIDE INDUCTION OF MICRONUCLEUS IN RED BLOOD CELLS OF OUTBRED WHITE MICE]. Tsitologiia 57: 452-458.

56. Prakash G, Hosetti BB, Dhananjaya BL (2014) Antimutagenic effect of dioscorea pentaphylla on genotoxic effect induced by methyl methanesulfonate in the Drosophila wing spot test. Toxicol Int 21: 258-263.

57. Sarac N (2015) Antioxidant, mutagenic, and antimutagenic activities of Tragopogon longirostis var. longirostis, an edible wild plant in Turkey. Indian J Pharmacol 47: 414-418.

58. Habibi E, Shokrzadeh M, Ahmadi A, Chabra A, Naghshvar F, et al. (2015) Genoprotective effects of Origanum vulgare ethanolic extract against cyclophosphamide-induced genotoxicity in mouse bone marrow cells. Pharm biol 53: 92-97.

13

How can Humans be Damaged from Sulfuric Acid?

Se Kwang Oh*, **Hee Jun Shin, Han You Lee and Hye Jin Chung**

Department of Emergency Medicine, College of Medicine, Soonchunhyang University, Korea

*****Corresponding authour:** Se Kwang Oh, Department of Emergency Medicine, College of Medicine, Soonchunhyang University, Korea, E-mail: 13744@hanmail.net

Abstract

Purpose: This study was conducted to identify the clinical characteristics associated with sulfuric acid injury evaluated in emergency department.

Method: This study was retrospective multicenter study with sulfuric acid injured patients who were visited in 3 emergency departments during 10 years in South Korea. Data were collected retrospectively from Jan 2006 to Dec 2015 on all sulfuric acid injuries presenting to the 3 emergency departments. Collected data were those of demographic, exposure site, injury mechanism, final diagnosis and hospital care.

Result: A total of 46 patients were enrolled. Most of the patients were male (88.5%). The face and eye were the most commonly injured body parts (53.4%) and most commonly injured mechanism was splashing injury (69.5%) in sulfuric acid burn patients. A total of 25 (54.3%) patients were identified as having lesions more than second degree burn.

Conclusion: sulfuric acid can cause severe burns to the skin. When working with sulfuric acid, have to wear acid proof protect clothing, goggle and glove. And it is need to pay close attention when working with sulfuric acid.

Keywords: Sulfuric acid; Chemical burns; Occupational injuries

Introduction

Sulfuric acid is a strong acidic compound in the state of viscous liquid that is colorless and odorless and has been used a lot for industrial and experimental purposes, for example manufacturing of phosphoric acid or fertilizer, petroleum industry, metal process, and battery manufacturing and even used at home for cleaning a drainpipe [1]. Also, it is used as a material for committing a terrorist act against others in addition to hydrochloric acid, because it causes fatal damages to human body as a strong acid. According to the researches that have been conducted so far, sulfuric acid, among various chemical substances that causes chemical damage is one of the causative agents that occupy the highest frequency following the hydrofluoric acid [2,3]. However, there are very few studies on major exposure mechanism of sulfuric acid damage, area of damage, and severity. Accordingly, this study was conducted to understand the exposure routes of sulfuric acid-damaged patients and the clinical features and contribute to the prevention and treatment of sulfuric acid damage later.

Material and method

Subjects and period

This study was conducted in patients who were injured by sulfuric acid among the chemical injury patients visited in Gumi Soonchunhyang university hospital, Bucheon Soonchunhyang university hospital and Ulsan university hospital emergency department, Korea, from Jan 2006 to Dec 2015 for 10 years.

Study method and contents

This study was done retrospectively by reviewing medical records and variables related to patients included age, gender, injured body part, mechanism of injury, diagnosis and disposition. We excluded from this study that compound chemical materials and unknown chemicals. Injured sites were classified and recorded as face, eye, hand, arm, leg, neck, trunk, respiratory system, digestive system and other body regions. And mechanism of injury was recorded as splash, explosion, contact, inhalation, ingestion and others. Additionally, diagnosis, hospitalization, discharge from hospital, and transfer of hospital were recorded after treatment in an emergency department.

Analytical methods

In statistical analysis, SPSS window 21.0 (SPSS Inc., Chicago, IL, USA) was used for data collect and continuous variable was indicated with mean (± standard deviation), and frequency and percentage were obtained for nominal variable and categorical variable.

Results

A total of 46 patients visited the 3 hospital emergency departments due to sulfuric acid injury during the study period. In gender, males (39 individuals: 84.7%) were more than females (7 individuals: 15.2%), average age was at 40.1 years, which suggested that those in their 40s (15 individuals: 32.6%) occupied the most, followed by those in their 30s (12: 26%), those in their 20s (9: 19.5%), those in their 50s (5: 10.8%), and those in their 60s (4: 8.6%) (Table 1). 22 patients were injured in two or more lesions and 24 patients were injured in one lesion. In injured site, face occupied the most at 22 individuals (30.9%)

among which, the number of those whose eyes were injured was 16 individuals (22.5%).

Characteristics	N (%)
No. of patients	
Gender	
Male	39 (84.7%)
Female	7 (15.2%)
AGE (years)	
<20	1 (2.1%)
20-29	9 (19.5%)
30-39	12 (26.0%)
40-49	15 (32.6%)
50-59	5 (10.8%)
>60	4 (8.6%)

Table 1: General characteristics of the patients.

To look at other injury sites, arm was injured in 10 individuals (14%), trunk in 6 (8.4%), leg in 5 (7.0%), hand in 4 (5.6%), respiratory system in 4 (5.6%), neck in 3 (4.2%) and digestive system in 1 (1.4%) (Table 2).

Exposure site	N (%)
Face	22 (30.9%)
Eye	16 (22.5%)
Arm	10 (14.0%)
Trunk	6 (8.4%)
Leg	5 (7.0%)
Hand	4 (5.6%)
Respiratory system	4 (5.6%)
Neck	3 (4.2%)
Digestive system	1 (1.4%)
Total	71

Table 2: Sulfuric acid exposure site.

In mechanism of injury, the number of those who injured from splash was 32 patients (69.5%), which occupied the most frequency, followed by explosion injury (9: 19.5%), direct contact (2: 4.3%), inhalation (2: 4.3%), and ingestion (1: 2.1%) (Table 3).

All patients injured sulfuric acid were unintentional injuries. In diagnosis for sulfuric acid injured patients, the number of those who had second degree chemical burn was 23 patients (37.7%), chemical conjunctivitis 18 patients (29.5%), first degree chemical burn 11 patients (18.0%), third degree chemical burn 2 patients (3.2%), and inhalation burn 2 patients (3.2%) (Table 4).

Injury Mechanism	N (%)
Splash	32 (69.5%)
Explosion	9 (19.5%)
Contact	2 (4.3%)
Inhalation	2 (4.3%)
Ingestion	1 (2.1%)
Total	46

Table 3: Classification of sulfuric acid exposure mechanism.

Diagnosis	N (%)
1st degree chemical burn	11 (18.0%)
2nd degree chemical burn	23 (37.7%)
3rd degree chemical burn	2 (3.2%)
Chemical conjuntivitis	18 (29.5%)
Chemical pneumonitis	2 (3.2%)
Etc.	5 (8.1%)
Total	61

Table 4: Diagnosis of sulfuric acid injured patients.

Disposition	Total (n=46)
Discharge from emergency room	28 (60.8%)
Admission	4 (8.6%)
Discharge against medical advice	5 (10.8%)
Transfer	9 (19.5%)

Table 5: Disposition of sulfuric acid injured patients.

Among the enrolled patients, the number of patients who discharged from hospital after treatment in an emergency department was 28 patients (60.8%), followed by 9 patients (19.5%) who were transferred to other hospitals, 5 patients (10.8%) who discharged against medical advice and 4 patients (8.6%) who were hospitalized in hospital (Table 5).

Discussion

About 25,000 chemical substances are commonly used for industrial or agricultural or household purposes and most of these materials may cause chemical damage [4]. Especially acidic or basic materials, among chemical substances are particularly harmful to human body and among which, sulfuric acid is one of the major materials that cause chemical burns due to acidity [5]. As a result of analyzing 2,930 accidents that were exposed to chemical substances and had occurred in Poland from 1999 to 2009, it was found that they were exposed to more than 200 chemical substances, and especially sulfuric acid, among non-flammable corrosive liquids occupied the second highest frequency following hydrochloric acid [3].

Shin et al. [2] analyzed the patients who were hospitalized to the emergency center for treating chemical damage occurred due to chemical accidents at industrial places for five years and reported that the high-frequency chemical damage-causing materials include hydrofluoric acid, compound chemicals, sulfuric acid, and magnesium in consecutive order. Sulfuric acid is one of the chemical materials that are the most commonly used. It is also used as basic raw material for chemical industry and further, used widely as material for fertilizers, explosives, and dyes. Sulfuric acid can cause severe damages to all areas of contact and if severe exposure occurs through breathing or ingestion, may cause systemic symptoms [6]. Sulfuric acid is a kind of strong acid, and if contacted with the skin, causes heat in tissues and coagulation necrosis, thus causing thrombosis in capillary and finally it may cause third-degree burns to the skin [7]. If contacted with the eye, it may cause blindness. Also, sulfuric acid is known to cause tissue damage by changing the pH in the areas of contact [8].

Chemical damage largely occurs during work. It is caused largely by chemical materials being splashed to the face or eye. And damage by sulfuric acid occurs a lot due to carelessness at workplaces or at home [9]. According to Bond et al. [10], at the places other than workplace, sulfuric burns occur the most while cleaning a pipeline.

In this study, splash injury caused by carelessness during work or experiment occupied the most and the major damaged areas are face and eye. Also, simple splash injury occupied most of the damage mechanism, and the patients who were damaged by second or higher-degree burns were observed as 25 patients in 46 in total and two patients were found to have third-degree burn, which indicates high severity. This is because if even a small amount of sulfuric acid touches the human body, it causes heat while reacting to the water in tissues, thus causing thermal burns. Also, even a low concentration of sulfuric acid may cause pain in the eye, increased secretion, and conjunctivitis and if highly concentrated sulfuric acid is splashed to the eye, may cause corneal burn, loss of eyesight, and even eyeball rupture [11,12].

Also, since skin burns caused by sulfuric acid often causes full-thickness skin burns accompanied with skin necrosis, skin incision or skin graft is often required [10]. Due to such characteristics, sulfuric acid is used a lot for deliberately damaging purposes against others as reported a lot in the recent press, and similar cases happened many times in foreign countries as well. According to the studies on 38 patients damaged by sulfuric acid that were carried out by Italian medical staffs in Bangladesh in 1998, 33 patients, who were females aged from 13 to 40 years and the major cause of damage was revenge or punishment between men and women, and face was the major area of damage and most of the patients underwent a surgical operation of skin expansion or flap or skin graft [13].

The inhalation of sulphur dioxide without direct contact with sulfuric acid may cause severe stimulus and caustic damage in the respiratory system and if sulfuric acid is inhaled in large amounts, it can be fatal due to pulmonary edema.

Benomran et al. [14] also reported on a 27-year-old male patient who died of bronchus by inhalation of sulphur dioxide occurred during sulfuric acid pipeline work and of severe pulmonary edema. Also in this study a 21-year-old male patient who suffered from chemical pneumonitis caused by inhalation of sulfuric acid was identified (Supplementary Table)

However, this study also has some limitations. This is a retrospective study that was based on the review of medical records. As it just relied on medical records to know a patient's clinical features and damage information, few can be known about the concentration of sulfuric acid and scope of damage. Moreover, the patients whose chemical substances that caused damages were not specified in medical records were excluded from the study. However, it is significant in that more various routes of sulfuric acid damage and extent of damage in many patients who are from three different areas can be known from this study. Most of the damages caused by sulfuric acid were due to careless splash injury during chemical substances-handling work and the areas of damage were largely face and eye, which occupied the highest frequency. In most cases, damages of second or higher-degree burn were observed and often hospital treatment was required. Sulfuric acid is one of the most common materials that cause chemical damage and may cause major burns and severe tissue damage. Therefore, close attention must be paid during sulfuric acid-transporting or handling work or experiment, and face shield, chemical goggle, and chemical glove also needs to be worn. And especially in an emergency department, if a sulfuric acid-damaged patient enters the hospital, skin and eye must be washed immediately by holding appropriate decontamination areas and equipment.

References

1. Moriarty TF (1979) Corrosive chemicals: acids and alkali. Drug Ther 3: 89.

2. Shin HJ, Oh SK, Yoo BD, Jun DH, Lee DH (2015) A Clinical Analysis of Patient Exposure to Sulfuric Acid Injured. J Korean Soc Clin Toxicol 13: 78-86.

3. Palaszewska-Tkacz A, Czerczak S, Konieczko K (2017) Chemical incidents resulted in hazardous substances releases in the context of human health hazards. Int J Occup Med Environ Health 21: 95-110.

4. Palao R, Monge I, Ruiz M, Barret JP (2010) Chemical burns: pathophysiology and treatment. Burns 36: 295-304.

5. Carlotto RC, Peters WJ, Neligan PC, Douglas LG, Beeston J (1996) Chemical burns. Can J Surg 39: 205-211.

6. Canadian Centre for Occupational Health and Safety (CCOSH). Sulfuric acid, Cheminfo.

7. Jelenko C 3rd (1974) Chemicals that 'burn'. J Trauma 14: 65-72.

8. Agency for Toxic Substances and Disease Registry (ATSDR) (1998) Toxicological Profile for Sulfuric Trioxide and Sulfuric Acid. US development of Health and Human Services. Atlanta, US.

9. Lusk PG (1999) Chemical eye injuries in the workplace. Prevention and management. AAOHN J 47: 80-7.

10. Bond SJ, Schnier GC, Sundine MJ, Maniscalco SP, Groff DB (1998) Cutaneous burns caused by sulfuric acid drain cleaner. J Trauma 44: 523-526.

11. National Library of Medicine (2016) Hazardous Substances Data Bank. Fact Sheet for sulfuric acid.

12. Jurkiewicz MJ (1990) Plastic surgery: principles and practice. Mosby, St Louis, USA, 1355-1410.

13. Faga A, Scevola D, Mezzetti MG, Scevola S (2000) Sulphuric acid burned women in Bangladesh: a social and medical problem. Burns 26: 701-709.

14. Benomran FA, Hassan AI, Masood SS (2008) Accidental fatal inhalation of sulfuric acid fumes. J Forensic Leg Med 15: 56-58.

14

Impurity Profiling of Street Methamphetamine Samples Seized in Kermanshah, Iran with Special Focus on Methamphetamine Impurities Health Hazards

Neda Amini[1], Afshar Etemadi-Aleagha[2] and Maryam Akhgari[3*]

[1]Department of Toxicology & Pharmacology, pharmacology & Toxicology Department, Faculty of pharmacy, Pharmaceutical Sciences Branch, Islamic Azad University (IAUPS), Iran

[2]Department of anesthesiology, Tehran University of Medical Sciences (TUMS), Amir Alam Hospital, Tehran, Iran

[3]Department Forensic Toxicology, Legal Medicine Research Center, Legal Medicine Organization, Tehran, Iran, *Corresponding author: Maryam Akhgari, Assistant professor of Forensic Toxicology, Department of Forensic Toxicology, Legal Medicine Research Center, Legal Medicine Organization, Tehran, Iran, Email: akhgari1349@yahoo.com

Abstract

Objective: Methamphetamine abuse remains a significant public health concern since its assent to peak popularity in Iran. Methamphetamine possesses one of the most domestic markets among other drugs of abuse in Kermanshah, Iran. Clandestine methamphetamine laboratories employ different methods and consequently a wide range of chemicals for the illicit production of methamphetamine. Yet there is limited information about active pharmaceutical ingredients in methamphetamine samples seized in Kermanshah, Iran. The current study aimed to identify active pharmaceutical ingredients and manufacturing by-products in methamphetamine samples seized in Kermanshah, Iran. As no organ in the body remains unscathed by methamphetamine and its impurities abuse, the other purpose of the present study was to discuss health effects associated with impure methamphetamine abuse in a brief review.

Methods: Analytical study was conducted on 53 methamphetamine samples using gas chromatography/mass spectrometry method. We reviewed the health outcomes of methamphetamine abuse and the evidences supporting pharmacological effects of methamphetamine impurities.

Results: Analysed methamphetamine samples contained methamphetamine, amphetamine, ecstasy, phenmetrazine, pseudoephedine, tramadol, benzaldehyde, acetic acid and other chemicals. Information has been discussed for common harmful effects of methamphetamine and its impurities abuse.

Conclusion: Illicit methamphetamine crystals contained different chemical impurities originated from manufacturing processes and active pharmaceutical ingredients deliberately added to them. The main prominent synthetic routes for methamphetamine synthesis are Leuckart and Nagai methods in Kermanshah, Iran. In addition to the chemical hazards present in methamphetamine laboratories, there are many hazards posed to anyone involved in direct and indirect contact with these contaminants.

Keywords: Methamphetamine; Illicit production; Forensic analysis; Impurity profiling; Methamphetamine impurity; Health hazards

Introduction

Methamphetamine (MA) was one of the most popular abused substances in the world during the past two decades. This highly addictive substance was introduced to Iranian drug black market in 2005 [1]. According to the United Nations Office on Drugs and Crime (UNODC) report, Iran ranked fifth behind Thailand in MA seizure between 2010-2012 [2]. Yearly increases in MA seizures reported by Iran's Drug Control Headquarters confirms that the availability of this substance is increasing [3]. Now, MA is the most common available amphetamine type stimulant (ATS) in Iran and its popularity is growing rapidly [4]. The growing demand for MA encourages drug makers to produce illicit forms of this substance in clandestine laboratories. These laboratories were discovered in Iran since 2008 [2]. Illegal manufacture of MA is an imperfect procedure resulting in the production of a chemical containing substantial amounts of impurities called Shesheh/Shishe (glass), Shabu, Dar Va Panjereh, Gach, Lachaki,

Ice and Crystal in Iran [5]. There are many chemical procedures for MA synthesis including phosphorous-Iodine (Moscow, Nagai, Hypo), Birch, and metal hydrogenation (Emde), using ephedrine and pseudoephedrine as precursors, and Reductive Amination from phenyl-2-propanone (P2P) [6].

The preparation of prescribed drugs is well controlled and should have the minimum impurities, however the goal of illegal preparation of substances is to make money with the minimum cost. Use of illicit methods for production and lack of quality control can contribute to the low quality of street drugs [7].

Illicit manufacturing of MA produces a large amount of waste materials including heavy metals, volatile, flammable and corrosive chemicals. Furthermore many drugs are used to "cut" or adulterate MA samples. Impurities in MA samples may have pharmacological and toxicological properties similar or different from proposed synthesized substance [8,9]. The presence of other active pharmaceutical ingredients in illegal street substances in Iran is worrying since they can modify or intensify the signs and symptoms of intoxication and fatal drug overdose [10].

Street MA is an impure cocktail that contains synthetic intermediates, byproducts and active pharmaceutical ingredients deliberately added to it depending on the synthetic procedures used and the capabilities of procedures to purify the end product.

It is believed that MA abuse has many negative health consequences. First reports of serious adverse health effects of amphetamines began in 1935. Low dose administration of amphetamine inhaler caused flushing, palpitation and high blood pressure [11]. The world medical literature reported 43 methamphetamine-associated deaths in a 35-year interval before controlled substances act in 1970 [12].

There are some studies concerning impurity profiling of MA samples in Iran. Also MA is among the most abused substances in many provinces in Iran such as Kermanshah [13]. According to a report, Iran's anti-narcotic police forces had seized 800 kg of illicit drugs in a two week period in Kermanshah in 2014 [14]. Thus MA abuse is one of the most social problems in Kermanshah, Iran. Authorities' attention is focusing more and more on the growing issue of MA abuse-associated health hazards in Iran, however information concerning the pharmacology of the MA impurities is very limited.

The main goal of the present study was to characterize impurities in MA samples seized in Kermanshah, Iran and also to discuss MA impurities health hazards in more details.

Materials and Methods

All chemicals and solvents were of analytical reagent grade obtained from Merck (Darmstadt, Germany). Standards for drugs were obtained from pharmaceutical companies, Tehran, Iran. Methamphetamine (MA) hydrochloride, amphetamine hydrochloride (AM), Methylenedioxymethamphetamine (MDMA) hydrochloride and pseudoephedrine hydrochloride were obtained from Lipomed Pharmaceutical (Arlesheim, Switzerland).

Qualitative and quantitative analyses were conducted on street MA samples. Included in the present study were 53 MA samples collected from anti-narcotic police seizures in Kermanshah, Iran during 30 December 2013 to 1 January 2015. Samples were referred to forensic toxicology laboratory, Kermanshah, Iran for systematic toxicological analysis using gas chromatography/mass spectrometry (GC/MS) method.

Laboratory analyses of samples were as follows:

Sample preparation

Five grams of MA samples were weighed out from each seizure. Samples were crushed well to a fine powder. Fifty milligrams of each sample was mixed in 1 mL of phosphate buffer solution (pH=10 and 0.1 M) and vortexed for 5 min. Each sample was mixed with 500 µL of ethyl acetate and vortexed for 10 min. The mixture was centrifuged for 5 min at 3000 rpm. Aqueous phase was frozen in a cooling bath and the organic phase (ethyl acetate) was separated for subsequent analysis. Inert substances, bulking agents and herbal constituents were not tested due to little interest in this study context.

Methanol (100 µL) was added to residues, and after mixing, 0.2 µL of sample was injected into GC/MS. All of the samples were analysed qualitatively, except for methamphetamine, amphetamine and

methylenedioxymethamphetamine. These three ingredients were analysed quantitatively. The linearity of the method was evaluated at five concentration levels ranging from 30-1500 ng/mL (y=5.54x10^{-2} X +1.8 × 10^{-1}) with r^2=0.9910 for MA, concentration levels ranging from 30-1500 ng/mL (y=3.171 x 10^{-4} X+2.33 × 10^{-3}) with r^2=0.9954 for AM and concentration levels ranging from 40-1500 ng/mL (y=1.09 × 10^{-2} χ + 1.574 × 10^{-1}) with r^2=0.9999 for MDMA. Limit of detection (LOD) was 10 ng/mL for all three analytes. Limit of quantitation (LOQ) was 30 ng/mL for MA and AM and 40 ng/mL for MDMA.

Gas chromatography/mass spectrometry (GC/MS) technique

GC/MS had been used as the mainstay of pharmaceutical analysis. An Agilent model 7890A gas chromatograph (Agilent Technologies, Sdn Bhd, Selangor, Malaysia) fitted with split/splitless injector and a HP5-MS capillary column (cross-linked 5% methyl phenyl silicone, 30 m length × 0.25 mm ID × 0.25 µm film thickness) was used. The capillary column was connected to a mass analyzer (MS 5975C) (Agilent Technologies) operated by electron impact (70 eV) in full scan mode (50-550 m/z). NIST, Wiley and MPW 2011 libraries were used for identification of precursors, intermediates, final products and active pharmaceutical ingredients.

Results

To detect pharmaceutical and non-pharmaceutical ingredients, precursors, intermediates and synthetic by-products in methamphetamine samples in Kermanshah, Iran, we analysed 53 MA samples using GC/MS technique. All of the samples were white crystals with different crystal shapes and sizes. GC/MS analysis showed that all of the samples contained MA and five of them contained amphetamine. The most frequent impurity in MA samples was phenyl-2-propanone followed by phenmetrazine and pseudoephedrine. Figure 1 shows the GC/MS chromatogram of one impure methamphetamine sample. Other impurities, frequency of their occurrence in seized samples and the reason for their presence are shown in Table 1. Quantitative analysis of samples showed that the range of MA, AM and MDMA contents in street MA samples was 15-33%, 9-11% and 2-4% respectively. It is important to say that not all impurities were present in all samples.

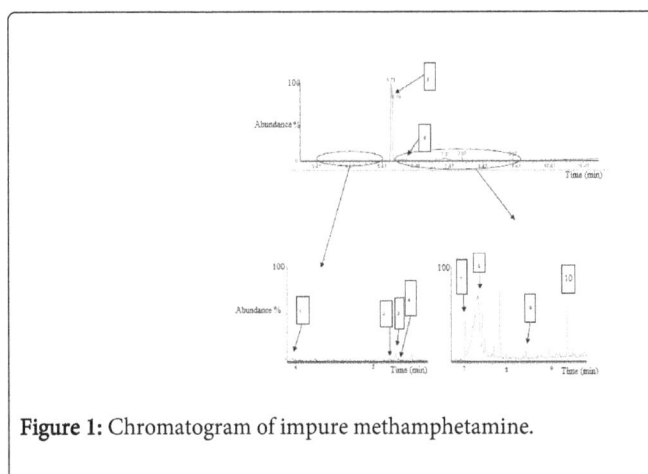

Figure 1: Chromatogram of impure methamphetamine.

Discussion

The purpose of the present study was to characterize the impurities in MA samples seized in Kermanshah, Iran. Furthermore this study discusses health consequences associated with direct and indirect contact with MA and its impurities.

According to the results of the study, all of the samples were in white crystalline form. This result was in agreement with those of Khajeamiri et al. [15]. Our study demonstrated that MA samples contained various types of precursors, intermediates, active pharmaceutical ingredients and other illicit drugs in combination with MA and AM. A wide variety of reagents and precursors are used in the production of ATS [6].

Acetic acid was detected in about 90% of samples. Acetic acid is used in the manufacture of MA using P2P as starting reagent [16]. Also acetates, such as acetic acid or lead acetate are used in cooking processes to precipitate MA as final product [17,18].

Potential reason for presence as impurity or additive	Frequency of occurrence No (%)	Impurity found
Used in the production of MA using P2P	50 (94.34)	Acetic acid
Intermediate reagent in the production of MA by the Leuckart or reductive amination methods	25 (47.17)	Phenyl-2-propanone
Conversion of ephedrine to phenmetrazine at GC high temperature	11 (20.75)	Phenmetrazine
Cutting agent in the production of ATS	10 (18.87)	N,N-Dimethylamphetamine
Indicative of Leuckart route used for MA production		
Used as precursor in MA synthesis	10 (18.87)	Pseudoephedrine
An intermediate in MA synthesis procedure from ephedrine and pseudoephedrine by Emde and Nagai methods	9 (16.98)	1,2-dimethyl-3-phenylaziridine
Starting material in the synthesis of	5 (9.43)	Benzaldehyde
P2P		
Deliberately added active pharmaceutical ingredient	5 (9.43)	Tramadol
Product of Nagai method, product of MA precipitation using acetic moiety	3 (5.67)	N-acetylmethamphetamine
Overlapping with areas of MA synthesis	2 (3.77)	Ecstasy
Produced as incomplete hydrolysis of MA in Leuckart reaction	1 (1.89)	N-Formylmethamphetamine
An intermediate in MA synthesis procedure from ephedrine and pseudoephedrine by Emde and Nagai methods	1 (1.89)	N-Benzyl 2-methylaziridine
ATS= Amphetamine-Type Stimulants; MA= Methamphetamine; P2P= Phenyl-2-Propanone		

Table 1: Impurities, frequency of their occurrence and the reason for their presence in seized methamphetamine samples, Kermanshah, Iran.

More than 20% of samples showed positive results for phenmetrazine. Ephedrine may be converted to phenmetrazine in the presence of formaldehyde contaminated solvents. According to the United Nations (UN) Convention of Psychotropic Substances, 1971 phenmetrazine is a controlled substance and can be abused for its mood elevating property [19]. This can be one of the reasons for adding this substance to MA samples.

Pseudoephedrine or ephedrine is used as precursors for illicit MA production. It can be used in its pure form or extracted from medicines called sympathomimetic decongestants used as cold or flu drugs [20].

The presence of N-formylmethamphetamine, P2P and benzaldehyde in seized MA samples supports more evidence for the use of Leuckart method as one of the most routine ways for the production of MA in Kermanshah, Iran.

About 18% of studied samples contained N,N-dimethylamphetamine (DMA). DMA is a cutting agent or adulterant added to MA or other ATS [11]. Li et al., 2006 reported that DMA is the products of pyrolysis at high temperatures using GC/MS analysis method [21].

The presence of benzaldehyde in about 10% of samples suggests that it was used as starting material for the production of P2P, which is converted to MA in Leuckart method [15].

Aziridine derivatives were detected in 17% of analysed samples. This is possibly due to the involvement of Nagai method for the production of MA [22].

N-acetyl methamphetamine was found in about 6% of samples. This substance is the product of the reaction of MA with ethylacetate. Precipitating of MA in acidic condition in the presence of acetates as solvent yields N-acetylmethamphetamine [14]. It can be produced from thermal decomposition of an unknown compound in the injection port of gas chromatography instrumentation too [23].

The origin of some of the impurities in MA samples in the present study is obscure. Tramadol was detected in about 10% of samples. To our knowledge this is the first report indicating the presence of tramadol in illicit MA samples. Tramadol has different chemical structure in comparison to ATSs and cannot be categorized as synthetic by-products. One possible explanation for the detection of other illicit drugs in MA samples is the common preparation places for these substances or adding them to MA samples deliberately.

There are reports from clinical toxicology and poison centers in Iran indicating increasing in the frequency of MA abuse [24]. Addiction to ATS is a serious public health problem with many negative consequences and complications [25]. Methamphetamine abuse can result in many direct and indirect health effects. They can be categorized as follows:

Adverse health consequences related to direct exposure to methamphetamine and its impurities

Neurologic side effects: Methamphetamine has lipophilic structure and can distribute in CNS following different routes of administration [26]. Methamphetamine abuse has terrible neurologic consequences. Chronic use of MA causes elevations of dopamine, serotonin and other monoamines. Mounting in dopamine level can change the function of central nervous system (CNS) which manifests as a range of neurologic disorders [27]. Intracranial hemorrhage is associated with methamphetamine-induced hypertension and tachycardia [28]. Basal ganglia and brainstem bleeding as well as ischemic stroke were reported in MA abusers [29,30]. Seizure, memory loss, aggression and impairment in attention, cognition, decision making and psychosis are other neurologic effects of MA abuse [31,32]. Chronic MA abuse causes toxic psychosis characterized by visual, auditory and tactile sensory hallucinations [33]. Methamphetamine toxicity has neuroimmune basis. Exposure to MA can affect adaptive and innate immunity; it can inhibit cascades of events which can alter cellular or behavior functions. High dose or repeated MA exposure alters the function of glial cells causing neuroinflammation, neural damage and behavioral impairments [34].

MA increases metabolism in the CNS and skeletal muscles resulting in an elevation in the brain and body temperature. This substance dysregulates body temperature and promotes heat generation and retention in the body by suppressing the mechanisms which facilitate temperature reduction, hence producing hyperthermia which can be fatal in untreated cases [35].

Phenmetrazine causes CNS stimulation, cardiotoxicity causing tachycardia, arrhythmias, hypertension and cardiovascular collapse. Myocardial ischemia, ventricular dysfunction and infarction can occur in sever poisoning [36].

N,N-dimethylamphetamine induces degeneration of nerve terminals in the mouse striatum. It has dopamine depleting effects [37].

Pseudoephedrine has CNS stimulant properties and can produce agitation, anxiety, restlessness, weakness and irritability. High doses cause severe sweating, fever, heart failure and asphyxiation leading to death [38].

When pseudoephedrine is used as precursors in MA synthesis, chloroephedrine is formed as an intermediate. This intermediate has sympathomimetic property and induces heart rate and mean arterial pressure increase in rats [39].

Ecstasy acts as a hallucinogenic amphetamine. It shows sympathomimetic responses like amphetamine. At high doses ecstasy induces severe hyperthermia. Fatal dysrhythmias, ventricular

fibrillation, asystole, rhabdomyolysis, hepatotoxicity, acute renal failure, subarachnoid hemorrhage, cerebral infarction and intracranial bleeding have been reported following ecstasy use. Chronic use of ecstasy may cause prominent damage to the serotonergic axons and nerve terminals [40].

Combination of different types of drugs as drug cocktails may be prepared to get an enhanced effect. Combination of MA and opioid drugs such as tramadol can be dangerous. Coadministration of tramadol and CNS stimulants such as MA increases the risk of seizure [41]. Tramadol inhibits the reuptake of serotonin in nerve terminals [42]. A build up of serotonin content can occur as a result of combined action tramadol and other serotonin reuptake inhibitors such as MA [43]. Serotonin toxicity has many health effects including hyperthermia, hypertension, tremor, diarrhea and confusion [44,45].

MA and ecstasy combination may have greater acute effects such as rhabdomyolysis and cardiac disease in comparison to the equivalent doses of each substance alone [46]. Detection of tramadol and ecstasy in MA samples seized in Kermanshah is an important issue to take into consideration that this cocktail can have negative health consequences for abusers. Diluents and adulterants such as talc can cause ischemia or hemorrhagic stroke after intravenous administration [30].

Acute lead poisoning was reported as a result of lead-contaminated MA abuse [32]. Abdominal pain, muscle weakness, seizure, coma and CNS damage are common side effects of lead poisoning [17].

α-Benzyl-N-methylphenethylamine (BNMPA) is an impurity of illicit MA with convulsant activity in experimental studies. This impurity exerts its convulsant activity through similar mechanism with MA and is a toxic substance for CNS [12].

Cardiovascular side effects: Chest pain, acute coronary syndrome, hypertension, tachycardia, cardiac dysrhythmia, cardiomyopathy, aortic dissection and myocardial toxicity due to the overstimulation of cardiac adrenergic receptors, endocarditis, myocardial ischemia and damage to the blood vessels of the brain were reported in MA abusers [11,47,48].

Cutaneous and soft tissue effects: Skin and soft tissue infections are common dermatologic effects of MA abuse. Formication is an abnormal skin sensation known as delusional paresthesias, similar to that of crawling of insects on or under the skin. Dehydration, sweating and escape of toxic wastes create a sensation on the nerve endings called formication. This phenomenon causes MA user to pick his/her skin obsessively with fingernails making open red sores (crank bug), most commonly on the face and arms. Skin sores may be infected by staph bacteria and if left untreated can cause dangerous sepsis or deeper abscess [49].

Acetic acid is very hazardous in case of skin, eye contact or inhalation and ingestion. It may be toxic (irritant and corrosive) to kidneys, mucous membranes and teeth. Respiratory tract irritation and bronchial infection are other health consequences of acetic acid inhalation [50]. P2P may be toxic to mucous membranes and upper respiratory tract and can cause eye, skin or respiratory system irritation [51].

Dental and oral cavity side effects: Teeth damage is caused by MA and its impurities due to their acidic or basic pH [7]. Many factors contribute to the production of "meth-mouth" including reduction of salivary flow as a result of indirect sympathomimetic activity of MA xerostomia, bruxism, consumption of soft drinks instead of water and poor oral hygiene. Also MA abusers suffer from broken or loose, blackened or stained teeth and gingivial inflammation [52,53].

Musculoskeletal side effects: Bone remodeling is under the control of the central nervous system. Also bone metabolism may alter as a result of CNS and hypothalamus stimulation by MA [54].

Bone mineral loss, bone fracture and osteoporosis due to MA abuse were reported in previous studies [55,56]. Kim et al. (2009) in a study conducted on 46 hospitalized male MA abusers found that the mean bone marrow density value was lower in MA abusers in comparison to control group [56]. Katsuragawa (1999) studied the effect of MA on the quality of calcaneus bone. Results showed that MA causes chronic effects on the metabolism of human skeletal system [55]. Luo et al. (2015) indicated that some essential elements such as magnesium and calcium deficiency can be connected with osteoporosis in persons who abuse MA [57].

Other side effects: Phosphine is a respiratory poison. It inhibits cellular respiration and results in multi-organ damage and death [58]. Phosphine gas is produced as a potentially toxic by-product during the production of MA by the hydroiodic acid/red phosphorous method [59]. There are case reports of accidental inhalation of phosphine in illicit MA production processes [60]. Chemicals and reagents such as phosphine in clandestine MA laboratories may be hazardous for law enforcement personnel during investigation of these MA cooking places [61].

Benzaldehyde is used as starting material in the production of P2P which is converted to MA in Leuckart method [16]. Chronic exposure to benzaldehyde may cause mutation [62].

Aziridine derivatives (1,2-dimethyl-3-phenylaziridine and N-Benzyl 2-methylaziridine) are produced as by-product in the manufacturing process of MA. Aziridines show their mutagenicity by electrophilic attack on DNA [63].

Adverse health consequences related to indirect exposure to methamphetamine and its impurities

Production of illicit drugs is associated with acute and chronic health consequences not only for persons with direct contact but also for those who live near secret laboratories. [17,60]. Hazardous chemicals enter the environment and surface waters as contaminants and can be harmful to ecosystem by producing adverse physiological and toxic effects [64,65].

MA surface residues may have potential health effects. MA has low vapor pressure and remains on surfaces for a long time. Exposure to these contaminants through oral or dermal contact is of great importance to the environment contamination especially for young children exposed to re-emitted MA from surfaces [66]. "Drug endangered children" are described as children who are exposed to MA manufacturing environmental contaminants as well as parental abuse [31].

In fact the following points should be emphasized; chronic abusers in whom tolerance to the drug has developed may use as much as 5000-15000 mg of methamphetamine per day [67] and consequently may consume MA impurities in relatively high quantities.

We recommend further studies on samples obtained from other provinces or different geographic areas in Iran to detect impurities of illicit MA. As illicit drug manufacturers use different methods and precursors for MA synthesis, it is important to perform continuous

analysis of illicit drugs and study the pharmacologic effects of their impurities. In addition, other added drugs and adulterants may change at different time intervals.

We should say that we have encountered some limitations to perform the present study. Sample collection from anti-narcotic police was very difficult due to the illegality of abused substances. One limitation to this study was that it was not possible to analyse all active pharmaceutical ingredients quantitatively. However, this limitation did not overshadow our main purpose.

Although substance abuse effects on the body vary depending on the composition and active pharmaceutical ingredients in addition to proposed drug, all poly substance abuse negatively impacts abusers' health. Also MA crystals profiling can give valuable information to develop proper detoxification therapeutic regimen in addiction treatment centers.

Acknowledgment

The authors would like to personnel of Legal Medicine Organization, Kermanshah, Iran and Dr. Farzaneh Jokar and Dr. Karim Ebrahim Najaf Abadi for cooperation during this study. The authors declare that there is no conflict of interests.

References

1. United Nations Office on Drugs and Crime (UNODC) (2007) World Drug Report. United Nations Publication, Vienna.

2. United Nations Office on Drugs and Crime (UNODC) (2014) Global Synthetic Drugs Assessment - Amphetamine-type stimulants and new psychoactive substances. United Nations Publication, Vienna.

3. United Nations Office on Drugs and Crime (UNODC) (2009) World Drug Report. United Nations Publication, Vienna.

4. Alam Mehrjerdi Z, Barr AM, Noroozi A (2013) Methamphetamine-associated psychosis: a new health challenge in Iran. Daru 21: 30.

5. Alam Mehrjerdi Z (2013) Crystal in Iran: methamphetamine or heroin kerack. Daru 21: 22.

6. Stojanovska N, Fu S, Tahtouh M, Kelly T, Beavis A, et al. (2013) A review of impurity profiling and synthetic route of manufacture of methylamphetamine, 3,4-ethylenedioxymethylamphetamine, amphetamine, dimethylamphetamine and p-methoxyamphetamine. Forensic Sci Int 224: 8-26.

7. Grobler SR, Chikte U, Westraat J (2011) The pH Levels of Different Methamphetamine Drug Samples on the Street Market in Cape Town. ISRN Dent 2011: 974768.

8. Rege B, Carter KM, Sarkar MA, Kellogg GE, Soine WH (2002) Irreversible inhibition of CYP2D6 by (-)-chloroephedrine, a possible impurity in methamphetamine. Drug Metab Dispos 30: 1337-1343.

9. Akhgari M, Jokar F, Bahmanabadi L, Etemadi Aleagha A (2012) Street-level heroin seizures in Iran: a survey of components. J Subs Use 17: 348-355.

10. Akhgari M, Jokar F, Etemadi Aleagha A (2011) Drug related deaths in Tehran, Iran: toxicological, death and crime scene investigations. Iran J Toxicol 5: 402-409.

11. Vearrier D, Greenberg MI, Miller SN, Okaneku JT, Haggerty DA (2012) Methamphetamine: history, pathophysiology, adverse health effects, current trends, and hazards associated with the clandestine manufacture of methamphetamine. Dis Mon 58: 38-89.

12. Moore KA, Mirshahi T, Compton DR, Poklis A, Woodward JJ (1996) Pharmacological characterization of BNMPA (alpha-benzyl-N-methylphenethylamine), an impurity of illicit methamphetamine synthesis. Eur J Pharmacol 311: 133-139.

13. Jalilian F, Motlagh FZ, Amoei MR, Hatamzadeh N, Gharibnavaz H, et al. (2014) Which one support (family, friend or other significant) is much

more important to drug cessation? A study among men Kermanshah addicts, the west of Iran. J Addict Res Ther 5:1.

14. Iranian Police Seize over 7 Tons of Illicit Drugs in 2 Weeks. October 29, 2014 - 17:03.

15. Khajeamiri AR1, Faizi M, Sohani F, Baheri T, Kobarfard F (2012) Determination of impurities in illicit methamphetamine samples seized in Iran. Forensic Sci Int 217: 204-206.

16. Dayrit FM, Dumlao MC (2004) Impurity profiling of methamphetamine hydrochloride drugs seized in the Philippines. Forensic Sci Int 144: 29-36.

17. Cole C, Jones L, McVeigh J, Kicman A, Syed Q, et al. (2010) A guide to adulterants, bulking agents and other contaminants found in illicit drugs (Review). Available from the Liverpool: Centre for public health, Faculty of Health and Applied Social Sciences, Liverpool John Moores.

18. Allen A, Cantrell TS (1989) Synthetic reductions in clandestine amphetamine and methamphetamine laboratories: A review. Forensic Sci Int 42: 183-199.

19. Wille SM, Lambert WE (2004) Phenmetrazine or ephedrine? Fooled by library search. J Chromatogr A 1045: 259-262.

20. Brzeczko AW, Leech R, Stark JG (2013) The advent of a new pseudoephedrine product to combat methamphetamine abuse. Am J Drug Alcohol Abuse 39: 284-290.

21. Li TL, Giang YS, Hsu JF, Cheng SG, Liu RH, et al. (2006) Artifacts in the GC-MS profiling of underivatized methamphetamine hydrochloride. Forensic Sci Int 162: 113-120.

22. Makino Y, Urano Y, Nagano T (2005) Investigation of the origin of ephedrine and methamphetamine by stable isotope ratio mass spectrometry: a Japanese experience. Bull Narc 57: 63-78.

23. Sekine H, Nakahara Y (1990) Abuse of smoking methamphetamine mixed with tobacco: II. The formation mechanism of pyrolysis products. J Forensic Sci 35: 580-590.

24. Sadeghi R, Agin K, Taherkhani M, Najm-Afshar L, Nelson LS, et al. (2012) Report of methamphetamine use and cardiomyopathy in three patients. Daru 20: 20.

25. Petit A, Karila L, Chalmin F, Lejoyeux M (2012) Methamphetamine Addiction: A Review of the Literature. J Addict Res Ther S1:006.

26. Hassan SF, Zumut S, Burke PG, McMullan S, Cornish JL, et al. (2015) Comparison of noradrenaline, dopamine and serotonin in mediating the tachycardic and thermogenic effects of methamphetamine in the ventral medial prefrontal cortex. Neuroscience 295: 209-220.

27. Rusyniak DE (2013) Neurologic manifestations of chronic methamphetamine abuse. Psychiatr Clin North Am 36: 261-275.

28. Inamasu J, Nakamura Y, Saito R, Kuroshima Y, Mayanagi K, et al. (2003) Subcortical hemorrhage caused by methamphetamine abuse: efficacy of the triage system in the differential diagnosis--case report. Neurol Med Chir (Tokyo) 43: 82-84.

29. Ogasawara K, Ogawa A, Kita H, Kayama T, Sakurai Y, et al. (1986) [Intracerebral hemorrhage and characteristic angiographic changes associated with methamphetamine--a case report]. No To Shinkei 38: 967-971.

30. Kelly MA, Gorelick PB, Mirza D (1992) The role of drugs in the etiology of stroke. Clin Neuropharmacol 15: 249-275.

31. McGuinness TM, Pollack D (2008) Parental methamphetamine abuse and children. J Pediatr Health Care 22: 152-158.

32. Miller MA, Kozel NJ (1991) Methamphetamine abuse: epidemiologic issues and Implications. National Institute on Drug Abuse Research.

33. Sanchez-Ramos J1 (2015) Neurologic Complications of Psychomotor Stimulant Abuse. Int Rev Neurobiol 120: 131-160.

34. Loftis JM, Choi D, Hoffman W, Huckans MS (2011) Methamphetamine causes persistent immune dysregulation: a cross-species, translational report. Neurotox Res 20: 59-68.

35. Matsumoto RR, Seminerio MJ, Turner RC, Robson MJ, Nguyen L, et al. (2014) Methamphetamine-induced toxicity: an updated review on issues related to hyperthermia. Pharmacol Ther 144: 28-40.

36. Phenmetrazine, Compound summary for CID 4762.

37. Ricaurte GA1, DeLanney LE, Irwin I, Witkin JM, Katz JL, et al. (1989) Evaluation of the neurotoxic potential of N,N-dimethylamphetamine: an illicit analog of methamphetamine. Brain Res 490: 301-306.

38. Salocks C, Kaley KB (2003) EPHEDRINE AND PSEUDOEPHEDRINE. Technical Support Document: Toxicology Clandestine Drug Labs: Methamphetamine 1.

39. Varner KJ, Hein ND, Ogden BA, Arsenault JR, Carter KM, et al. (2001) Chloroephedrine: contaminant of methamphetamine synthesis with cardiovascular activity. Drug Alcohol Depend 64: 299-307.

40. Hahn IH. MDMA Toxicity.

41. Interactions with Methamphetamine (Tramadol).

42. Nazarzadeh M, Bidel Z, Carson KV (2014) The association between tramadol hydrochloride misuse and other substances use in an adolescent population: Phase I of a prospective survey. Addict Behav 39: 333-337.

43. Iravani FS, Akhgari M, Jokar F, Bahmanabadi L (2010) Current trends in tramadol-related fatalities, Tehran, Iran 2005-2008. Subst Use Misuse 45: 2162-2171.

44. Alam-Mehrjerdi Z, Mokri A, Dolan K (2015) Methamphetamine use and treatment in Iran: A systematic review from the most populated Persian Gulf country. Asian J Psychiatr .

45. Nisijima K, Shioda K, Iwamura T (2007) Neuroleptic malignant syndrome and serotonin syndrome. Prog Brain Res 162: 81-104.

46. Yuki F, Rie I, Miki K, Mitsuhiro W, Naotaka K, et al. (2013) Warning against co-administration of 3,4-methylenedioxymethamphetamine (MDMA) with methamphetamine from the perspective of pharmacokinetic and pharmacodynamic evaluations in rat brain. Eur J Pharm Sci 49: 57-64.

47. Hawley LA, Auten JD, Matteucci MJ, Decker L, Hurst N, et al. (2013) Cardiac complications of adult methamphetamine exposures. J Emerg Med 45: 821-827.

48. Islam MN, Jesmine K, Kong Sn Molh A, Hasnan J (2009) Histopathological studies of cardiac lesions after long term administration of methamphetamine in high dosage--Part II. Leg Med (Tokyo) 11 Suppl 1: S147-150.

49. Formication; aka, speed bumps, meth sores, crank bugs.

50. Material Safety Data Sheet. Acetic acid MSDS, chemicals and laboratory equipments.

51. Safety data sheet, phenyl acetone (exempt preparation).

52. Wang P, Chen X, Zheng L, Guo L, Li X, et al. (2014) Comprehensive dental treatment for "meth mouth": a case report and literature review. J Formos Med Assoc 113: 867-871.

53. Shetty V, Mooney LJ, Zigler CM, Belin TR, Murphy D, et al. (2010) The relationship between methamphetamine use and increased dental disease. J Am Dent Assoc 141: 307-318.

54. Tomita M, Katsuyama H, Watanabe Y, Okuyama T, Fushimi S, et al. (2014) Does methamphetamine affect bone metabolism? Toxicology 319: 63-68.

55. Katsuragawa Y (1999) Effect of methamphetamine abuse on the bone quality of the calcaneus. Forensic Sci Int 101: 43-48.

56. Kim EY, Kwon do H, Lee BD, Kim YT, Ahn YB, et al. (2009) Frequency of osteoporosis in 46 men with methamphetamine abuse hospitalized in a National Hospital. Forensic Sci Int 188: 75-80.

57. Luo R, Zhang S, Xiang P, Shen B, Zhuo X, et al. (2015) Elements concentrations in the scalp hair of methamphetamine abusers. Forensic Sci Int 249: 112-115.

58. Solgi R, Abdollahi M (2012) Proposing an antidote for poisonous phosphine in view of mitochondrial electrochemistry facts. J Med Hypotheses Ideas 6: 32-34.

59. Salocks C, Kaley KB (2003) Technical Support Document: Toxicology Clandestine Drug Labs: Methamphetamine 1.

60. Martyny JW, Arbuckle ShL, McCammon Jr ChS, Esswein EJ, Erb N, et al. (2007) Chemical concentrations and contamination associated with clandestine methamphetamine laboratories. J Chem Health Saf 14: 40-52.

61. Burgess JL (2001) Phosphine exposure from a methamphetamine laboratory investigation. J Toxicol Clin Toxicol 39: 165-168.

62. Hazardous Substance Fact Sheet, Benzaldehyde. New Jersy Department of Health and Senior Services.

63. Kanerva L, Keskinen H, Autio P, Estlander T, Tuppurainen M, et al. (1995) Occupational respiratory and skin sensitization caused by polyfunctional aziridine hardener. Clin Exp Allergy 25: 432-439.

64. Nowicki P, Klos J, Kokot ZJ (2014) Trends of Amphetamine Type Stimulants DTR Mass Load in Poznan Based on Wastewater Analysis. Iran J Public Health 43: 610-620.

65. Kates LN, Knapp CW, Keenan HE (2014) Acute and chronic environmental effects of clandestine methamphetamine waste. Sci Total Environ 493: 781-788.

66. Poppendieck D, Morrison G, Corsi R (2015) Desorption of a methamphetamine surrogate from wallboard under remediation conditions. Atmos Environ 106: 477-484.

67. Derlet RW, Heischober B (1990) Methamphetamine. Stimulant of the 1990s? West J Med 153: 625-628.

15

Inhibition of Soluble Epoxide Hydrolase as a Novel Approach to High Dose Diazepam Induced Hypotension

Arzu Ulu[1], **Bora Inceoglu**[1], **Jun Yang**[1], **Vikrant Singh**[2], **Stephen Vito**[1], **Heike Wulff**[2] **and Bruce D Hammock**[1*]

[1]*Department of Entomology and Nematology, and Comprehensive Cancer Center, University of California, Davis, USA*

[2]*Department of Pharmacology, School of Medicine, University of California, Davis, USA*

[*]**Corresponding author:** Dr. Bruce D Hammock, Department of Entomology and Nematology, and Comprehensive Cancer Center, University of California, Davis, USA, E-mail: bdhammock@ucdavis.edu

Abstract

Context: Hypotension is one of the dose limiting side effects of benzodiazepines (BZDs), in particular of diazepam (DZP) which is still widely used in the clinic. Currently, only one FDA approved antidote exists for BZD overdose and novel approaches are needed to improve management of DZP overdose, dependency and withdrawal.

Objective: Here, we hypothesized that increasing bioactive lipid mediators termed epoxy fatty acids (EpFAs) will prevent hypotension, as was shown previously in a murine model of LPS-induced hypotension. Therefore, we first characterized the time and dose dependent profile of DZP induced hypotension in mice, and then investigated the reversal of the hypotensive effect by inhibiting the soluble epoxide hydrolase (sEH), an enzyme that regulates the levels of EpFAs.

Materials and Methods: Following baseline systolic BP recording using tail cuffs, mice were administered a sEH inhibitor (TPPU) before DZP and BP was monitored. Blood and brain levels of DZP and TPPU were quantified to examine distribution and metabolism. Plasma EpFAs levels were quantified to determine TPPU target engagement.

Results: In this murine model, DZP induced dose dependent hypotension which was more severe than midazolam. The temporal profile was consistent with the reported pharmacokinetics/pharmacodynamics of DZP. Treatment with TPPU reversed the hypotension resulting from high doses of DZP and decreased the sEH metabolites of EpFAs in the plasma demonstrating target engagement.

Discussion and Conclusion: Overall, these findings demonstrate the similarity of a murine model of DZP induced hypotension to clinical observations in humans. Furthermore, we demonstrate that stabilization of EpFAs by inhibiting sEH is a novel approach to overcome DZP-induced hypotension and this beneficial effect can be enhanced by an omega three diet probably acting through epoxide metabolites of the fatty acids.

Keywords: Soluble epoxide hydrolase inhibitors; Diazepam; Midazolam; Hypotension; EETs; DHETs

Introduction

Benzodiazepines (BZDs) are the most frequently prescribed psychoactive agents that are used to treat a number of conditions including anxiety, insomnia, seizures and alcohol dependence [1,2]. They are among the drugs of first choice for several epileptic conditions because of their rapid onset of activity, high efficacy and favorable risk to benefit ratio. BZDs are allosteric modulators of the GABA$_A$ chloride channel complex (gamma aminobutyric acid), which increase the affinity of this receptor channel to the neurotransmitter GABA [1]. The BZD binding site of the GABA channel is a well exploited target with a number of registered BZD drugs, which have different potencies and toxicities.

Although BZDs have been extremely useful in the treatment of major diseases, the dose limiting adverse effects such as dependence, tolerance, hypotension, and loss of consciousness leave room for improvement on the current standard of care of BZDs [3,4].

Occasionally, BZDs are used in relatively high doses such as antidotes for pesticide or nerve gas poisoning or following overdose. Thus, an antidote for BZDs becomes necessary to prevent lethality [5,6]. In contrast to the availability of multiple BZD drugs the only FDA approved antidote for an overdose of BZDs is flumazenil. Flumazenil competitively inhibits ligand binding at the BZD binding site inside the GABA$_A$ channel [7]. Expectedly, use of flumazenil may predispose patients to increased sensitivity to seizures or necessitate resedation [8,9].

A rapid and significant decrease in BP is one of the most pronounced side effects of BZDs such as diazepam (DZP). The mechanism of the hypotensive effect of BZDs is largely unknown. While some studies suggest that BZDs have a vasodilatory effect, which may involve binding to GABA receptors, others suggest that BZDs affect peripheral vascular resistance through a decrease in muscle sympathetic nerve activity [10]. This hypotensive effect requires close monitoring and intervention since it could lead to fainting, decreased blood oxygen levels and reduced availability of oxygen to the brain. Because flumazenil use has limitations, an alternative approach to safely treat this overdose related toxicity could be positive modulation of BP.

Agents that can be co-administered with BZDs without affecting their potency and pharmacokinetics while reducing fatal hypotension could be tremendously useful in the treatment of cases of overdose and make the BZDs safer for susceptible patient populations such as elderly people and patients with cardiovascular disease already taking anti-hypertensives. Soluble epoxide hydrolase inhibitors (sEHIs) are known to modulate BP. The sEH is a α/β hydrolase fold enzyme that metabolizes a biologically important group of endogenous lipid mediators, namely epoxy fatty acids (EpFAs). These EpFAs have numerous physiological roles such as regulation of vascular resistance and blood flow [11-14], and depending on the context either raise or lower blood pressure (BP) [14-16].

In addition to BP regulating effects, the modest anticonvulsant effects of sEH inhibitors seem to depend on or be related to GABAergic signaling [17]. Systemic inhibition of sEH or intracerebroventricular (i.c.v.) administration of EpFAs, specifically those derived from arachidonic acid selectively delay the onset of GABA antagonist induced but no other types of seizures [17]. Therefore, taking advantage of these properties of the EpFAs and sEHIs we asked if DZP induced hypotension could be prevented by inhibiting sEH. We also demonstrate that this murine model is suitable to examine new agents that block hypotension induced by BZDs.

Materials and Methods

Animals and treatments

All animal protocols were approved by the University of California Davis Animal Use and Care Committee, and experiments were carried out in compliance with the National Institutes of Health Guide for the use and care of laboratory animals. Upon arrival to the vivarium, 7 week old mice (Swiss Webster mice, Charles River Laboratories, Wilmington, MA) were acclimated to their new housing environment for one week and kept under a 12 hour light/dark cycle with free access to food and water.

DZP (5 mg/mL, Hospira, Inc., Lake Forest, IL) was dissolved in 40% propylene glycol, 10% ethanol and saline. TPPU (1-trifluoromethoxyphenyl-3-(1-propionylpiperidin-4-yl) urea) was synthesized [18], purified and characterized in-house (a kind gift of Dr Sing Lee from UC Davis) and was dissolved in PEG400 to obtain a clear solution. Mice were injected (i.p.) either with DZP alone at 1, 3 or 10 mg/kg or in combination with TPPU at 3 mg/kg i.p. one hour before administration of DZP at the doses indicated. Midazolam (Hospira, Inc., Lake Forest, IL) was administered at 1.8 and 10 mg/kg doses by intramuscular route using saline as vehicle. Animals that served as controls were given the corresponding vehicle solutions, PEG400 for TPPU or 40% propylene glycol, 10% ethanol in saline for DZP and saline for midazolam injections.

BP measurements

Systolic BP (SBP) was measured using a tail cuff volume pressure recording system (8-channel CODA, Kent Scientific, CT) with minor modifications. In our study we selected the tail cuff method instead of direct measurements for BP for several key reasons. Direct measurement methods require either surgery or sedation of the animals which could interfere with the effect of DZP and lead to misinterpretation of the data. Surgical implantation of telemetry probes often cause inflammation which may interfere with the study. Since we are interested in quantification of anti-inflammatory EpFAs, an increase in inflammatory markers such as prostaglandins would potentially affect our results after DZP administration. Moreover, we performed acute treatments and measurements which do not require long term monitoring of BP. Collection of heart rate data was initially not considered as one of the parameters mainly because DZP is known not to influence it [10].

Briefly, restrained animals were maintained on warm heating pads. During the measurements a cloth was placed on the restrainers to maintain heat and to provide a calm environment for the mice. A baseline measurement of 20 cycles was recorded for each animal before any treatment is given. After obtaining a baseline, animals were injected with either PEG400 or TPPU and SBP was measured for another 20 cycles to obtain the change in BP post-PEG400 or TPPU.

One hour after administration of PEG400 or TPPU, DZP was administered and changes in BP were monitored for one hour or 120 cycles. In other experiments SBP was monitored for extended durations by placing the mice into the tail cuff and recording a 20 min period at the beginning of every hour or for the durations indicated in the figure legends.

DZP quantification in tissue and plasma

DZP was quantified in plasma and brain samples by LC/MS analysis, which was performed with a Waters Acquity UPLC (Waters, NY, USA) and TSQ Quantum Access Max mass spectrometer (MS) (Thermo Fisher ScientificTM, Waltham, MA, USA). Sample preparation and LC/MS conditions are detailed in the supplementary data.

Quantification of EpFAs and TPPU

Bioactive lipid mediators also known as oxylipins or TPPU (see LC/MS chromatogram on Figure S 2) from treated animals were extracted from plasma using solid phase extraction and quantified using the QTRAP4000 LC/MS/MS system as described previously [19] with a minor modification, which included a shorter acquisition time to focus on only the most relevant EpFAs and their diol metabolites (26 analytes).

Statistical analysis

All data are reported as mean ± standard error of the mean. To determine differences in BP among the groups repeated measures one-way ANOVA was performed, followed by pairwise comparisons using a post hoc test (i.e. Bonferroni), all of which were performed on Graph Pad Prism software. P values less than 0.05 were considered statistically significant.

Results

Characterization of the murine model of DZP induced hypotension

To determine if BZDs have a hypotensive effect on mice, we tested multiple doses of DZP and midazolam using NIH Swiss mice (Figures 1-3). DZP treatment led to hypotension in mice in a dose dependent manner (Figure 1A-C). Repeated measures one-way ANOVA revealed an overall significant blood pressure lowering effect (F=30, P<0.01) with significant differences among those treated with different doses of DZP (P<0.01) except for DZP 10 mg/kg versus DZP 3 mg/kg (P>0.05).

Following an acclimation period, 15 min of BP recordings prior to any treatment were assigned as the baseline for each animal. The average baseline SBP was 113 ± 2 (mean ± SEM, n=48 mice) throughout the study. In parallel to observations in patients, all doses of DZP treatment led to a decrease in BP, with the lowest dose displaying a shorter duration of effect. At the higher doses of 3 and 10 mg/kg animals experienced a more prominent and sudden drop in BP within 5 min after administration of DZP (Figure 1B and 1C) and the hypotensive effect lasted significantly longer. For several individual

DZP treated mice the SBP was at or under the limit of detection (60 mmHg) of the tail cuff volume-pressure recording system and these were recorded as 60 mmHg and are included in the data set. At the 3 mg/kg DZP dose several periods of more intense hypotension were consistently observed, while at the 10 mg/kg dose the BP was reduced maximally and remained low throughout the rest of the 90 min recording period. Overall, hypotension induced by 3 and 10 mg/kg of DZP lowered SBP by approximately half of the baseline with a longer recovery period, while 1 mg/kg of DZP led to 10-20% decrease from baseline with a 10 min recovery time.

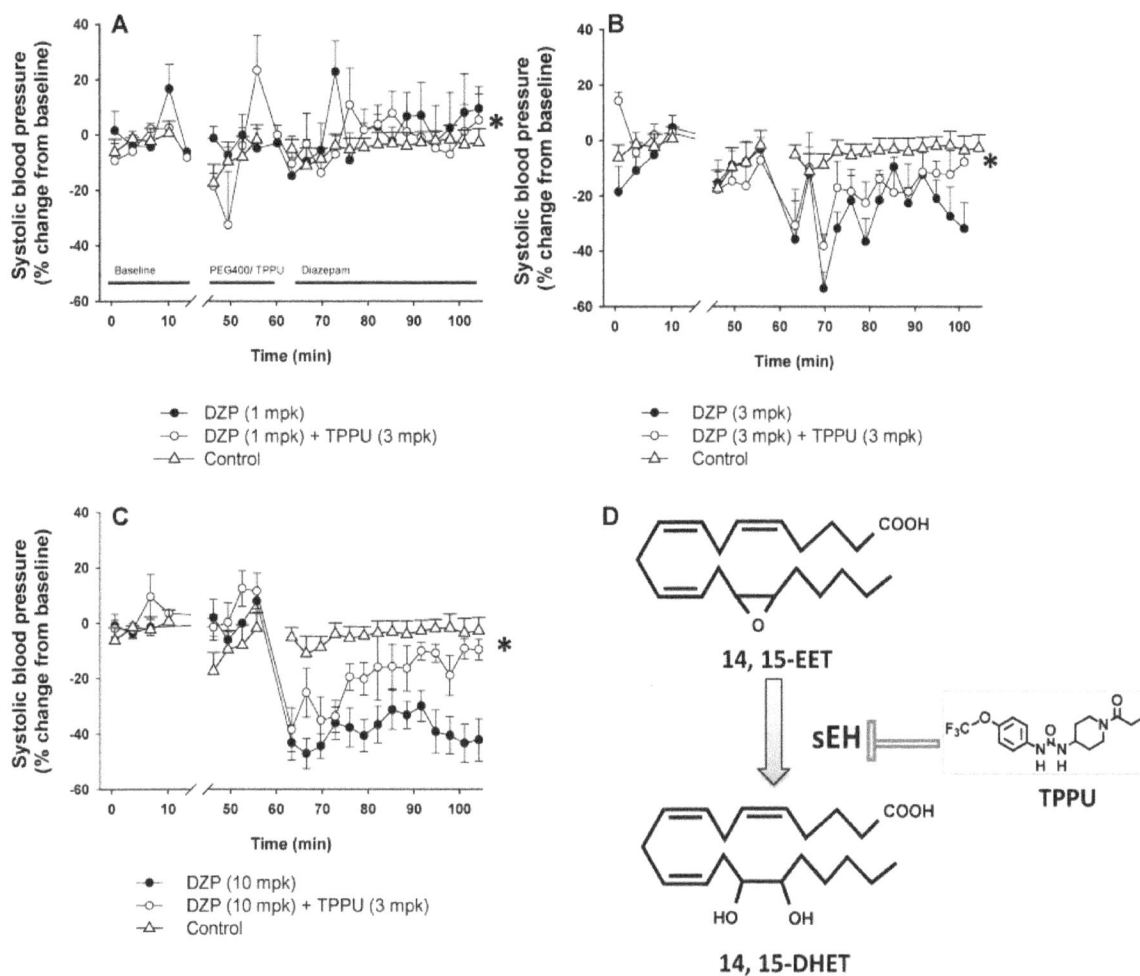

Figure 1: DZP induced hypotension is dose dependent and reversible by TPPU. Dose dependent effects of DZP on blood pressure are displayed for A. 1 mg/kg, B. 3 mg/kg and C. 10 mg/kg doses. Upon obtaining baseline BP (data before the break on the x-axis), mice were administered TPPU (i.p., 3 mg/kg) or vehicle (PEG400) 1 h before injection of DZP at varying dosages. Post-PEG400 or TPPU blood pressure was recorded for 20-23 cycles (between 45-60 min). Then, DZP was administered and BP was recorded following 5 min after DZP injections. Timeline of the experiment is illustrated on panel A. Data are mean ± SEM, n=6/group. D. Lipid epoxides such as EETs are endogenous chemical mediators known to return high blood pressure to normotensive levels. EETs are rapidly converted to DHETs by soluble epoxide hydrolase (sEH). This degradation is blocked by TPPU.

To further understand the duration of DZP induced hypotension mice treated with the 3 and 10 mg/kg DZP and were intermittently monitored over a period of 24 h (Figure 2 and 3). At 5 and 6 h post DZP, BP was still below baseline in mice treated with 3 and 10 mg/kg

DZP and there was full recovery at 24 h post treatment. In addition to the first 100 min after DZP (Figure 1), we performed another repeated measures one-way ANOVA that included data collected on all time points from baseline to 24 hours. This analysis revealed a significant difference among the treatment groups (F=140.7, P<0.01). Pairwise comparisons showed a significant difference between DZP 10 mg/kg versus DZP 3 mg/kg and between animals treated with DZP versus DZP+TPPU within each DZP dose group (P<0.01).

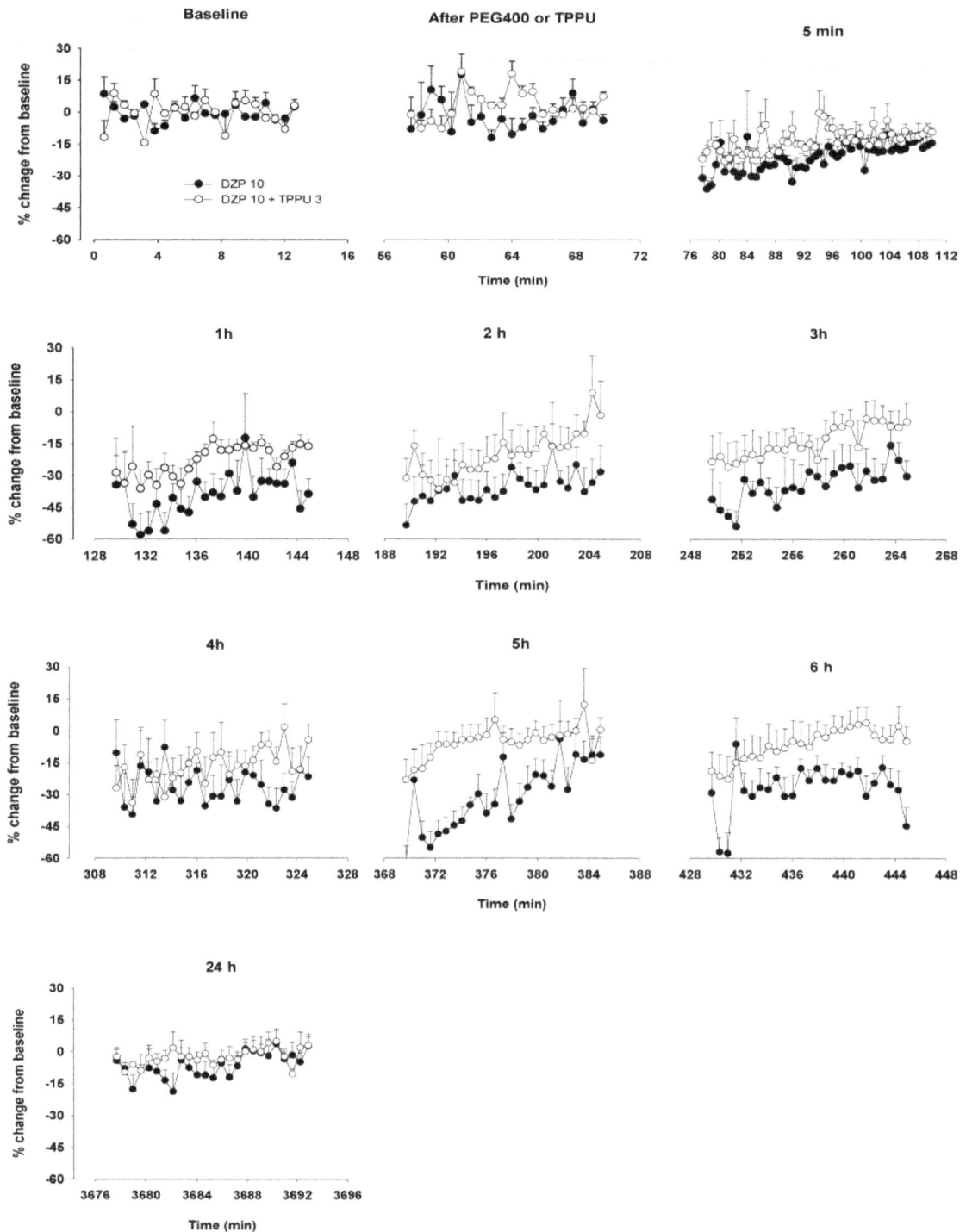

Figure 2: DZP induced hypotension lasts for at least 6 h. Time dependent effects of DZP at 3 mg/kg dose with or without TPPU on blood pressure (n=6 per group). Upon obtaining baseline BP, mice were administered TPPU (i.p., 3 mg/kg) 1 h before injection of DZP. Blood pressure was recorded at baseline, 45 min after TPPU or PEG400 administration, at 5 min after DZP (3 mgkg) and then at 1, 2, 3, 4, 5 and 24 h. Data are mean ± SEM, n=6/group.

To validate the utility of the model we tested another BZD, midazolam (Figure 4). Two doses of midazolam were selected. The first dose was 1.8 mg/kg midazolam (Figure 4A) in mice which is roughly equivalent to the human dose at 1 mg/kg [20]. The second dose was 10-fold higher than the human equivalent dose (Figure 4B).

Midazolam led to significant changes in BP at both doses (P<0.01, Figure 4). The recovery from midazolam occurred between 1-2 h after midazolam was administered, suggesting a faster recovery than following DZP, which is consistent with the shorter half-life of midazolam as compared to DZP.

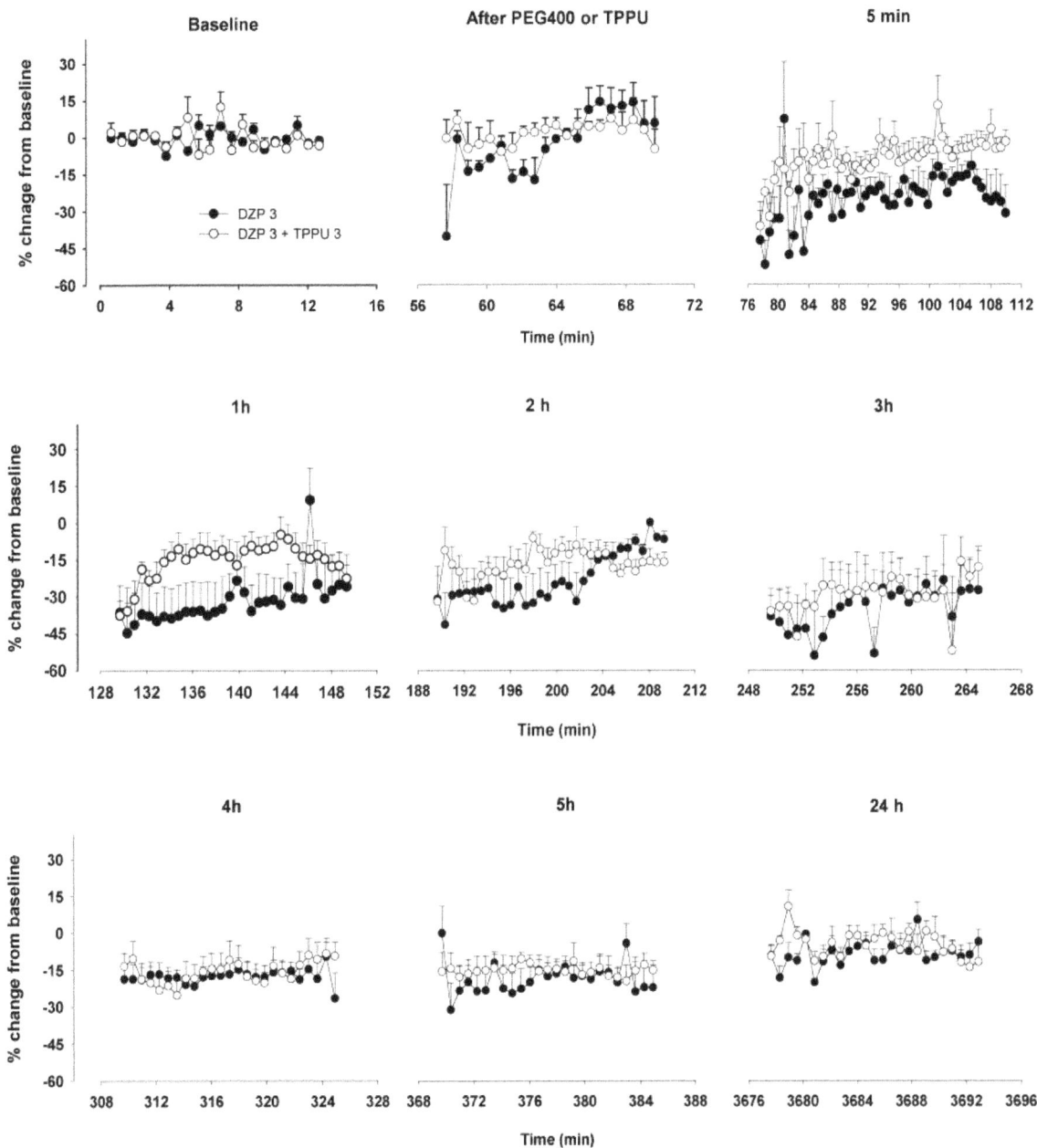

Figure 3: Time dependent effects of DZP at 10 mg/kg dose with or without TPPU on blood pressure (n=6 per group). Upon obtaining baseline BP, mice were administered TPPU (i.p., 3 mg/kg) 1 h before injection of DZP at varying dosages. Blood pressure was recorded at baseline, at 45 min after TPPU or PEG400 administration, at 5 min after DZP (10 mg/kg) and then at 1, 2, 3, 4, 5, 6 and 24 h. Data are mean ± SEM, n=6 / group.

Inhibition of sEH reverses the hypotensive effect of DZP

To test if inhibition of sEH will normalize BP, we first investigated the effect of the vehicles used to formulate DZP and TPPU. These

vehicle treatments by themselves did not lead to significant changes in BP. TPPU alone or when administered together with the DZP vehicle under physiologic conditions (i.e. without DZP) did not elicit any significant changes (P=0.56). These data reiterate the proposed homeostatic role of EpFAs and sEH inhibitors in the absence of an underlying pathological condition [14,15].

A high dose of TPPU (3 mg/kg) was administered 45 min prior to all three doses of DZP treated animals and BP was recorded for an hour. At the lowest dose (1 mg/kg), DZP showed a slight hypotensive effect (P=0.3, as compared to baseline BP) and accordingly TPPU was the least effective in these mice. TPPU did not prevent the sudden drop in BP 5 min after administration of DZP at higher doses (3 and 10

mg/kg DZP). However, animals treated with TPPU recovered significantly faster from hypotension compared to those treated with DZP alone (Figure 1, P<0.001). This reversal of SBP with TPPU treatment was maximal at about 30 min after administration of DZP. In addition, when we evaluated the area under the curve (AUC) of the BP-time course, we found that the AUC for the BP in the DZP plus TPPU treatment group was significantly higher than the AUC in the group treated with DZP alone (P<0.05). These data suggest that TPPU is indeed effective in normalizing BP at higher doses of DZP.

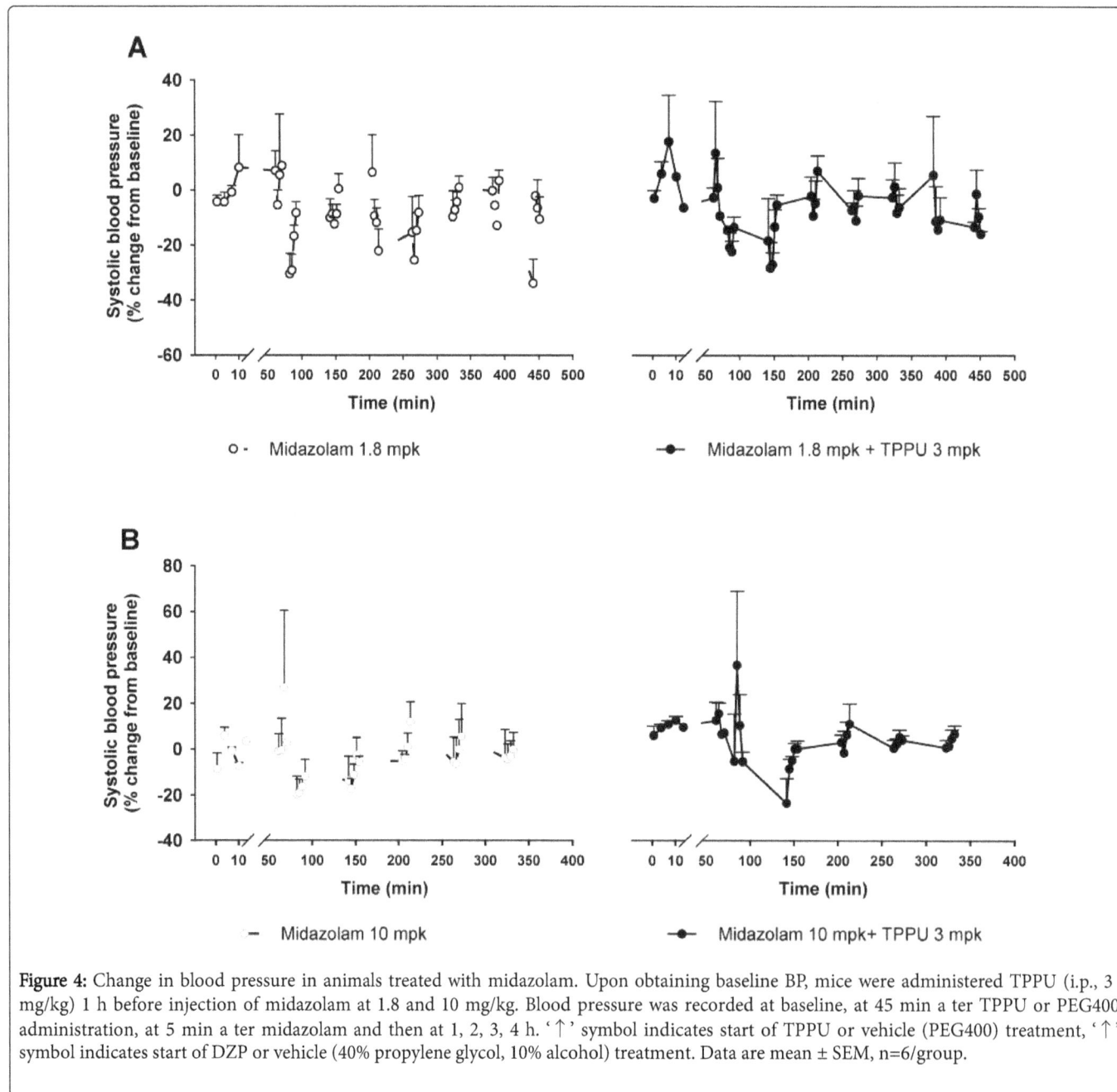

Figure 4: Change in blood pressure in animals treated with midazolam. Upon obtaining baseline BP, mice were administered TPPU (i.p., 3 mg/kg) 1 h before injection of midazolam at 1.8 and 10 mg/kg. Blood pressure was recorded at baseline, at 45 min a ter TPPU or PEG400 administration, at 5 min a ter midazolam and then at 1, 2, 3, 4 h. '↑' symbol indicates start of TPPU or vehicle (PEG400) treatment, '↑' symbol indicates start of DZP or vehicle (40% propylene glycol, 10% alcohol) treatment. Data are mean ± SEM, n=6/group.

Treatment with Midazolam also resulted in significant changes in BP in the repeated measures ANOVA analysis (F=71.9, P<0.01). While administration of midazolam led to significant hypotension at both doses (P<0.05), TPPU was effective only when administered with the

low dose of midazolam (P=0.004 for midazolam 1.8 mg/kg versus midazolam 1.8 mg/kg+TPPU) (Figure 4).

Tissue and plasma levels of DZP and TPPU

Next we quantified plasma and brain levels of both compounds (Table 1). For DZP at the highest dose, an immediate and a delayed time point of 5 and 60 min were selected. For the TPPU receiving groups, these same time points corresponded to 50 and 105 min post administration of TPPU. The brain levels of DZP were significantly higher than plasma at both time points (P<0.05) with a brain-to-plasma ratio of 3.5 ± 0.3 (mean ± SEM, n=24), which is in line with previous reports [21,22]. Consistent with previous reports [21], both tissue and plasma levels of DZP decreased at least 3 fold at 1 h after dosing. TPPU co-administration did not change plasma and brain levels of DZP.

In addition, tissue and plasma levels of TPPU were at least 10 times higher than the IC50 for murine sEH (IC50: 2 nM [18]), suggesting a near complete inhibition of sEH. We observed three times higher levels of TPPU in the brain than in the plasma at both time points, which is consistent with effective penetration through the blood-brain barrier.

TPPU treatment with or without DZP modulates the plasma biomarkers of sEH inhibition

Treatment with TPPU at a 3 mg/kg dose should inhibit nearly all enzyme activity [18]. Based on previous work using i.p. or oral administration TPPU has a plasma elimination half-life of >24 h [18,23,24]. Moreover, TPPU was also quantified from saline perfused mouse brain and demonstrated to have significant blood brain barrier penetration [17], in keeping with what we are finding in this study (Table 1). We therefore expected TPPU to change both plasma and brain levels of the EpFAs and as a surrogate examined plasma levels of the EpFAs and tested if DZP administration following TPPU lead to pharmacokinetic interference between these two compounds.

	[TPPU] (µM)	
Time after TPPU administration	Brain	Plasma
50 min (5 min after DZP)	32.8 ± 3.4	11.8 ± 0.6
105 min (1 h after DZP)	27.8 ± 2	10 ± 0.3
Time after DZP administration	[DZP] (µM)	
	Brain	Plasma
5 min- DZP 10 mpk	15 ± 3	3 ± 0.8
5 min- DZP 10 mpk+TPPU	15 ± 3	7 ± 2
1 h- DZP 10 mpk	1 ± 0.1	0.4 ± 0.05
1h- DZP 10 mpk+TPPU	1 ± 0.1	0.4 ± 0.03

Table 1: Tissue and plasma levels of TPPU and DZP in mice.

To examine target engagement by TPPU, we quantified the EETs (epoxyeicosatrienoic acid) and EpOMEs (epoxyoctadecenoic acid) from plasma. These cytochrome P450 enzyme generated bioactive lipids are highly responsive to sEH inhibition. DZP alone after 5 min did not elicit any significant changes in the levels of biomarker EpFAs, when compared to vehicle controls (P>0.05). The EETs and EpOMEs are substrates of the sEH enzyme and are metabolized to DHETs and DiHOMEs by the sEH activity.

The plasma and tissue levels of EpFAs are usually in the low nM range and in vivo their half-life is in the order of several seconds because of the sEH activity, although in vitro they are fairly stable [25,26]. Therefore the ratio of epoxides to diols is used as biomarkers of target engagement in studies with sEH inhibitors [12,15,27].

In mice treated with both DZP and TPPU, both the EETs and EpOMEs increased approximately 2-3 fold with significant decreases in their corresponding degradation products the DHETs and DiHOMEs, leading to 7-10 fold higher epoxide to diol ratio at both time points (Figure 5). In addition to P450 metabolites of arachidonic acid, we observed an increase in some of the cyclooxygenase and lipoxygenase metabolites of arachidonic acid after administration of diazepam, suggesting a trend towards increased inflammation upon DZP administration.

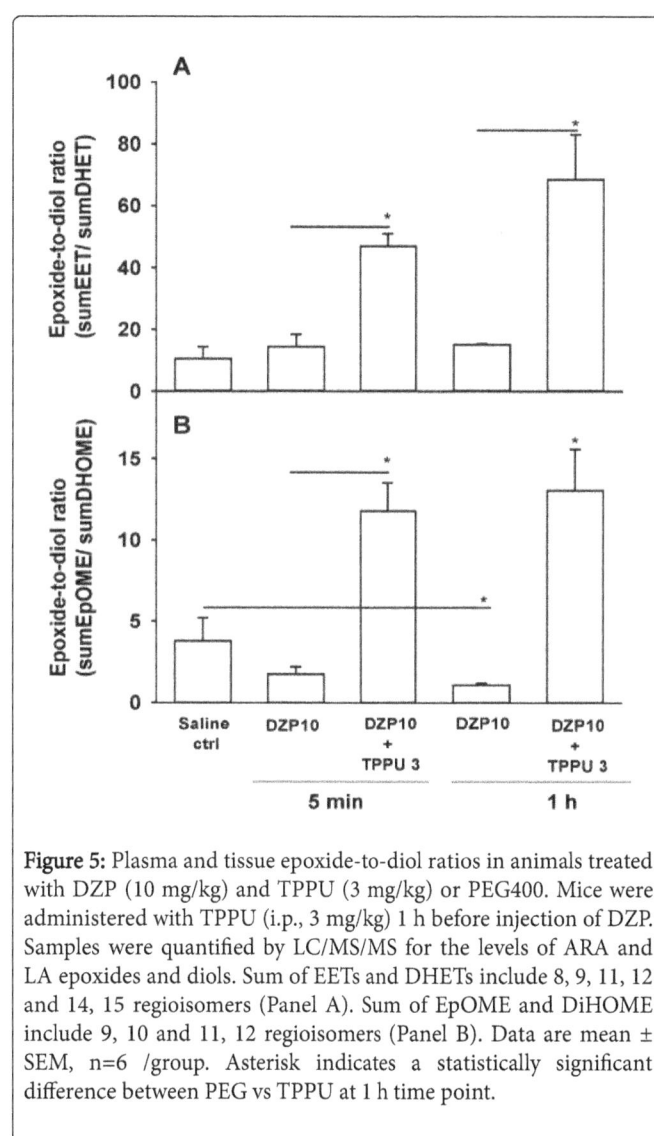

Figure 5: Plasma and tissue epoxide-to-diol ratios in animals treated with DZP (10 mg/kg) and TPPU (3 mg/kg) or PEG400. Mice were administered with TPPU (i.p., 3 mg/kg) 1 h before injection of DZP. Samples were quantified by LC/MS/MS for the levels of ARA and LA epoxides and diols. Sum of EETs and DHETs include 8, 9, 11, 12 and 14, 15 regioisomers (Panel A). Sum of EpOME and DiHOME include 9, 10 and 11, 12 regioisomers (Panel B). Data are mean ± SEM, n=6 /group. Asterisk indicates a statistically significant difference between PEG vs TPPU at 1 h time point.

Discussion

We established a murine model to study the hypotensive effects of DZP and midazolam and to test whether this adverse effect could be reversed by sEH inhibition. Our findings on BZD induced hypotension are consistent with reports from patients, although the murine model seems less sensitive to the hypotensive effects of DZP. However, this method provides a rapid and sufficiently stringent approach to investigate anti-hypotensive compounds. The main finding of this study is that sEH inhibition leads to a faster recovery from the hypotensive effect of DZP.

The BZD drugs have a range of potencies and toxicities based on their affinity to the GABA channel subtypes and pharmacokinetic properties including, onset and duration of action, rate of absorption and presence of active metabolites. Due to their euphoric effects, they are also drugs of abuse. The estimated number of emergency room visits in the US, involving nonmedical use of BZDs was reported to be about 270, 000 in 2008 [28]. However, current options for management of BZD overdose are limited. Flumazenil is a selective BZD antagonist and therefore the drug of choice in BZD overdose [29]; however, it was reported to cause seizures, resedation and cardiac arrhythmias, in some cases within minutes of its administration [30,31]. Additionally, it has a short half-life and requires repetitive dosings to obtain the desired effect. Therefore, its use is limited. Naloxone is also used in BZD overdose even though it is an opioid antagonist [32]. While other vasoactive substances (catecholamine, phosphodiesterase inhibitors, etc.) are available to treat hypotension in shock, cardiac arrest or calcium channel blocker toxicity [33,34], these are not the first line of choice in the treatment of BZD overdose. Therefore, novel approaches are needed to target hypotension associated with BZDs.

Dose dependent effects of treatments with BZDs

In our study, DZP caused a dose dependent decrease in BP (Figure 1), which is consistent with previous studies [35]. Hypotension induced by both doses of DZP lasted well beyond the short plasma elimination or brain disappearance half-life of DZP, which is reported to be about 8 min each following i.v. administration in mice [21]. In contrast, the two major bioactive metabolites of DZP, desmethyl DZP and oxazepam have a brain disappearance half-life of approximately 3 h following 2.85 mg/kg DZP administration, and oxazepam given alone has a brain disappearance half-life of up to 5 h. Midazolam induced hypotension is rarely encountered at clinically used doses but it may elicit hypotension at high doses or when administered with opioids [36]. Data here are consistent with the characteristics of midazolam.

Effect of TPPU on BZD induced hypotension

While pretreatment with a sEH inhibitor did not cause an immediate effect on normalizing BP after DZP injection, the time to recovery from the hypotensive effect of DZP was significantly shortened. Supporting this observation, at later time points we still obtained statistically significant differences in BP between mice treated with DZP alone and mice treated with DZP and TPPU (Figure 2 and 3).

The sEH inhibitor used here is CNS permeable [17]. In line with previous findings, in this study TPPU crossed the blood brain barrier with a ~3.5 time's higher concentration in the brain than in plasma. While the tissue levels of DZP and TPPU were comparable at early time points, TPPU levels remained high for a longer time. This likely contributed to the faster recovery of animals that were treated with DZP plus TPPU. Most importantly, plasma and brain levels of both DZP and TPPU from mice that received both compounds were nearly identical to those receiving individual compounds at either time point. This observation implies that there was no significant pharmacokinetic interaction between these two agents, a desired property in combinatorial treatments.

The sEH inhibitors seem to normalize BP rather than modulating it in a single direction. Anti-hypotensive and anti-hypertensive effects of sEH inhibitors are well documented in various models [12,14]. When hypertension is induced by Angiotensin II the sEH inhibitors lower systolic BP, while in models of hypotension induced by systemic LPS elicited sepsis, they elevate BP from less than 40 mmHg (undetectable by tail cuff method) to normal range [14]. Dietary supplementation of ω-3 fatty acids or infusion of one of the EpFA regioisomers, the 19,20-EpDPE with an implanted mini-pump both enhance the efficacy of TPPU supporting the hypothesis that sEH inhibitors stabilize the levels of EpFAs which in turn regulate BP [16,26,37]. Reducing the hypotensive side effect of DZP should allow higher doses of BZDs like midazolam and diazepam to be used. In particular, there seems to be no negative functional interaction between GABA agonists and sEH inhibitors. Specifically the anti-convulsant effect of DZP is slightly enhanced by sEH inhibitor co-administration. In addition, sEH inhibitor may positively regulate the synthesis of an unidentified endogenous GABA agonist, possibly a neurosteroid [17]. Given the apparently large therapeutic window of sEH inhibitors and the apparent lack of negative side effects [38-40] these compounds may find use in reducing the hypertensive side effects is several drug classes. One of the other outcomes associated with the effects of sEH inhibitors on the nervous system is their anti-depressant effects. Although we have not assessed such functional outcomes in our current study, we have reported a strong and relatively quick anti-depressant effect of sEH inhibitors in different murine models of depression, where we observed remarkable increases in the tissue levels of sEH in the brain as compared to control animals [41]. The increase in the brain sEH levels also reflected itself in postmortem brain samples obtained from depressed patients. These results suggested a key role for sEH in the pathogenesis of depression. Future studies are underway to characterize sedative effects of sEH inhibitors.

Conclusions

Overall, our study demonstrates that the sEH inhibitor TPPU does not interfere with the PK of DZP but can be beneficial to treat cases of BZD induced hypotension. The observation that TPPU is most effective at the highest doses of DZP suggests the endogenous substrates, EpFAs are homeostatic molecules. Such EpFAs include P450 metabolites of omega-3 fatty acids suggesting that an omega-3 fatty acid rich diet can potentially enhance the anti-hypotensive effects of TPPU.

Sources of Funding

This work was supported by the NIEHS grant R01 ES002710, NIEHS Superfund Research Program grants P42 ES004699, the CounterAct Program, National Institutes of Health Office of the Director (NIH OD), and the National Institute of Neurological Disorders and Stroke, Grant Number U54 NS079202, NIEHS grant U24 DK097154 and National Institute of Arthritis and Musculoskeletal and Skin Diseases R21AR062866.

Acknowledgments

We would like to thank Mrs. Louisa Lo for her extensive and thorough administrative assistance and help with manuscript editing.

References

1. Mohler H (2011) The rise of a new GABA pharmacology. Neuropharmacology 60: 1042-1049.

2. Greenfield LJ Jr (2013) Molecular mechanisms of antiseizure drug activity at GABA_A receptors. Seizure 22: 589-600.

3. Ochoa JG, Kilgo WA (2016) The Role of Benzodiazepines in the Treatment of Epilepsy. Curr Treat Options Neurol 18: 18.

4. Wu W, Zhang L, Xue R (2016) Lorazepam or diazepam for convulsive status epilepticus: A meta-analysis. J clin neurosci p S0967-5868: 00704-00703.

5. Marrs TC (2003) Diazepam in the treatment of organophosphorus ester pesticide poisoning. Toxicol Rev 22: 75-81.

6. Bailey AM, Baker SN, Baum RA, Chandler HE, Weant KA (2014) Being prepared: emergency treatment following a nerve agent release. Adv Emerg Nurs J 36: 22-33.

7. Licata SC, Rowlett JK (2008) Abuse and dependence liability of benzodiazepine-type drugs: GABA(A) receptor modulation and beyond. Pharmacol Biochem Behav 90: 74-89.

8. Seger DL (2004) Flumazenil--treatment or toxin. J Toxicol Clin Toxicol 42: 209-216.

9. Bartlett D (2004) The coma cocktail: indications, contraindications, adverse effects, proper dose, and proper route. J Emerg Nurs 30: 572-574.

10. Kitajima T, Kanbayashi T, Saito Y, Takahashi Y, Ogawa Y, et al. (2004) Diazepam reduces both arterial blood pressure and muscle sympathetic nerve activity in human. Neurosci Lett 355: 77-80.

11. Neckar J, Kopkan L, Huskova Z, Kolar F, Papousek F, et al. (2012) Inhibition of soluble epoxide hydrolase by cis-4-[4-(3-adamantan-1-ylureido)cyclohexyl-oxy]benzoic acid exhibits antihypertensive and cardioprotective actions in transgenic rats with angiotensin II-dependent hypertension. Clin Sci (Lond) 122: 513-525.

12. Imig JD, Zhao X, Zaharis CZ, Olearczyk JJ, Pollock DM, et al. (2005) An orally active epoxide hydrolase inhibitor lowers blood pressure and provides renal protection in salt-sensitive hypertension. Hypertension 46: 975-981.

13. Loch D, Hoey A, Morisseau C, Hammock BO, Brown L (2007) Prevention of hypertension in DOCA-salt rats by an inhibitor of soluble epoxide hydrolase. Cell Biochem Biophys 47: 87-98.

14. Liu JY, Qiu H, Morisseau C, Hwang SH, Tsai HJ, et al. (2011) Inhibition of soluble epoxide hydrolase contributes to the anti-inflammatory effect of antimicrobial triclocarban in a murine model. Toxicol Appl Pharmacol 255: 200-206.

15. Schmelzer KR, Kubala L, Newman JW, Kim IH, Eiserich JP, et al. (2005) Soluble epoxide hydrolase is a therapeutic target for acute inflammation. Proc Natl Acad Sci U S A 102: 9772-9777.

16. Ulu A, Harris TR, Morisseau C, Miyabe C, Inoue H, et al. (2013) Anti-inflammatory effects of omega-3 polyunsaturated fatty acids and soluble epoxide hydrolase inhibitors in angiotensin-II-dependent hypertension. J Cardiovasc Pharmacol 62: 285-297.

17. Inceoglu B, Zolkowska D, Yoo HJ, Wagner KM, Yang J, et al. (2013) Epoxy fatty acids and inhibition of the soluble epoxide hydrolase selectively modulate GABA mediated neurotransmission to delay onset of seizures. PLoS One 8: e80922.

18. Rose TE, Morisseau C, Liu JY, Inceoglu B, Jones PD, et al. (2010) 1-Aryl-3-(1-acylpiperidin-4-yl)urea inhibitors of human and murine soluble epoxide hydrolase: structure-activity relationships, pharmacokinetics, and reduction of inflammatory pain. J Med Chem 53: 7067-7075.

19. Yang J, Schmelzer K, Georgi K, Hammock BD (2009) Quantitative profiling method for oxylipin metabolome by liquid chromatography electrospray ionization tandem mass spectrometry. Anal Chem 81: 8085-8093.

20. Reagan-Shaw S, Nihal M, Ahmad N (2008) Dose translation from animal to human studies revisited. FASEB J 22: 659-661.

21. Kaur P, Kim K (2008) Pharmacokinetics and brain uptake of diazepam after intravenous and intranasal administration in rats and rabbits. Int J Pharm 364: 27-35.

22. Fenyk-Melody JE, Shen X, Peng Q, Pikounis W, Colwell L, et al. (2004) Comparison of the effects of perfusion in determining brain penetration (brain-to-plasma ratios) of small molecules in rats. Comp Med 54: 378-381.

23. Liu JY, Lin YP, Qiu H, Morisseau C, Rose TE, et al. (2013) Substituted phenyl groups improve the pharmacokinetic profile and anti-inflammatory effect of urea-based soluble epoxide hydrolase inhibitors in murine models. Eur J Pharm Sci 48: 619-627.

24. Ulu A, Appt S, Morisseau C, Hwang SH, Jones PD, et al. (2012) Pharmacokinetics and in vivo potency of soluble epoxide hydrolase inhibitors in cynomolgus monkeys. Br J Pharmacol 165: 1401-1412.

25. Inceoglu B, Jinks SL, Ulu A, Hegedus CM, Georgi K, et al. (2008) Soluble epoxide hydrolase and epoxyeicosatrienoic acids modulate two distinct analgesic pathways. Proc Natl Acad Sci U S A 105: 18901-18906.

26. Ulu A, Stephen Lee KS, Miyabe C, Yang J, Hammock BG, et al. (2014) An omega-3 epoxide of docosahexaenoic acid lowers blood pressure in angiotensin-II-dependent hypertension. J Cardiovasc Pharmacol 64: 87-99.

27. Ulu A, Davis BB, Tsai HJ, Kim IH, Morisseau C, et al. Soluble epoxide hydrolase inhibitors reduce the development of atherosclerosis in apolipoprotein e-knockout mouse model. J Cardiovasc Pharmacol 52: 314-323.

28. Cai R, Crane E, Poneleit K, Paulozzi L (2010) Emergency department visits involving nonmedical use of selected prescription drugs in the United States, 2004-2008. J Pain Palliat Care pharmacother 24: 293-297.

29. Djordjevic S, Jovic-Stosic J, Kilibarda V, Segrt Z, Perkovic-Vukcevic N (2016) Determination of flumazenil in serum by liquid chromatography-mass spectrometry: Application to kinetics study in acute diazepam overdose. Vojnosanit pregl 73: 146-51.

30. Veiraiah A, Dyas J, Cooper G, Routledge PA, Thompson JP (2012) Flumazenil use in benzodiazepine overdose in the UK: a retrospective survey of NPIS data. Emerg Med J 29: 565-569.

31. Gerak LR, France CP (2012) Quantitative analyses of antagonism: combinations of midazolam and either flunitrazepam or pregnanolone in rhesus monkeys discriminating midazolam. J Pharmacol Exp Ther 340: 742-749.

32. Galea S, Worthington N, Piper TM, Nandi VV, Curtis M, et al. (2006) Provision of naloxone to injection drug users as an overdose prevention strategy: early evidence from a pilot study in New York City. Addict Behav 31: 907-912.

33. Kanagarajan K, Marraffa JM, Bouchard NC, Krishnan P, Hoffman RS, et al. (2007) The use of vasopressin in the setting of recalcitrant hypotension due to calcium channel blocker overdose. Clin Toxicol (Phila) 45: 56-59.

34. Overgaard CB, Dzavík V (2008) Inotropes and vasopressors: review of physiology and clinical use in cardiovascular disease. Circulation 118: 1047-1056.

35. de Morais HH, Barbalho JC, de Holanda Vasconcellos RJ, Landim FS, da Costa Araujo FA, et al. (2015) Comparative study of hemodynamic changes caused by diazepam and midazolam during third molar surgery: a randomized controlled trial. Oral Maxillofac surg 19: 267-273.

36. Frolich MA, Arabshahi A, Katholi C, Prasain J, Barnes S (2011) Hemodynamic characteristics of midazolam, propofol, and dexmedetomidine in healthy volunteers. J Clin Anesth 23: 218-223.

37. Zhang G, Panigrahy D, Mahakian LM, Yang J, Liu JY, et al. (2013) Epoxy metabolites of docosahexaenoic acid (DHA) inhibit angiogenesis, tumor growth, and metastasis. Proc Natl Acad Sci U S A 110: 6530-6535.

38. Imig JD (2015) Epoxyeicosatrienoic acids, hypertension, and kidney injury. Hypertension 65: 476-482.

39. Kodani SD, Hammock BD2 (2015) The 2014 Bernard B. Brodie award lecture-epoxide hydrolases: drug metabolism to therapeutics for chronic pain. Drug Metab Dispos 43: 788-802.

40. Morisseau C, Hammock BD (2013) Impact of soluble epoxide hydrolase and epoxyeicosanoids on human health. Annu Rev Pharmacol Toxicol 53: 37-58.

41. Ren Q, Ma M, Ishima T, Morisseau C, Yang J, et al. (2016) Gene deficiency and pharmacological inhibition of soluble epoxide hydrolase confers resilience to repeated social defeat stress. Proc Natl Acad Sci U S A 113: E1944-52.

16

In-vitro Evaluation of Antimicrobial Branded Herbal Formulations for their Efficacy

Faheem Jan[1], Ifthekhar Hussain[2], Naveed Muhammad[3*], Muhammad Adnan Khan[4], Mazhar Ali Khan[1], Muhammad Taj Akbar[1] and Waqas Ahmad[5]

[1]Department of Microbiology, Hazara University, Mansehra, Pakistan

[2]Department of Pharmacy, Hazara University, Havelian Campus, Abbottabad, Pakistan

[3]Department of Phamacy, Abdul Wali Khan University Mardan, KPK, Pakistan

[4]Microbiologist BF- Biosciences Ltd Lahore Pakistan

[5]Faculty of Pharmacy University of Sargodha, Sargodha, Pakistan

*Corresponding author: Naveed Muhammad, Department of Pharmacy, Abdul Wali Khan University Mardan, KPK, Pakistan, E-mail: drnaveedrph@gmail.com

Abstract

In the present research work forty six herbal antimicrobial branded products were investigated for their antibacterial/antifungal activities using well diffusion method. Those herbal products were collected from local market which were manufactured by well-known herbal manufacturer and have clear recommendations against various microbial infections. These antimicrobial products were tested on the basis of pathogeneses caused by different microorganisms as indicated on the label. Among the tested branded formulations, only nine herbal preparations exhibited better antimicrobial activities, while rest of herbal formulations were devoid of antimicrobial effect. B34 and B30 demonstrated antibacterial activity when tested against *Salmonella paratyphi* B18 was the only product, which showed activity against *Pseudomonas aeruginosa* The pathogenic fungi *Candida albican* that causes various infections was sensitive to herbal products like B42, B41, B43 and B14 as like to their sensitivity to antifungal drug (Griseofulvin). The results of the present study indicated the poor quality of herbal products being sold in the market with very high label claims. Only 9 out of 46 sampled products with antimicrobial label claimed qualify to some extent for medicinal use. As any health authority (DRA/MOH) in Pakistan does not regulate the herbal products, there was no control or check on the manufacturers and prescriber of these medicines. All the tested products contained herbs, which had proven data for their antimicrobial activity, still most of them failed to produce any pharmacological results.

Keywords: Antimicrobial; Branded herbal formulations; Antibacterial and antifungal

Introduction

In last few years exploring of herbs used for medicinal purposes, which may be safe, economical and easily available to the consumers as well as resistance of disease, causing organisms should be minimum or no development of resistance. The efficacy of more plant species has been determined through scientific validation but most herbal remedies used may cause serious toxic effects and also drug-drug interaction because these herbal remedies may not undergo careful scientific evaluation. Ongoing researches are required to explain the pharmacological activities of many herbal remedies being used [1]. As the environmental conditions, such as the type of soil and cultivation, methods may affect the natural composition of the constituents in a plant so the ingredient that may cause a specific antimicrobial effect is not known. The antimicrobial activity of most plants have been determined but majority of them have not been evaluated properly [2]. A source of antimicrobial activity has been reported from many plants therefore these plants may be used as a source of effective and powerful drugs in different countries of the world [3]. Ointments containing Aloe vera, Neem and Turmeric exhibited broad spectrum anti-bacterial and anti-fungal activitites against *E. coli, S. aureus, Pseudomonas aeruginosa B. subtilis .A. ruius .A. nigri and P. notatum*

[4]. Medicinal plant parts may be collected either in small quantities for use by the local communities and folk healers or in larger quantities for many herbal manufacturers for extracts as raw drugs because they possess different medicinal properties [5]. The main objectives of the current study were, to evaluate the antimicrobial branded herbal formulations for their efficacy and awareness of the public about blind use of these herbal formulations.

Materials and Methods

This research study was performed at the Department of Microbiology, Hazara University, Mansehra, Pakistan. All the experimental equipment and materials were supplied by the said department.

Samples collection

Forty six herbal branded formulations were purchased from the local market.

Apparatus used

Pre sterilized glass petri dishes, Metallic borer, volumetric flask, Pyrex A (Germany), Sanyo labo autoclave, MLS-3780, S,NO-2Y0301 Phase, Company Sanyo electric co, Ltd Made in Japan, Streamline

Horizontal laminar flow cabinet, ESCO. En 1822.1 class H 13. HEPA filters, ISO 14644.1 Class 4. IEC 61010-1, US Federal standard 209E Class 10, Uni-Bloc SHIMADZU. Capacity Maximum 220 g and Minimum 10mg. SHIMADZU corporation made in Japan, Irmeco hybridization Oven. Digital constant temperature tank (China). Item-Model VRN-360. RPM 60-230 +10, Gemmy industrial corp (Taiwan).

In vitro antimicrobial studies of selected herbal branded formulations

The herbal branded formulations were tested by Agar Well Diffusion Techniques as described by [6]. Different concentrations of the extract were used for testing. For the agar well diffusion method, Mueller Hinton agar plates were seeded with standard inoculation of the microorganisms being tested. Herbal branded formulations were studied for their antimicrobial activity against the selected experimental microorganisms.

Applications of herbal medicines

Wells of 6 mm diameter were prepared in the plates with a sterile metal borer and five, 10, 15, 20, 25 and 100 microlitres of the already prepared test samples were pipette directly into the wells. These plates were incubated overnight at 37°C [7]. The antimicrobial potential of test compound was determined on the basis of diameter of zone of inhibition around the wells [8]. The test was carried out in triplicate and the mean zones of inhibition were calculated. For each bacterial strain, controls were included that comprised of sterile water (in the case of the aqueous extract) or ethanol (in the case of the ethanolic extract). Other wells were supplemented with 10 µg ciprofloxacin. Griseofulvin antifungal discs were used as standard drug. The zones of inhibition were then measured after 24 hrs incubation period. All the experiments were conducted in triplicate [9]. In case, ethanol was used as solvent, calculated the effective zone size of the test samples the zone size of the negative control (ethanol) was subtracted from the total zone of inhibition size.

Results

Antibacterial effects against *Escherichia coli*

Twenty-eight herbal products were tested for their antibacterial activity against *E. coli* All the tested products were clinically used against all pathogenic condition caused by *E. coli*. The manufacturer of these tested herbal formulations claim that these herb are used for various infections. It is clear that the drops of B14 has maximum inhibitory activity against this gram negative bacterium with zone of inhibition 25 mm. The syrup B8 showed weak activity against *E. coli* with mean zone of inhibition 7 mm. B11 and B41 also showed activity against the tested bacterium with zone of inhibition 15 and 13 mm respectively. The antibacterial effects of these products were compared with standard broad spectrum antibacterial drug (ciprofloxacin) having 26 mm zone size. It was very surprising to note that twenty four tested products failed to show antibacterial activity although the label of all these products indicated that these products were being used in various bacterial infections (Table 1).

S.No	Test samples	Resistant	Sensitive	Zones of inhibition
1	B1 (syrup)	R	-	-
2	B2 (syrup)	R	-	-
3	B14 (drops)	-	S	25 ± 1.23 mm
4	B3 (syrup)	R	-	-
5	B32 (syrup)	R	-	-
6	B18 (syrup)	R	-	-
7	B33 (syrup)	R	-	-
8	B26 (syrup)	R	-	-
9	B28 (syrup)	R	-	-
10	B5 (syrup)	R	-	-
11	B6 (syrup)	R	-	-
12	B11 (syrup)	-	S	15 ± 2.13 mm
13	B27 (syrup)	R	-	-
14	B23 (syrup)	R	-	-
15	B7 (syrup)	R	-	-
16	B8 (syrup)	-	S	7 ± 1.34 mm
17	B9 (syrup)	R	-	-
18	B44 (syrup)	R	-	-
19	B24 (syrup)	R	-	-
20	B12 (syrup)	R	-	-
21	B43(Oil)	R	-	-
22	B29 (Powder)	R	-	-
23	B11 (Tablet)	R	-	-
24	B12 (Ointment)	R	-	-
25	B38 (Ointment)	R	-	-
26	B45 (Ointment)	R	-	-
27	J B11 (Ointment)	R	-	-
28	B41 (Ointment)	-	S	13 ± 2.87 mm
	Ciprofloxacin (standard)	-	S	26 ± 0.09 mm

Table 1: Antibacterial potential of various herbal branded formulations against *Escherichia coli*.

Antibacterial effects against *Staphylococcus aureus*

Twenty-seven herbal formulations were tested against S. aureus. Out of tested samples only B11 exhibited antibacterial effects against S. aureus with zones of inhibition 20 mm and rest of samples were devoid of antibacterial effect (Table 2).

S.No	Test samples	Resistant	Sensitive	Zones of inhibition
01	B1 (syrup)	R	-	-
02	B16 (syrup)	R	-	-
03	B32 (syrup)	R	-	-
04	B17 (syrup)	R	-	-
05	B18 (syrup)	R	-	-
06	B19 (syrup)	R	-	-
07	B22B21 (syrup)	R	-	-
08	B28(syrup)	R	-	-
09	B5 (syrup)	R	-	-
10	B6 (syrup)	R	-	-
11	B11 (syrup)	-	S	20 ± 2.87 mm
12	B24 (syrup)	R	-	-
13	B7(syrup)	R	-	-
14	B8 (syrup)	R	-	-
15	B9 (syrup)	R	-	-
16	B44 (syrup)	R	-	-
17	B10 (syrup)	R	-	-
18	B32 (syrup)	R	-	-
19	B23 (syrup)	R	-	-
20	B43(Oil)	R	-	-
21	B21 (Ointment)	R	-	-
22	B37 (Cream)	R	-	-
23	B38 (Ointment)	R	-	-
24	B45 (Ointment)	R	-	-
25	B24(Ointment)	R	-	-
26	B2(Ointment)	R	-	-
27	B41 (Ointment)	R	-	-
	Ciprofolxacin (standard)	-	S	26 ± 0.08 mm

Table 2: Antibacterial potentials of various herbal branded formulations against *Staphylococcus aureus*.

Antibacterial effects against *Salmonella paratyphi*

Five herbal products were tested against *S.paratyphi* as the labels of these products indicated that these products are recommended in the treatment of *S. paratyphi* infections. Out of tested products *B34* and *B30* exhibited significant effect against tested bacteria. The zone of inhibition of *B34* and *B30* are 19 and 17 mm, respectively (Table 3).

S.No	Test samples	Resistant	Sensitive	Zones of inhibition
01	B30 (syrup)	-	S	17 ± 2.87 mm
02	B31 (syrup)	R	-	-
03	B32 (syrup)	R	-	-
04	B33 (syrup)	R	-	-
05	B34 (syrup)	-	S	19 ± 1.34 mm
	Ciprofloxacin (standard)	-	S	24 ± 0.07 mm

Table 3: Antibacterial potentials of various herbal branded formulations against *S. paratyphi*.

Antibacterial effects against *Shigella dysenteriae*

Fifteen herbal branded formulations were tested for their antibacterial effects against *Shigella dysenteriae*. Among the tested products only B11 showed significant activity had mean zones of inhibition 19 mm and rest of antimicrobial products showed resistance. The activity of the test samples were compared with Standard anti-bacterial drug with zone of inhibition 20 mm (Table 4).

S.No	Test samples	Resistant	Sensitive	Zones of inhibition
1	B1 (syrup)	R	-	-
2	B1 (syrup)	R	-	-
3	B3 (syrup)	R	-	-
4	B18 (syrup)	R	-	-
5	B26 (syrup)	R	-	-
6	B5 (syrup)	R	-	-
7	B6 (syrup)	R	-	-
8	B11 (syrup)	-	S	19 ± 1.23 mm
9	B27 (syrup)	R	-	-
10	B7(syrup)	R	-	-
11	B8 (syrup)	R	-	-
12	B29 (Powder)	R	-	-
13	B9 (syrup)	R	-	-
14	B10 (syrup)	R	-	-
15	B45 (tablet)	R	-	-
	Ciprofloxacin (standard)	-	S	20 ± 0.06 mm

Table 4: Antibacterial potentials of various herbal branded formulations against *Shigella dysenteriae*.

Antibacterial effect against *Pseudomonas aeruginosa*

Twenty-five herbal formulations were tested against *P. aeruginosa*. These formulations are indicated against *P. aeruginosa* infections. Among the tested samples only B18 was active with mean zone of inhibition 12 mm (Table 5).

S.No	Test samples	Resistant	Sensitive	Zones of inhibition
01	B1 (Syrup)	R	-	-
02	B15 (syrup)	R	-	-
03	B16 (syrup)	R	-	-
04	B17 (syrup)	R	-	-
05	B18 (Syrup)	-	S	12 ± 1.25 mm
06	B19 (syrup)	R	-	-
07	B20 (syrup)	R	-	-
08	B21 (syrup)	R	-	-
09	B33 (Syrup)	R	-	-
10	B26 (syrup)	R	-	-
11	B28 (syrup)	R	-	-
12	B27 (syrup)	R	-	-
13	B24 (syrup)	R	-	-
14	B44 (syrup)	R	-	-
15	B34 (syrup)	R	-	-
16	B23 (syrup)	R	-	-
17	B25 (syrup)	R	-	-
18	B25 (syrup)	R	-	-
19	B43 (Oil)	R	-	-
20	B29 (Powder)	R	-	-
21	B33 (Ointment)	R	-	-
22	B37 (Cream)	R	-	-
23	B41 (Ointment)	R	-	-
24	B12 (Ointment)	R	-	-
25	B41 (Ointment)	R	-	-
	Ciprofloxacin (standard)	-	S	14 ± 0.14 mm

Table 5: Antibacterial potential of various herbal branded formulations against *Pseudomonas aeruginosa*.

Antibacterial effects against *Salmonella typhimurium*

None of the tested formulations were effective against *Salmonella typhimurium* (Table 6).

S.No	Test samples	Resistant	Sensitive	Zones of inhibition
1	B1 (Syrup)	R	-	-
2	B11 (Syrup)	R	-	-
3	B7 (Syrup)	R	-	-

Table 6: Antibacterial potential of various herbal branded formulations against *Salmonella typhimurium*.

Antifungal activity against *Candida albicans*

Ten herbal branded formulations were tested for the determination of their antifungal activity. Out of the tested products four products showed activity against *Candida albicans* with zone of inhibition 26 mm, 5 mm, 4 mm and 6 mm respectively. Surprisingly B14 showed better result than Griseofulvin the standard anti-fungal drug (Table 7).

S.No	Test sample	Resistant	Sensitive	Zone of inhibition
1	B23	R	-	-
2	B35	R	-	-
3	B14	-	S	26 ± 1.23 mm
4	B37	R	-	-
5	B38		S	5 ± 2.14 mm
6	B45 Marham	R	-	-
7	B46	R	-	-
8	B40	R	-	-
9	B43		S	4 ± 0.82 mm
10	B41		S	6 ± 1.23 mm
	Griseofulvin (standard)		S	17 ± 0.11 mm

Table 7: Antifungal activity against *Candida albican*.

Discussion

The scope of present study is to evaluate the antimicrobial activity of various herbs in the form of final dosage form. Herbal products are available in different dosage form like syrups, capsules, tablets, powder, ointments, emulsions and herbal teas. A number of herbal manufacturing companies have surfaced and established well equipped manufacturing units throughout Pakistan. Some of them are enjoying a very good business position while others are struggling. Botanical medicine has become a topic of increasing global importance, with both medicinal and economic implications. The numerous reports of adverse effects and widespread sale of adulterated products and misleading health claims of these products demand proper regulations on botanical medicine [10]. Depending on the particular country and existing legislation, herbal products used for diagnosis, cure, mitigation, treatment, or prevention of diseases are normally regulated as drugs. However, in some countries, including the United States, botanical products are marketed as "dietary supplement". Other countries treat the herbal preparations as drugs, and to be registered these products need to be tested to prove their safety and clinical efficacy. However, so far, few programs have been established to study the safety and efficacy of herbal medicines as originally proposed by the WHO Guidelines for the assessment of herbal medicines [11,12]. Currently, no organization or government body regulates the manufacture or certifies the labeling of herbal preparations. This means there is no assurance that the amount of the herb contained in the bottle or even from dose to dose, is the same as what is stated on the label. However, it is still important to ask companies that are making standardized herbal products the basis for their product's guarantee. It is still important to consult a doctor or an expert in herbal medicine for the recommended doses of any herbal products [13]. Drug regulatory agency (DRA) of Pakistan has recently been established and is in process of completing its structure. The tasks assigned to DRA were previously carried out by Ministry of Health of Pakistan (MOH), which has been dissolved. Affairs related to drugs/ medicines are governed by Drug Act of Pakistan 1976 with few amendments. But Drug Act of Pakistan 1976 only addresses the Allopathic medicines, while the Herbal/ Unani/ Homeopathic medicines do not qualify the definition of drug as per Drug Act. A drug may be any substance or mixture of substance that is manufactured, sold, stored, offered, for sale or represented for internal or external use in the treatment, mitigation, prevention or diagnosis of disease, an abnormal physical state or the symptoms thereof in human being or animals or the restoration, correction or modification of organic function in human being or animals. Not being a substance exclusively used or prepared for use in accordance with the Ayurvedic, Unani, Homeopathic or Biochemical system of treatment except those substances and in accordance with such condition as may be prescribed [14,15]. Tables 8-12 shows list of herbal products purchased from the market and their ingredients (herbs). Literature review in Table 1 shows all these herbs have a strong research data for their pharmacological activities. Almost every sample product contains one or more herbs having reported antimicrobial activity supporting the label claims of these products. But the present study shows that only few products have shown promising results against the selected strains.

Medicine name	Manufacturer	Ingredients used
B1	Aftab Qarshi	Pomegranate bark, *Clitoria ternatea, Curcuma zerumbet, Foeniculum vulgare*
B2	Dawakhana Hakim Ajmal Khan	Rosa damascene mil, *Foeniculum vulgare, Polygonumbistora, Helicteres isora, Phyllanthus, Amomum subulatum*
B3	Falcon Herbal Lab	*Rosa damascene, Cinnamomum zeylanicum, Hyssopus Officinalis, Kamoon sufaid, Mangifera indica,* Danheel, Grape seed, *Menthasylvestris, Coriandrumsativum,* Sodium bicarbonate, Satelimon, Turang, Sirkadesi, *Punica granatum, Pruns domestica, Foeniculum vulgare,* Sodium chloride, QandSufaid.
B4	Qarshi	*Acacia arabica* wild, *Punica granatum, Foeniculum vulgare, Myrtus communis*
B5	Wasay Lab	*Mentha sylvestris, Peucedanum graveolens, Foeniculum vulgare, Cinnamomum zeylanicum, Rawand khatai, Myrtus communis, Polygonumbistora*
B6	Al-Majid Herbal	As in B5
B7	Mumtaz Dawakhana	*Ptychotis ajowan, Punica granatum, Wrightia tinctoria, Bombax malabaricum, Cypreuss carious, Plantago major, Mentha sylvestris, Myrtus communis, Punica granatum, Ptychotis ajowan, Foeniculum vulgare, Tajqalmee, Ocimum gratissim, Tamarix gallica, Polygonumbistora*
B8	Mumtaz Dawakhana	*Mentha sylvestris, Carcuma cassia,* Post taranj, *Amomum subulatum, Rosa damascene,* Samakdana
B9	Master Unani	*Amomum subulatum, Hyssopus officinalis, Mentha sylvestris, Punica granatum,* Namaksiah, *Ptychotis ajowan, Cinnamomum zeylanicum, Myristica fragrano, Valeriane offecinalis, Mentha sylvestris, Camphor.*
B10	Ashraf Lab	*Acacia arabica, Punica granatum, Myrtus communis, Psidium guajava, Cydonia oblonga, Pyrus malus.*
B11	Qarshi	*Punica granatum, Mentha sylvestris, Amomum subulatum, Citrus limonum* *Valeriana officinalis, Rosa damascene, Coriandrum sativum, Pistacia vera*
B12	Falcon	*Foeniculum vulgare, Ptychotis ajowan, Mentha sylvestris, Coriandrum stivum, Cinnamomum tamala, Amomum subulatum, Apium graveolens, Mentha sylvestris,* Qandsufaid
B13	(Al-majid herbal pharma)	*Glycyrrhiza glabra, Ocimum gratissim,* Ispaghol husk, *Pistacia lentiscum,* Tokhm-e bartang, *Phyllanthus, Ptychotis ajowan*

Table 8: List of herbal formulations used for the treatment of GIT disorders. (Colitis due to dysentery, diarrhea, gastritis and enteritis, acute and chronic dysentery, useful for intestinal ulcers, Cholera. For watery and bloody diarrhea and gastrointestinal weakness and cramps, gastralgia, peptic ulcer).

Medicine name	Manufacturer	Ingredients used
B14	Qarshi	*Camphora officinarum, Mentha pipriata oil, Ptychotis ajowan oil, Foeniclum vulgare oil, Pistacia terebinthus oil, Populus euphratica* oil

B15	Ashraf Lab	*Ptychotis ajowan, Curcuma Longa, Urginea indica, Foenicullum vulgare, Mentha arvensis, Ephedra vulgaris, Adhatoda vasica, Calotropis gigantea, Lobelia, Polygala senega, Papaver somniferum, Glycyrrhiza glabra, Rhus succedanea, Linum usitatissimum, Piper cubeba, Piper longum, Zingiber officinale.*
B16	Qarshi	*Ephedra vulgaris,* Ammoniichloridum, *Glycyrrhiza glabra, Adhatoda vasica*
B17	Ashraf lab	*Glycyrrhiza glabra, Cichorium intybus, Tinospora cordifolia, Hyssopus officinalis, Viola odorata, Polygala senega, Ephedra vulgaris, Scilla serrata, Sisymbrium irio, Ficus carica, Ptychotis ajowan, Bombyx mori*
B18	Qarshi	*Ephedra vulgaris, Papaver somniferum, Glycyrrhiza glabra, Adhatoda vasica, Rhus succedanea, Achyranthus aspera, Mentha piperita*
B19	AftabQarshi	*Adhatoda vasica, Glycyrrhiza glabra, Adiantum capillus-veneris, Ptychotis ajowan, Ephhedra vulgaris.*
B20	Riazdawakhana	*Adhatodavasica, Calotropis, Curcuma longa, Ephedra, Eucalyptus, Foeniculumvulgare, Foeniculumvulgare, Lyceum barbarum, Menthe arvensis, Papaversomniferum, Pimpinellaanisum, PtychotisajowanScilla, Trigonellafoenumgraecum.*
B22	Ashraf Lab	*Ehphedra vulgaris, Glycyrrhizaglabra, Polygala senega, Adhatodavasica, Plumbicarbonas, Papaversomniferum, Menthaarvensis, Foeniculumvulgare, Lobelia nicotianaefolia.*
B11	New Pak	*Adhatodavasica, Hyssopusofficinalis, Althoeraofficinalis, Zizyphussativus, Ficuscarica, Adiantumcapillus-veneris, Piper betle, Glycyrrhizaglabra, Viola odorata, Malvasylvestris, Sande, Cordiamyxa, Ephedra vulgaris.*
B23	AftabQarshi	*Onosmabrcateatum, Hyssopusofficinalis, Viola odorata, Rhus succedanea, Cordiamyxa, Ephedra vulgaris, Glycyrrhizaglabra, Zizyphussativus, B25B24, Foeniculumvulgare.*
B25	AftabQarshi	*Morusnigra.*
B25	Falcon	*Morusnigra (extract), Glycyrrhizaglabra.*

Table 9: List of herbal formulations used for Respiratory Tract Infections (RTIs).

B26	Otogen	*Small caltrops, Sanataium white, Coriandrumsativum, Carbonate of potash, Postassinitras, Tinosporiacordifolia, Cucumber.*
B27	MumtazDawakhana	B27 juice, Sugarcane vinegar, *Potassium carbonate,* Peter Salt, *Helmintholithusjudiacus, Ptychotisajowan*
B28	Ashraf lab	*Emblicaofficinalis, Terminaliachebula (raw), Terminaliablerica, Vitexnegundo, Artemisia absinthium, Meliaazadirach , Alhagimaurorum, Azadirachtaindica, Azadirachtaindica, Centaureasolsitialis, Citrulluscolocynthis, Sphaeranthusindicus, Tephrosapurpurea, Fagoniacretica, Smilexofficinalis, Swertiachirata, Fumariaofficinalis, Achilleamillefolium, Zizyphussativus*
B29	Qarshi	*Calcined oyster shell, Datura alba, Rheum emodi, Zingibarofficinale* 34.4mg.

Table 10: List of herbal formulations used for Urinary Tract Infections (UTIs)

B30	AftabQarshi	*Caesalpinabonducella, Foeniculumvulgare, Sisymbriumirio, Glycyrrhizaglabra, Vicisvinifera, Fumariaofficinalis, Ficuscarica,* Ammonium chloride, *Tinsporacardifilia,* Miers,Alum,*Ptychotisajowan.*
B31		
B32	Ashraf	*Tinosporiacardifolia, Cichoriumintybus, Nymphaea alba , Azadiracchtaindica, Fumariaofficinalis,Pterocarpussantalinus, Glycyrrhizaglabra, Foeniculumvulgare, Sphaeranthushirtus, Ext glycyrrhiza, Berbreisaristata,* Ammonium chloride.
B33	Qarshi	*Tinosporacordifolia, Meliaazadirachta, Swertiachirata, Glycyrrhizaglabra, Sisymbriumirio , Ptychotisajowan, Fumariaofficinalis, Solanumnigram*
B34	Qarshi	*SisymbriumIrio, Zizyphus Vulgaris, Glycyrrhizaglabra, FicusCarica, AmomumSublatum, Oyster shell, Zinc Murakab, Foeniculumvulgare.*

Table 11: Medicines used for treating different type of temperatures.

Aafaqee	Al-shifadawakhana.	Graphites, *Calendula,* Canthris, Hydrastis, Sulphur, Carbovrg, Glycerin, Vasline.

B35	Kent Homoeopathic Pharmacy	Berb. Equif, *Calendula,MatricariarecutitaEchinacea angustfolia, Emblicaofficinalis, Hydrocotyleasiatica,* Kali brom, *Thujaoccidentalis.*
B37	Q-Sons	*Hydrocotyleasiatica, Echinacea angustfolia, Emblicaofficinalis, Calendula, Thujaoccidentalis.*
B38	Unanifakiri	Sat loban, *Camphor*, Borax, *Plumbimonoxidum*, Kashgharisufaida, *Menthasylvestris*, Kanreet, Gadalfaza, *Ptychotisajowan.*
B46B39	Hamdard	*Camphoraofficinarums , Oleum eucalypti, Thymol, Oleum turpentine, Ferula gummosa,* Chlorophyll col
B40	JalilJildiUnaniDawakhana	Sulphur, *Psoralea corylifolia,* Copper Sulphate, Hydrargyri subchloridum, Sulsufaid.
B41	AL-Chemist	Jastphool, Boric acid, *Styrax benzoin, Ptychotisajowan, Menthasylvestris, Cinnamomumcamphora,* Nees, Vasline.
Musaffi	AftabQarshi	*Swertiachirata, Fumariaofficinalis, Sphaeranthushirtus, Zizyphus vulgaris, Fagoniaarbica, Artemisia absinthium, Meliaazadirachta, Lowsonia alba*
B24	Qarshi	*Tinosporacardifolia, Fumariaofficinalis, Swertiachirata, Sphaeranthushirtus, Artemisia vulgaris, Terminaliachebula, Tephrosiapurpurea, Zizphus vulgaris, Meliaazadirachta, Lycopodiumclavatum*
B44	Ashraf Lab	*Pterocarpus Santalinus, Azadirachtaindica, Fumariaindica, Swertiachirata, Smilax china,Smilaxofficinalis, Sphaeranthusindicus, Tephrosiapurpurea,* Cassia tora *(seeds), Prunusdomestica, Ipomoea turpethum, Terminaliachebula (raw), Cassia angustifolia, Cuscutareflexa, Zizyphussativus, Artemisia absinthium*

Table 12: Medicines used for different types of skin disease

Conclusion

The results of the present study indicated the poor quality of herbal products being sold in the market with very high label claims. Only 9 out of 46 sampled products with antimicrobial label claimed qualify to some extent for medicinal use. As any health authority (DRA/MOH) in Pakistan does not regulate the herbal products, there was no control or check on the manufacturers and prescriber of these medicines. All the tested products contained herbs, which had proven data for their antimicrobial activity, still most of them failed to produce any pharmacological results. We can conclude any of the following reasons.

1.These products had not been produced by the professional people.

2. They had not been processed properly.

3. Selection of herbal ingredients was not proper. Quality assurance played important role to monitor such shortcomings.

4. Common extraction processes for herbal product manufacturing were decoction, distillation, infusion, maceration and percolation. These processes need trained employees and appropriate equipment. Any deficiency in provision of both of these may lead to poor quality.

Recommendations

It is necessary to identify and rectify these problems immediately. Following recommendations were made based on present study:

1. Proper legislation must be done to regulate the manufacturing and prescription of Herbal/ Unani/Homeopathic medicines.

2. Only qualified pharmacists must be allowed to supervise the manufacturing of such products. The role of Botanist/Phytochemist is necessary for proper identification of herbs and their extraction process.

3. The herbal manufacturing industries should be issued manufacturing licenses as is done in case of pharmaceutical industries.

a. Herbal manufacturing industries should be forced to establish well equipped quality control labs to ascertain the efficacy and safety of their products.

4. Quality assurance is required to monitor all the activities related to identification, collection, drying, transportation, storage, and extraction of herbs, manufacturing of herbal product, stability of formulation, quality control and marketing.

5. As the properties of soil to soil vary it is impossible to procure or collect herbs with similar phytoconstituents every time, every industry must have its own Research and Development department (R&D).

References

1. Dhamija HK, Ankit SC (2011) Herbs Now in arena of hyperlipidaemia, Der Pharmacia Sinica 2: 51-59.

2. Balandrin MF, Klocke JA, Wurtele ES, Bollinger WH (1985) Natural plant chemicals: sources of industrial and medicinal materials. Science 228: 1154-1160.

3. Srivastava J, Lambert J, Vietmeyer N (1996) Medicinal plants: An expanding role in development," World Bank Technical Paper 320.

4. Pandey A, Jui VJ, Patil AA, Joshi RN, Kuchekar BS (2010) Formulation and evaluation of anti-bacterial and anti-fungal activity of a B46 containing Aloe-vera, Azadirachtaindica and Curcuma- longa. J Chem Pharm Res, 2: 182-186.

5. Uniyal SK, Singh KN, Jamwal P, Lal B (2006) Traditional use of medicinal plants among the tribal Candida albicans and Neisseria gonorrhea communities of ChhotaBhangal, Western Himalayan. J EthnobiolEthnomed 2: 14-21 2006.

6. Perez C, Paul M, Bazerque P (1990) An antibiotic assay by the agar well diffusion. MethodActa Biology and Medicine 15: 113-115.

7. Sumitra S, Sharma SK (2005) Antibacterial Activity of Essential Oil and Root extract of Eucalyptus teriticornis. Indian Journal of Natural Products 21: 6-17.

8. Barkatullah I, Muhammad N, Muhammad, Lubna T (2012) Antimicrobial evaluation, determination of total phenolic and flavoniod contents in Zanthoxylumarmatum DC. Journal of Medicinal Plants Research 6: 2105-2110.

9. Marcus DM, Grollman AP (2002) Botanical medicines--the need for new regulations. N Engl J Med 347: 2073-2076.

10. Bulletin of the World Health Organization (1993) Research guidelines for evaluating the safety and efficacy of herbal medicine 1-86.

11. Akerele O (1993) Summary of WHO guidelines for the assessment of herbal Medicines.HerbalGram28: 13-19.

12. Blumenthal M, Brusse WR, Goldberg A, Gruenwald J, Hall T, et al. (1998) The Complete German Commission E Monographs: Therapeutic Guide to Herbal Medicines. The American Botanical Council, USA.

13. http://tnsop.net/doc/pdf/philippineculture__ph--filer--toledo-cebu--herbal-medicine.html

14. Akhtar S (1976) The Drug Act 1976 Act No xxx1of 1976 with Drug Rules. National Law book house 1- turner road Lahore. B to Z printers Lahore, Pakistan.

15. Barkatullah, Ibrar M, Muhammad N, Ur- Rehman I, Rehman MU (2013) Chemical Composition and Biological Screening of Essential Oils of Zanthoxylumarmatum DC Leaves. J ClinToxicol 3: 172

17

Neutrophil to Lymphocyte Ratio as a Predictor of Endoscopic Damage in Caustic Injuries

Seyit Uyar*

Antalya Training and Research Hospital, Antalya, Turkey

*****Corresponding author:** Seyit Uyar, Antalya Research Hospital, Antalya, Turkey, E-mail: seyituyar79@hotmail.com

Abstract

Context: The endoscopic degree of injuries is the main finding for further management of caustic ingestions. However, if endoscopy cannot be performed quickly, clinicians decide on treatment and follow-up goals according to the signs and symptoms of the patient. The aim of this study was to determine the association of white blood cells (WBC), C-reactive protein (CRP) and neutrophil-lymphocyte ratio (NLR) with the degree of caustic injury and to evaluate whether NLR is able to predict the severity of injuries.

Materials and methods: A retrospective evaluation was made of a total of 190 patients with a mean age of 38.6 years. WBC, neutrophil, lymphocyte and CRP values and endoscopic findings of all patients at hospital admission were retrieved from hospital files. The association between WBC, NLR, CRP and endoscopic findings was evaluated.

Results: Endoscopy was normal in 28 of 119 patients (23.5%) and most patients (42 of 119 (35.3%) had only gastric involvement. NLR was significantly higher in patients with injuries than normal patients (p=0.010), whereas WBC and CRP not. NLR was also significantly higher in patients with both esophagus and gastric injuries compared to patients with no organ involvement (p<0.001). NLR, WBC and CRP were weakly correlated to the grade of involvement. In the ROC analysis, the AUC value was 0.914 (95% CI (0.85-0.96, p<0.001)) and the cut-off value for NLR was 8.71 with sensitivity of 90% and specificity of 91.7% for discriminating injuries as grade 0-1-2 from 3-4.

Conclusions: Higher NLR values showed widespread and severe involvement of caustic ingestion. NLR also seems to be a more reliable method to make a distinction between severe and mild injuries. It is an easily derived and inexpensive marker of inflammation and might guide the management of patients before endoscopic evaluation in emergency departments.

Keywords: Neutrophil; Inflammation; Carcinoma; Lymphocyte; Leukocytosis

Introduction

Caustic injuries remain a medical problem, which can cause serious damage to the gastrointestinal tract. Altough mainly seen in children, these injuries can also be seen in adults, both intentionally and accidentally [1]. Caustic ingestion may cause esophageal and gastric superficial edema, erythema, erosions, ulcerations, necrosis and ultimately perforation in the early period [2]. Patients with perforation have to be diagnosed without any loss of time, as immediate surgical intervention may be required [3]. Late sequelae of caustic injuries include strictures in the esophagus and stomach, gastric outlet obstruction, mucosal metaplasia and carcinoma [4]. These complications of caustic injuries are detected with upper gastrointestinal endoscopy and endoscopic findings are the major predictor of the formation of late complications [2,5]. However, endoscopy is not always feasible especially in developing countries where these events are common. The laboratory tests [6], computed tomography [7] and endoscopic ultrasound [8] were used for this purpose in different studies. White blood cell count (WBC), C-reactive protein (CRP), and arterial blood gas analysis are laboratory tests used in a few studies for prediction of degree of caustic injury and of late

sequeles. For example, Cheng et al. evaluated arterial blood gas analysis in caustic ingestions and concluded that arterial pH<7.22 or base excess<-12 indicate severe esophageal injury and the need for emergency surgery [9].

The neutrophil-lymphocyte ratio (NLR) is a method which is cost effective and readily available and could be an important measure of systemic inflammation [10]. It is used as an inflammatory marker in various diseases such as cancer, inflammatory disorders, hypertension, diabetes, obesity, hyperlipidemia and vascular diseases [10,11]. Elevated NLR levels are associated with poor survival and increased morbidity in various chronic conditions [12]. Elevated NLR levels have been associated with poor survival of patients undergoing coronary bypass surgery [13] and any cancer survival studies have also shown that NLR can be a significant predictor of overall and disease-specific survival of patients [14-16].

The aim of this study was to determine the WBC, NLR and CRP values of patients with corrosive injuries and to assess the correlation of these acute phase parameters with organ involvement and the degree of injury. It was also evaluated whether NLR could predict the endoscopic degree of caustic injuries.

Methods

A retrospective evaluation was made of patients with a diagnosis of corrosive ingestion admitted to the University of Health Sciences Antalya Training and Research Hospital between 2008 and 2016. WBC, neutrophil, lymphocyte and CRP values and the endoscopic findings of all patients at hospital admission were retrieved from hospital files. Since CRP of all patients were not tested, totally 67 patients were evaluated for CRP. Patients were excluded if endoscopy had not been applied, or if endoscopy was applied after 96 hours and without laboratory tests within the first six hours of hospital admission. Patients under the age of 18 years were also excluded from the study. The association between WBC, NLR, CRP and endoscopic findings was evaluated. The endoscopic classification of caustic injuries is shown in Table 1 [17].

Grade	Features
Grade 0	Normal
Grade 1	Superficial mucosal edema and erythema
Grade 2	Mucosal and submucosal ulcerations
Grade 2A	Superficial ulcerations, erosions, exudates
Grade 2B	Deep discrete or circumferential ulcerations
Grade 3	Transmural ulcerations with necrosis
Grade 3A	Focal necrosis
Grade 3B	Extensive necrosis
Grade 4	Perforations

Table 1: Endoscopic classification of caustic injuries.

The study protocol was applied in accordance with the principles of the Declaration of Helsinki. Approval for the study was granted by the Local Research Institutional Ethics Committee.

Results

A total of 190 patients (58 male, 61 female) with a mean age of 38.6 ± 15 years (range, 18-79 years) were evaluated. The median WBC count was 9 $10^3/mm^3$ (2.8-31 $10^3/mm^3$), median CRP level was 3 mg/dL (1-174 mg/dL), median neutrophil count was 5.6 $10^{\wedge 3}/mm^3$ (1.3-27.9 $10^3/mm^3$), median lymphocyte count was 2.1 $10^3/mm^3$ (0.4-5.2 $10^3/mm^3$) and median NLR was 2.7 (0.8-32.8). Endoscopy was normal in 28 of 119 patients (23.5%). Involvement was only esophageal in 12 (10.1%) patients, only gastric in 42 (35.3%) and both esophageal and gastric in 37 (31.1%) (Table 2).

Of the esophagus involved patients, 30 (61.2%) were grade 1, 15 (30.6%) were grade 2a, 3 (6.1%) were grade 2b, and 1 (2)% was grade 3a. Of the gastric involved patients, 55 (69.6%) were grade 1, 8 (10.1%) were grade 2a, 6 (7.6%) were grade 2b, 7 (8.8%) were grade 3a, 2 (2.5%) were grade 3b, and 1 (1.2%) was grade 4 (Table 2).

Age (years), mean ± sd		
38.6 ± 15		
Gender, n (%)	Male	58 (48.7)

	Female	61 (51.3)
WBC ($10^3/mm^3$), median (min-max)		9 (2.8-3.1)
	Neutrophil	5.6 (1.3-27.9)
	Lymphocyte	2.1 (0.4-5.2)
NLR, median (min-max)		2.7 (0.8-32-8)
CRP (mg/dL), median (min-max)		3 (1-174)
Caustic ingestion characteristics		
Organ involvement, n (%)	None	28 (23.5)
	Esophagus	12 (10.1)
	Stomach	42 (35.3)
	Esophagus+stomach	37 (31.1)
Grade of esopahgeal injury (n: 49), n (%)	Grade 1	30 (61.2)
	Grade 2a	15 (30.6)
	Grade 2b	3 (6.1)
	Grade 3a	1 (2)
	Grade 3b	0
	Grade 4	0
Grade of gastric injury (n: 79), n (%)	Grade 1	55 (69.6)
	Grade 2a	8 (10.1)
	Grade 2b	6 (7.6)
	Grade 3a	7 (8.8)
	Grade 3b	2 (2.5)
	Grade 4	1 (1.2)

WBC: white blood cell, NLR: neutrophil-lymphocyte ratio, CRP: C-reactive protein

Table 2: Patient demographic characteristics, involved organs and endoscopic grade of the injury.

The comparisons of the WBC, NLR and CRP values between injured and non-injured patients are shown in Table 3. WBC (9.1(2.8-31) vs. 8.75(6.7-15.5), p=0.573) and CRP (3(1-174) vs. 3(1-39), p=0.166) values were not significantly different in both group. NLR (2.9(1.02-32.8) vs. 2.2(0.8-11.8), p=0.010) was significantly higher in injured patients than normals. with organ involved than non-involved patients NLR (5(1.4-32.8) vs. 2.2(0.8-11.8), p<0.001) was significantly higher in patients with esophagus and gastric involvement compared to non-involved patients.

	Injured patients	Non-injured patients	p*
CRP (mg/dL)	3 (1-174)	3 (1-39)	0, 166
n	n:52	n:15	

WBC (10^{33}	9, 1 (2, 8-3, 1)	8, 75 (6, 7-15, 5)	0, 473
n	n:91	n:28	
NLR	2, 9 (1, 02-32, 8)	2, 2 (0, 8-11, 8)	0, 010
n	n:91	n:28	
Comparison of NLR values according to location of injury			
Esophagus (n:12)	2, 7 (1, 4-14, 8)		0, 199
Stomach (n:42)	2, 29 (1, 02-26)	2, 2 (08-11, 8)	0, 283
Esophagus+ Esophagus (n: 37)	5 (1, 4-32, 8)		0, 001

Table 3: Comparison of WBC, NLR and CRP values between injured and non-injured patients and comparison of NLR values according to location of injury.

There were no significant differences between patients with only esophagus or stomach involvement compared to non-involved patients in terms of NLR (Table 3).

All the variables (WBC (r=0.43, p=0.006), NLR (r=0.43, p<0.001) and CRP (r=0.29, p=0.019)) were determined to be weakly correlated to the grade of involvement (Table 4).

	Grade of injury	
	r*	p
NLR	0.43	<0.001
WBC (10^3/mm^3)	0.25	0.006
CRP (mg/dL)	0.29	0.019
*Spearman's rho		
WBC: white blood cell, NLR: neutrophil-lymphocyte ratio, CRP: C-reactive protein		

Table 4: Correlation between endoscopic grade of injury and NLR, WBC and CRP values.

ROC analysis was applied for the prediction of the grade of caustic injuries as 0 *vs.* 1-2-3-4 and as 0-1-2 *vs.* 3-4. The AUC (area under curve) value was 0.66 (95% CI (0.57-0.75, p=0.003) for prediction of the prsence of injury (Figure 1A) and the cut-off value for NLR was 2.56 with a sensitivity of 59.34% and specificity of 64.29% (Table 5).

	AUC	Cut-off value	Sensitivity (%)	Specificity (%)
NLR (Grade 0 *vs.* 1-2-3-4)	0.66, 95% CI (0.57-0.75, p=0.003)	2.56	59.34	64.29
NLR (Grade 0-1-2 *vs.* 3-4)	0.914, 95% CI (0.85-0.96, p<0.001)	8.71	90	91.7

Table 5: Estimates of NLR for discrimination of grade of caustic injuries.

Number of patients with NLR ≤ 2.56 was 55 and it was 64 for NLR>2.56. For discrimination of the grade of injuries as 0-1-2 from

3-4, the AUC value was 0.914 (95% CI (0.85-0.96, p<0.001)) (Figure 1B) and the cut-off value for NLR was 8.71 with sensitivity of 90% and specificity of 91.7% (Table 5). Number of patients with NLR >8.71 was 18.

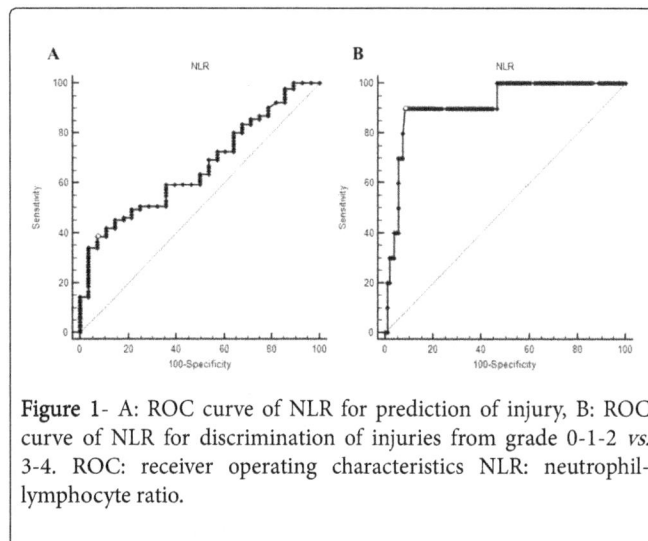

Figure 1- A: ROC curve of NLR for prediction of injury, B: ROC curve of NLR for discrimination of injuries from grade 0-1-2 *vs.* 3-4. ROC: receiver operating characteristics NLR: neutrophil-lymphocyte ratio.

Discussion

Caustic injuries may lead to irreversible catastrophic complications. Endoscopy is the gold standard for evaluation of caustic ingestions, but it can take time to apply. The initial signs and symptoms of patients are the main factors which determine the treatment and follow-up goals in emergency clinics before endoscopy. Betalli et al. reported that the presence of symptoms was the strongest predictor of severe esophageal lesions in a multi-centre observational study of a pediatric population [18]. Endoscopy is usually recommended in the first 12-48 hours after caustic ingestion [2] and is reliable for up to 96 hours after the injury [17]. The degree of injury determined on endoscopy is the major finding for patient management and prediction of complications. Generally, grade 0 and 1 lesions do not develop sequelae and morbidity and mortality also increase as the degree of injury increases [17]. Patients with grade 1 or 2A injury are permitted oral intake earlier and are generally discharged within days with antacid therapy. Patients with grade 2 or 3 injury however, are more severe cases and may need closer observation and may stay longer in hospital [2]. In the current study, the endoscopic findings of 28 patients (23.5%) were normal and most of the patients (42/119) had gastric involvement. Only 1 patient had a grade 4 gastric injury and a total of 10 patients had grade 3 injury of the esophagus or stomach.

Studies on laboratory values are limited in caustic injuries. In this study, the WBC and CRP values of patients in injured and non-injured group were not significantly different, whereas NLR was significantly higher in injured patients. While the NLR values were not different in the involvement of the esophagus or stomach separately, it was significantly higher in patients with both esophagus and stomach damaged than those of the patients with no organ involvement (p<0.001). In a paediatric population study, WBC count was found significantly more frequent in children with high-grade injury than low-grade injury [19]. The comparison groups were designed differently from ours and mean age of patients was 3.4 in that study. However, in a similar study by Chen et al. [20] found that there was no statistically significant difference in terms of WBC and CRP values between high-grade and low-grade injuries. In another study in patients with median age 22 years (min:2-max:61), WBC count was higher in high-grade injured patients [21]. Kaya et al. and Chen et al. reported that WBC count could not predict the severity of esophageal injury in these studies; however Hovanond et al. stated that WBC count was an independent predictor for high-grade injury. The prognostic relevance of leukocytosis was suggested another report by Rigo et al. [22]. They suggested that a WBC count $\geq$ 20.000 cells/m^3 should be considered a predictor of a poor outcome. There is no study evaluating NLR value and caustic injuries in the literature.

Although it was a weak correlation, WBC, NLR and CRP values were significantly correlated to the grade of injury in our study. AUC value was less than 80% for NLR greater than 2.56 for discrimination of grade 0 from 1-2-3-4 in ROC analysis. NLR greater than 8.71 was a significantly good diagnostic marker for the differentiation of mild and severe caustic injuries (grade 0, 1, 2 *vs.* 3, 4) [AUC:0.914, 95% CI (0.85-0.96, p<0.001)]. This is a valuable finding for primary physicians in Emergency Departments to be able to plan further management of the patient. However, the number of patients with severe injury (n=10) and NLR>8.71 (n=18) was low. Because, caustic injuries are mostly seen in developing countries and endoscopy is not readily available and emergency endoscopic grading is the main factor reflecting patient survival and functional outcome [17]. In a study by Cabral et al., most patients with mild injuries (grade I-IIIa) were managed with medical treatment (10/158 patients underwent surgery), whereas most of the patients with severe injuries (grade IIIb-IV) were managed surgically (78/84 patients underwent surgery) [23]. Therefore, according to the results of the current study, patients with NLR values >8.71 need closer observation and further evaluation compared to those with lower values.

Due to its retrospective design, our study has some limitations. All patients had complete blood count test, whereas only 67 of 119 patients had CRP values. Although we excluded the patients with laboratory tests that had not evaluated in the six hours, the exact timing of the caustic damage was not assessed because the data for all patients were not complete. Number of patients with severe injury was low according to mild-moderate patients in our study. This is the first study evaluating NLR in caustic injuries which was used for diagnosis and predictor of course in many diseases.

In conclusion, NLR has a significant association with organ involvement and grade of involvement. It is an easily derived, inexpensive and widely available marker of inflammation. Elevated NLR levels may be a marker of severe caustic injuries and widespread involvement. Thus, it could be an effective guide for the management of patients before endoscopic evaluation in Emergency Departments. However, further prosective controlled studies with larger populations are needed in this subject.

References

1. Patrick R, Shawn M (2016) Foreign Bodies, Bezoars, and Caustic Ingestions, In: Mark Feldman, Lawrence S. Friedman, Lawrence J. Brandt (Eds). Sleisenger & Fordtran's Gastrointestinal & Liver diseases. 10th edition, Saunders Elseiver Science, USA 2016, pp 426-438.

2. Contini S, Scarpignato C (2013) Caustic injury of the upper gastrointestinal tract: a comprehensive review. World J Gastroenterol 19: 3918-3930.

3. Cattan P, Munoz-Bongrand N, Berney T, Halimi B, Sarfati E, et al. (2000) Extensive abdominal surgery after caustic ingestion. Ann Surg 231: 519-523.

4. McAuley CE, Steed DL, Webster MW (1985) Late sequelae of gastric acid injury. Am J Surg 149: 412-415.

5. Poley JW, Steyerberg EW, Kuipers EJ (2004) Ingestion of acid and alkaline agents: outcome and prognostic value of early upper endoscopy. Gastrointest Endosc 60: 372–377.

6. Katzka DA (2001) Caustic Injury to the Esophagus. Curr Treat Options Gastroenterol 4: 59-66.

7. Ryu HH, Jeung KW, Lee BK (2010) Caustic injury: can CT grading system enable prediction of esophageal stricture? Clin Toxicol (Phila). 2010;48: 137-142.

8. Chiu HM, Lin JT, Huang SP (2004) Prediction of bleeding and stricture formation after corrosive ingestion by EUS concurrent with upper endoscopy. Gastrointest Endosc 60: 827–833.

9. Cheng YJ, Kao EL (2003) Arterial blood gas analysis in acute caustic ingestion injuries. Surg Today 33: 483-485.

10. Imtiaz F, Shafique K, Mirza SS (2012) Neutrophil lymphocyte ratio as a measure of systemic inflammation in prevalent chronic diseases in Asian population. Int Arch Med 5: 2.

11. Balta S, Celik T, Mikhailidis DP (2016) The Relation Between Atherosclerosis and the Neutrophil-Lymphocyte Ratio. Clin Appl Thromb Hemost 22: 405-411.

12. Isaac V, Wu CY, Huang CT (2016) Elevated neutrophil to lymphocyte ratio predicts mortality in medical inpatients with multiple chronic conditions. Medicine (Baltimore) 95: e3832.

13. Gibson PH, Croal BL, Cuthbertson BH (2007) Preoperative neutrophil-lymphocyte ratio and outcome from coronary artery bypass grafting. Am Heart J 154: 995-1002.

14. Walsh SR, Cook EJ, Goulder F, Justin TA, Keeling NJ (2005) Neutrophil-lymphocyte ratio as a prognostic factor in colorectal cancer. J Surg Oncol 91: 181-184.

15. Sarraf KM, Belcher E, Raevsky E, Nicholson AG, Goldstraw P, et al. (2009) Neutrophil/lymphocyte ratio and its association with survival after complete resection in non-small cell lung cancer. J Thorac Cardiovasc Surg 137: 425-428.

16. Sharaiha RZ, Halazun KJ, Mirza F (2011) Elevated preoperative neutrophil:lymphocyte ratio as a predictor of postoperative disease recurrence in esophageal cancer. Ann Surg Oncol 18: 3362-3369.

17. Zargar SA, Kochhar R, Mehta S, Mehta SK (1991) The role of fiberoptic endoscopy in the management of corrosive ingestion and modified endoscopic classification of burns. Gastrointest Endosc 37: 165-169.

18. Betalli P, Falchetti D, Giuliani S (2001) Caustic Ingestion Italian Study Group. Caustic ingestion in children: is endoscopy always indicated? The results of an Italian multicenter observational study. Gastrointest Endosc 68: 434-439.

19. Kaya M, Ozdemir T, Sayan A (2010) The relationship between clinical findings and esophageal injury severity in children with corrosive agent ingestion. Ulus Travma Acil Cerrahi Derg 16: 537-540.

20. Chen TY, Ko SF, Chuang JH (2003) Predictors of esophageal stricture in children with unintentional ingestion of caustic agents. Chang Gung Med J 26: 233-239.

21. Havanond C, Havanond P (2007) Initial signs and symptoms as prognostic indicators of severe gastrointestinal tract injury due to corrosive ingestion. J Emerg Med 33: 349-353.

22. Rigo GP, Camellini L, Azzolini F, Guazzetti S, Bedogni G, et al. (2002) What is the utility of selected clinical and endoscopic parameters in predicting the risk of death after caustic ingestion? Endoscopy 34: 304-310.

23. Cabral C, Chirica M, de Chaisemartin C (2012) Caustic injuries of the upper digestive tract: a population observational study. Surg Endosc 26: 214-221.

18

Oral Application of Charcoal and Humic Acids to Dairy Cows Influences *Clostridium botulinum* Blood Serum Antibody Level and Glyphosate Excretion in Urine

Henning Gerlach[1], Achim Gerlach[2], Wieland Schrödl[1], Bernd Schottdorf[3], Svent Haufe[4], Hauke Helm[5], Awad Shehata[1,6*] and Monika Krüger[1]

[1]*Institute of Bacteriology and Mycology, Faculty of Veterinary Medicine, University of Leipzig, An den Tierkliniken 29, D-04103 Leipzig, Germany*

[2]*Waldstraße 78, D-25712 Burg, Germany*

[3]*Carbon Terra GmbH Gutermannstrasse 25, D-86154 Augsburg, Germany*

[4]*WH Pharmawerk Weinböhla GmbH, Poststr. 58, D-01689 Weinböhla, Germany*

[5]*Südholzring 2, D-25693 Gudendorf, Germany*

[6]*Avian and Rabbit Diseases Department, Faculty of Veterinary Medicine, Sadat City University, Egypt*

***Corresponding author:** Dr. Shehata A, Institute of Bacteriology and Mycology, Veterinary Faculty, University of Leipzig, An den, Tierkliniken 29, D-04103 Leipzig, Germany, E-mail: shehata@vetmed.uni-leipzig.de

Abstract

The present study was initiated to investigate the influence of oral application of charcoal, sauerkraut juice and humic acids on chronic botulism in dairy cows. A total of 380 Schleswig Holstein cows suffering from chronic botulism were fed daily with 400 g/animal charcoal for 4 weeks (1-4 weeks of study), 200 g/animal charcoal (5-10 weeks of study), 120 g/animal humic acid (11-14s week of study), 200g charcoal and 500 ml Sauerkraut juice/animal (13-16 weeks of study), 200 g charcoal and 100 mL Aquahumin/animal (15-18s week of study), 100 g charcoal and 50 mL Aquahumin (19-22 weeks of study) followed by 4 weeks without any supplementation. Bacteriological and immunological parameters investigated included *C. botulinum* and botulinum neurotoxins (BoNT) in faeces, *C. botulinum* ABE and CD antibodies, positive acute phase proteins (APPs) haptoglobin and LPS-binding protein (LBP) using serum ELISA, negative APP paraoxanase by its enzymatic activity and glyphosate in urine by ELISA. Neither BoNT nor *C. botulinum* was detected in feacal samples. From week six until four weeks before the end of the study, there was a significant reduction in antibody levels. All supplementation, except low doses of charcoal (200g / animal) alone, led to a significant reduction of *C. botulinum* ABE and CD antibody levels. There also was a significant reduction of glyphosate in urine following supplementation with a combination of 200g charcoal plus either 500 mL sauerkraut juice or humic acid. Haptoglobin, paraoxanase and LBP were significantly increased by the 24th week of the study. The positive APPs and *C. botulinum* antibodies were significant negative correlations. In conclusion, a charcoal-sauerkraut juice combination and humic acids could be used to control chronic botulism and glyphosate damage in cattle.

Keywords Humic acids; Peripartual cases; *C. botulinum*

Introduction

In recent years, an increased frequency of a new form of bovine botulism has been observed. This form of botulism differs from regular food-born botulism by its slow and chronic development with various unspecific symptoms. This protracted form may develop when small, sub-lethal amounts of BoNT are taken up and/or absorbed over several days or are generated in the hind gut [1,2]. Clinical symptoms of chronic botulism are most often peripartual cases with indigestion (constipation alternating with diarrhea), non-infectious acute laminitis, ataxia and stiff stilted gait, impossibility to get up (paralysis), apathy, engorged veins, positive venous pulse, edema in legs, udder, and dew-lap, retracted abdomen, forced respiration and unexpected death. The prevalence of C. botulinum in cattle can be determined by detection of botulinum neurotoxins (BoNTs) and/or *C. botulinum* vegetative bacteria or spores in the gastrointestinal tract or organs (liver, kidney, lungs and muscles [1,3,4]. A second way to verify chronic botulism is with specific antibodies for BoNTs [3,5,6] detected

natural specific antibodies in wild canine species, horses and dairy cows.

C. botulinum is an ubiquitous Gram-positive, spore forming, obligatory anaerobic bacterium that inhabits soil, dust and organic matter such as feces of animals and man, slaughterhouse wastes, residues of biogas plants, and bio-compost. It generates eight highly toxic neurotoxin isoforms (BoNT A-H) that are the most toxic substances known [7-12]. All isoforms, together with the related tetanus neurotoxin (TeNT) secreted by *C. tetani*, are Zn2+-endoproteases. The immunologically distinct neurotoxins (A-H) of *C. botulinum* are homologous proteins consisting of a heavy and light chain linked by an essential disulfide bridge. The light chain blocks the release of acetylcholine at the neuromuscular junction. Human cases are mostly caused by types A, B, or E, while animal diseases are mostly caused by types C and D [1,13,14]. Several C. botulinum strains produce two neurotoxins [11]. Physiological differences are used to divide *C. botulinum* strains into 4 physiological groups; group I, consisting of *C. botulinum* A and proteolytic strains of *C. botulinum* B and F; group II, consisting of *C. botulinum* E and nonproteolytic strains of *C. botulinum* B and F; group III, consisting of *C. botulinum*

C and D; and group IV, consisting of *C. argentinense* (BoNT G). Neurotoxigenic strains of other Clostridium species such as *C. butyricum*, (BoNT E, group V) and C. baratii (BoNT F, group VI) have also been identified [14]. BoNTs are produced as a 150 kDa single polypeptide chain. The protein is post-translationally proteolyzed to form a dichain in which the heavy chain (HC, 100 kDa) and light chain (LC, 50 kDa) are linked through a disulfide bond. HC is composed of two 50 kDa domains, with the N-terminal half involved in translocation and the C-terminal half involved in binding with nerve cells. BoNTs bind specifically to neuronal cells, enter the cytoplasm, and then cleave core proteins involved in the vesicular fusion machinery (SNARE proteins) by its metalloprotease activity to block the release of neurotransmitters. When BoNTs are produced by the bacteria, the BoNTs are found in complexes associated with protective proteins (progenitor toxins). These are the nontoxic, nonhemagglutinin (NTNH, 130 kDa) and several nontoxic hemagglutinins (NTHAs). BoNTs cannot penetrate intact skin, but the toxin is absorbed from mucosal surfaces or wounds. In foodborne and intestinal botulism, botulinum toxins are produced from *C. botulinum* and other BoNT producing Clostridia, which colonize the lumen of the intestine where the toxins are absorbed from the digestive tract. BoNT binds through a double-receptor system consisting of a protein receptor and acidic lipid-gangliosides with its heavy chain domain [15,16].

The upper or small intestine is the most important site for absorption of BoNTs [17,18] but other mucous membranes also are able to absorb BoNTs [19]. BoNT complexes probably do not dissociate in the digestive tract. The whole toxin complex seems to be absorbed from the intestine into the lymphatics in the rat ligated duodenum loop assay. Molecular dissociation occurs immediately after BoNT complexes, designated progenitor toxins, are absorbed into the lymphatics [20]. Botulinum progenitor toxins are found in three forms with molecular masses of 900 kDa (LL toxin for type A), 500 kDa (L toxin for types A, B, C, D and G) and 300 kDa (M toxin for types A, B, C, D, E and F). The M toxin consists of BoNT and NTNHA with no hemagglutination activity, whereas the L toxin consists of BoNT, NTNHA and NTHA. The LL toxin is a dimer of L toxin [21]. NTNHA protects the BoNT from acidity and proteases in the digestive tract. NTHAs play an essential role in the effective absorption of the type C progenitor toxins to the small intestine. NTHA exists as subcomponents; HA-70, HA-33 and HA-17 [21]. The HAs of BoNT/A and B could disrupt the human epithelial intercellular junction through species-specific interaction with E-cadherin to presumably facilitate BoNT transport via the paracellular route [22-24]. NTHAs of BoNT A may bind to 9 different glycan sites of gut epithelial cells. Thus NTHA mediated absorption could be prevented by galactose and its derivates [25].

Treatment of BoNT intoxication is accomplished using specific polyclonal and monoclonal antibodies. Antitoxins given within 24 hour of the onset of disease can lower the death rate from botulism and shorten duration of the symptoms [16]. Antibodies only neutralize non-bounded BoNTs. Other possibilities for treatment could be peptide based inhibitors that mimic amino acid motives of the SNARE proteins to inhibit the catalytic part (endopeptidase) of the BoNT [15]. One obstacle for the endopeptidase inhibitors is how to deliver the molecules into the intoxicated nerve cells. Another way of treatment is mimicry of receptors. Binding of BoNTs to nerve cells in a two-step process is generally accepted. Binding to gangliosides is followed by high affinity binding to a protein receptor(s) [26]. Synaptotagmin has been proposed as the protein receptor for BoNT/A, /B, /E, and /G [15,27]. Aptamers, unique oligonucleotides with high affinity for their (proteins or small molecule) targets, are the newest treatment possibilities [16]. All of the above mentioned methods are mostly too expensive for food animals and cheaper methods are necessary. Neuvonen and Olkkola (1988) used charcoal to treat intoxications in humans. In the present study, *C. botulinum* types ABE and CD blood serum antibodies, feacal BoNTs and *C. botulinum* spores from 40 dairy cows in 4 different lactation states (10 each group) were investigated for 26 weeks [28]. The cows were supplemented with charcoal and humic acids in different doses to evaluate their BoNT binding capacity. Parallel haptoglobin [29] and LPS binding protein [30], as positive acute phase proteins (APPs), and paraoxanase [31,32] as negative APP were investigated. Urine was tested each 4 weeks for glyphosate to demonstrate the glyphosate neutralizing capacity of charcoal and humic acids, and to show a possible connection between glyphosate and chronic botulism.

Material and Methods

Animals and supplementations

A Schleswig Holstein dairy cow farm of about 380 cows with average milk production of 9000 L per year showed clinical symptoms of chronic botulism (flock stiff stilted gait, paresis, apathy, engorged veins on tarsus, positive venous pulse, mucous saliva, reduced tail tonus, small wounds in the udder region) in 10-15% of the cows and 60% of the cows suffered from Dermatitis digitalis (mortellaro). The entire animal population was involved in the various charcoal (CC) (≤ 8 mm diameter) and powdery humic acid (WH67) or sauerkraut juice (SJ) and liquid humic acid (Aquahumin) supplement. Each treatment represented 10 identical cows of the 1st, 2nd, and 3rd lactation and the dry cows group for the full time of the investigation. Their last polyvalent clostridial vaccination (Covexin, Intervet) was on 01.11.2012. The treatment regime with CC, SJ and/or humic acids was changed every 4 weeks (supplementation periods) in Table 1 and given as part of the total mixed ratio (TMR).

Date	SP1*	SP2	SP3	SP4	SP5	SP6	SP7
	11.11.2012-08.12. 2012	9.12.2012-20.01. 2013	21.01.2013– 17.02.2013	18.02.2013-17.03.20 13	18.03.2013-31.03.20 13	01.04.2013-14.04. 2013	15.04.2013-14.05.2 013
Supplements	400 g CC1	200 g CC	200 g CC+ 500 mL SJ2	120 g HA3	200 g CC+100mL AH4	100 g CC+50mL AH	Without supplements

*Supplementation period, 1CC=Charcoal (Carboligni, Schottdorf, Germany), 2SJ=Sauerkraut juice (KronprinzKonserven, Meldorf, Germany), 3HA=humic acids WH67 (PharmawerkWeinböhla, Germany), 4AH=Aquahumin (Pharmawerk Weinböhla, Germany).

Table 1: Overview at the various times of supplementation.

	06.01.2013	20.01.2013	17.02.2013	03.02.2013	03.03.2013	17.03.2013	31.03.2013	01.04.2013
Paresis	2/40	2/40	3/40	3/40	2/40	2/40	2/40	2/40
Cystitis	2/40	2/40	2/40	1/40	4/40	1/40	3/40	3/40
Diahrea	5/40	0/40	3/40	7/40	0/40	5/40	0/40	2/40
Viscus saliva	0/40	0/40	0/40	0/40	1/40	2/40	1/40	4/40
endometritis	0/40	1/40	0/40	0/40	0/40	0/40	0/40	0/40
Ataxia	0/40	0/40	0/40	0/40	0/40	0/40	0/40	1/40

Table 2: Clinical estimation of cows at the various sampling points.

The TMR was composed of grass and maize silage (glyphosate concentration not tested), concentrated mixed feed (1.93 mg/kg glyphosate), ground grains (0.51 mg/kg glyphosate), wheat straw (0.03 mg/kg glyphosate) and alfalfa hay (0.02 mg/kg glyphosate). After 31.03.2013, 10 kg draff/cow (0.01 mg/kg glyphosate) was fed. At each sampling point, each of the 40 treated cows was evaluated for clinical symptoms (Table 2).

Collection of samples

Blood, faeces and urine were analyzed 7 times at 4 week intervals with one exception (200 g CC over 6 weeks). Blood specimens were taken from the Vena coccygenamediana, coagulated blood centrifuged at 3000 x g for 15 min and the serum samples were stored at -20°C. Faeces were taken from Ampulla recti and spontaneous urination was sampled and stored at -20°C. All specimens were quickly cooled and sent to the laboratory.

Glyphosate testing of urine

Urine samples were diluted 1:20 with distilled water (aqua distillated, Braun, Germany) and tested for glyphosate by ELISA (Abraxis, USA) according to the manufacturer's instructions. Test validation was done with Gas Chromatography-Mass Spectroscopy (GC-MS) by Medizinsches Labor Bremen (Germany). The correlation coefficient between the two tests was 0.96 (Data not shown).

Analysis of free BoNT/A-E and C. botulinum spores in faeces

Preparation of faeces for detection of BoNT/A-E

Faecal samples were diluted 1:3 in PBS (Dulbecco, pH 7.4) containing 0.1% Triton X-100, 0.1% Tween 20 and 10 mM EDTA. The samples were thoroughly mixed and frozen at -20°C. After thawing, the diluted samples were centrifuged at 7000 x g for 15 min and the clarified supernatants were analyzed with BoNT-ELISA.

Indirect detection of C. botulinum spores

Rumen fluid and faecal samples were diluted 1:10 in RCM (0.5 g in 4.5 ml), vigorously mixed, and heated at 80°C for 10 min. Samples were incubated at 37°C for 7 d under anaerobic conditions and subsequently stored at -20°C until tested. After thawing, the sample was centrifuged at 7.000 x g for 15 min and the clear supernatant was analyzed for the type-specific soluble antigens of C. botulinum types A-E by ELISA.

BoNT-ELISA

BoNT/A-E were determined by an ELISA developed in our institute [2]. The standard volume was 100 µl per well and the standard incubation condition was 1 h at room temperature (1 h at RT) on a microtiter plate shaker (400 rpm). The coating buffer was 0.1 M NaHCO3 and the wash solution (WS) was 0.9% NaCl with 0.05% Tween 20 (Sigma-Aldrich, Taufkirchen, Germany). All washing steps were done in a Nunc-Immuno-Washer 12 (Nunc, Wiesbaden, Germany). After coating the ELISA wells with capture antibodies (3 mg/ml, BoNT-immunoaffinity purified-IgG from rabbits against BoNT/A-E, Institute of Bacteriology and Mycology, University of Leipzig, Germany) overnight at 4-6°C, they were incubated with 150 ml per well of 1% gelatin from cold water fish skin (Sigma-Aldrich, Taufkirchen, Germany) in 0.9% NaCl solution for 1 h at RT. The wells were washed twice with WS and loaded with the prepared faecal samples diluted 1:2 in 20 mMTris, pH 8.0, assay buffer [adjusted with 1 M HCl] containing 0.9% NaCl, 5 mM EDTA, 1% gelatin from cold water fish skin, 0.2% bovine serum albumin, 0.1 mg/ml rabbit IgG from normal serum and 0.2% Tween 20 (chemicals from Sigma-Aldrich or Fluka, Taufkirchen, Germany). After incubation, the wells were washed five times with WS and loaded with the detection antibodies conjugated with HRP and diluted in assay buffer. C. botulinum types A and B were detected with 2.5 mg/ml horse [Fab]2 from IgG against C. botulinum A and B (Novartis Vaccines and Diagnostics Co, Marburg, Germany). Types C and D were detected with 0.1 mg/ml of IgG from rabbits developed against BoNT/C and D (Institute of Bacteriology and Mycology, University of Leipzig). Type E was detected with 2.5 mg/ml IgG from horses against C. botulinum type E (WDT, Garbsen, Germany).

After incubation at RT, the plates were washed four times with WS and the HRP activity was determined by adding 100 µl/well of 2 mM H2O2 and 1 mM 3, 30, 5, 50-TMB. The substrate reaction was stopped with 1 M H2SO4 (50 µl/well) and the optical density (OD) was measured with an ELISA-reader at 450 nm. The sensitivity, specificity, precision, limit of detection, and range of quantification were determined previously. Cross reactivity of antibodies with *C. tetani, C. perfringens, C. sporogenes, C. sordellii, C. novyi, C. butyricum,* Bacillus cereus, Streptococcus agalactiae, Streptococcus zooepidemicus, Staphylococcus aureus, Staphylococcus epidermidis, Escherichia coli, Proteus vulgaris, Proteus mirabilis, Pseudomonas aeruginosa, Candida albicans and Candida krusei were all negative.

Evaluation of BoNT-ELISA

The relative units (RU) were calculated from the measured OD values as follow: (sample-OD minus twice the value of the control-OD [BoNT-negative sample of bovine faeces]) multiplied by 1000 and dilution factors per minute substrate incubation time.

Analysis of C. botulinum antibodies using ELISA

Solid phase antigen for ELISAs

C. *botulinum* types A (7272), B (7273), C (2300), D (2301), and E (2302) obtained from the National Collection of Type Cultures (NCTC) were used for preparation of ELISA antigens. Culture supernatant from *C. sporogenes* and *C. perfringens* (Isolated and identified by the Institute of Bacteriology and Mycology, Faculty of Veterinary Medicine, Leipzig University) served as a control antigen to study cross reactivity. All strains were cultured in reinforced Clostridial medium (RCM; Sifin, Berlin, Germany) and incubated anaerobically at 37°C for 7 days followed by freezing at 25°C. Supernatants were checked for BoNT-type with type specific ELISA [9]. After thawing and mixing, the culture suspension was centrifuged at 10,000 g for 15 min and the clear supernatant was separated. BoNT-proteins in the supernatants were detoxified with 20 mM formaldehyde (four additions weekly) and incubated at 37°C. Active formaldehyde groups were blocked by the addition of 100 mM lysine and 100 mM glycine in 100 mMTris/HCl (pH 8.0) solution and incubated at RT for 24 h. Complete detoxification was verified with the mouse test by Dr. F. Gessler (Miprolab, Göttingen, Germany), data not shown. The antigen preparation was washed with PBS (pH 7.4) and concentrated by ultrafiltration at a molecular weight cut-off of 50 kDa (viva- vivaspin 20, Sartorius Stedim Biotech, Göttingen, Germany). The protein concentration was measured with a spectral photometer (MBA 2000) and its integrated software (PerkineElmer, Norwalk, Connecticut, USA) and adjusted with PBS to 1 mg/ml.

Detection of IgG anti C. botulinum antibodies by ELISA

ELISA plates were coated with 100 ml/well of detoxified antigen from C. botulinum (1 mg/ml in 0.1 M NaHCO3) and incubated overnight at 4-6°C. Coated plates were washed twice with 0.9% NaCl containing 0.05% Tween 20 (Sigma-Aldrich, Taufkirchen, Germany) followed by 135 µl of blocking solution (1% bovine case) mixed with 15 ml diluted serum sample (1:10 in 50 mMTris buffer, pH 8, containing 0.9% NaCl, 10 mM EDTA, 1% yeast extract, 1% BSA, 20% RCM and 1% Tween 20) and incubated for 1 h at RT on a microtiter plate shaker. After washing four times, IgG from rabbits against bovine IgG (Fc) conjugated with horse radish peroxidase (HRP) (Dianova, Hamburg, Germany) diluted 1:20,000 in assay buffer (50 mM Tris pH 7.4, 0.9% NaCl, 0.2% yeast extract, 0.1% BSA, 0.1% bovine Casein, 2% RCM and 0.1% Tween 20) was added to each well and incubated 1 h at RT.

HRP activity was determined by adding 100 ml/well of 3 mM H2O2 and 1 mM 3, 3′, 5,′5- tetramethylbenzidine (TMB) in 0.2 M citrate-buffer (pH 4.0). The substrate reaction was stopped with 1 M H2SO4 (50 µl/well) and the optical density (OD) was measured with an ELISA-reader at 450 nm. RCM without *C. botulinum* antigen served as a control antigen to determine the degree of non-specific solid phase binding of immunoglobulin on each sample (control OD). The control OD value was subtracted from each antigen specific OD value to calculate the Anti- *C. botulinum* IgG level relative to an internal laboratory standard (pooled blood samples from >3000 cows) that was defined as 100 percent.

Haptoglobin analysis

The Hp concentration in blood serum was determined by ELISA as described by Schroedl et al. [33]. Briefly, the coating antibody was IgG from rabbit anti-Hp (DAKO, Hamburg, Germany), which was diluted 1:3000. The standard was bovine plasma in which the Hp concentration was determined with a standardized colorimetric assay for bovine Hp (Tridelta Development Ltd., Greystones, Co. Wicklow, Ireland) and further checked against purified bovine Hp. The standard concentration ranged from 3 to 200 ng ml-1. The samples were diluted 1:1000 and 1:50000 in assay buffer (50 mMTris-HCl with pH 8.0, 0.15 M NaCl, 10 mM EDTA, 0.1% Tween 20 and 0.2% bovine casein, all from Sigma-Aldrich, Taufkirchen, Germany). The detection antibody was polyclonal IgG (rabbit) anti-Hp (DAKO, Hamburg, Germany) conjugated with horseradish peroxidase. The detection antibody was diluted 1:10000 in assay buffer. The detection limit, including the dilution factor of 1000, was 1 µg ml-1.

LBP analysis by ELISA

The LBP coating antibody was affinity purified monoclonal IgG2a (mouse) anti-LBP-human (mAb-Abi-202) at 1.2 µg/ml. The standard LBP-range in the ELISA was 0.3 to 20 ng/ml human LBP (LBP-standard serum). The samples were diluted 1:1,000 and higher. The assay buffer for dilution of the standard and plasma samples was 50 mM Tris HCl (pH 8.0), 0.15 M NaCl, 10 mM EDTA, and 0.1% Tween 20 (v/v). The detection antibody was affinity purified monoclonal IgG1 (mouse) anti-LBP-human conjugated with horseradish peroxidase (mAb-Abi-204) diluted 1:6,000 in assay buffer. The two mAbs and the standard serum were provided by Prof. Ch. Schuett, Institute of Immunology, and University of Greifswald, Germany.

Paraoxanase analysis

Paraoxonase/arylesterase activity was measured spectrophotometrically using paranitrophenyl acetate (PNPA) as a substrate. A stock solution was prepared using 1M Hepes buffer (pH 7.5), 400 mM p-nitrophenyl acetate in DSMO and 100 mM CaCl2. The working buffer contained 10 mM CaCl2, 10 mMHepes, and 2 mM p- nitrophenyl acetate in 50 mL distilled water. Blood serum specimens (25 µL) diluted 1: 10 in distilled water were applied to microtiter plates and 200 µL of the working buffer were added. After 3 s shaking, the optical density was measured at 405 nm wave length (t0) and remeasured 10 min later (t1). The paraoxanase activity in U/mL is calculated with the following equation:

Paraoxonase activity = (t1-to) x serum dilution x1000 = (t1-to) x10x1000 = units/L

Statistical analysis

The statistical analysis was carried out with GraphPad Prism 4 (GaphPad Software, La Jolla, USA). A two-way analysis of variance followed by unpaired Student t-test was used to identify significant differences between means.

Results

Effect of supplementation on glyphosate in urine

A significant reduction in glyphosate excretion (P<0.0001) was only seen at the 14th and 18th week of the study (Figure 1).

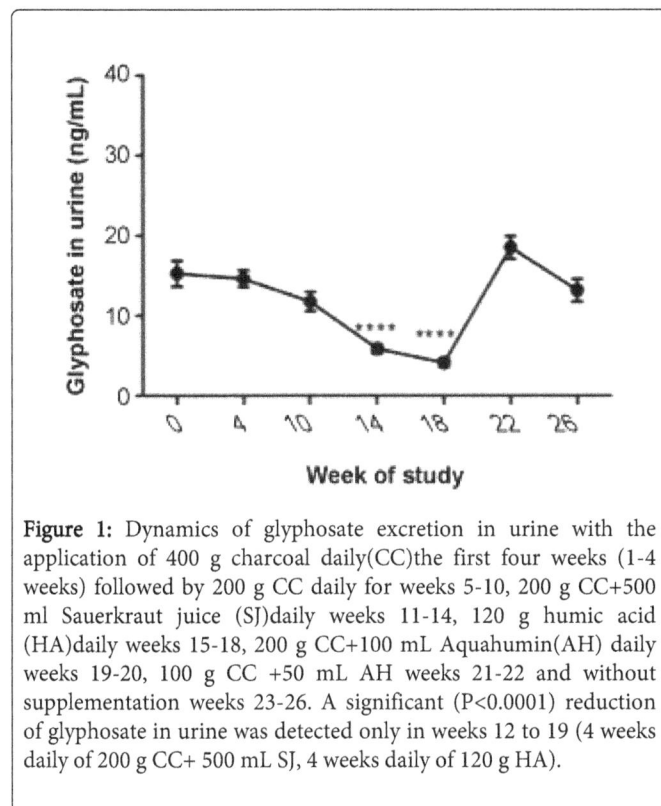

Figure 1: Dynamics of glyphosate excretion in urine with the application of 400 g charcoal daily(CC)the first four weeks (1-4 weeks) followed by 200 g CC daily for weeks 5-10, 200 g CC+500 ml Sauerkraut juice (SJ)daily weeks 11-14, 120 g humic acid (HA)daily weeks 15-18, 200 g CC+100 mL Aquahumin(AH) daily weeks 19-20, 100 g CC +50 mL AH weeks 21-22 and without supplementation weeks 23-26. A significant (P<0.0001) reduction of glyphosate in urine was detected only in weeks 12 to 19 (4 weeks daily of 200 g CC+ 500 mL SJ, 4 weeks daily of 120 g HA).

The combination of CC (200 g) and SJ (500 ml) as well as HA (120 g) reduced glyphosate in urine significantly.

Botulinum neurotoxin (BoNT) and C. botulinum in faeces

No BoNT or C. botulinum was detected in feacal samples.

Detection of C. botulinum IgG antibodies in blood serum

The dynamic effects of different supplementations on *C. botulinum* ABE and CD blood serum antibody levels over 24 weeks are shown in Figure 2.

Daily supplementation with CC and/or humic acids initiated at week 6 significantly reduced antibody levels (P<0.01 at week 6, P<0.001 for weeks 8-24, and P<0.05 for week 26. The effect of different supplements on *C. botulinum* CD blood serum antibody levels over the 26 weeks is shown in Figure 3.

Supplementation with daily 400 g CC significantly decreased CD antibody (P<0.01) while a daily application of 200 g CC allowed the

CD antibody level to increase. A highly significant (P<0.001) reduction in CD antibody was detected only after two weeks supplementation with 200 g CC plus 500 mL SJ. Antibody reduction was constant from week 4 to 24; however, four weeks after finishing supplementation (week 26), CD antibodies increased.

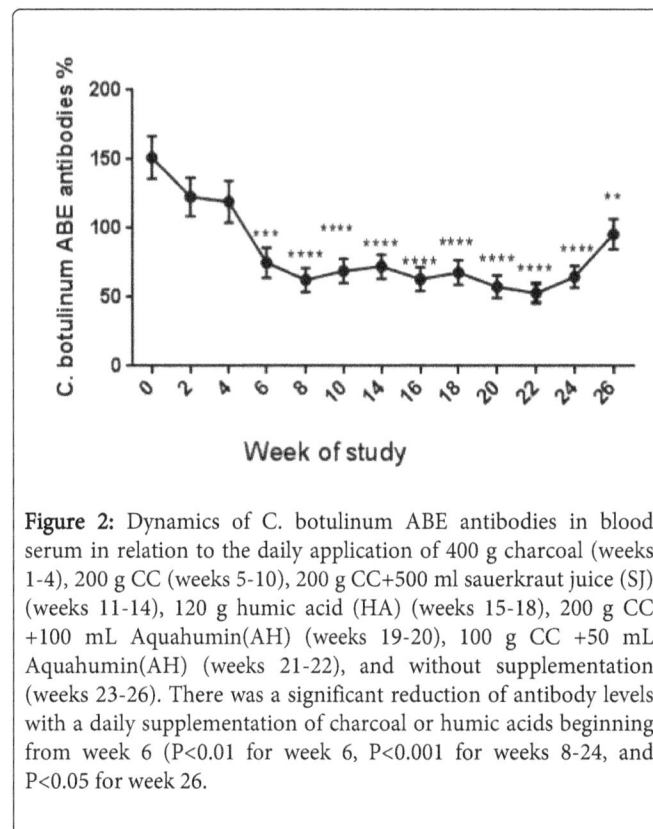

Figure 2: Dynamics of C. botulinum ABE antibodies in blood serum in relation to the daily application of 400 g charcoal (weeks 1-4), 200 g CC (weeks 5-10), 200 g CC+500 ml sauerkraut juice (SJ) (weeks 11-14), 120 g humic acid (HA) (weeks 15-18), 200 g CC +100 mL Aquahumin(AH) (weeks 19-20), 100 g CC +50 mL Aquahumin(AH) (weeks 21-22), and without supplementation (weeks 23-26). There was a significant reduction of antibody levels with a daily supplementation of charcoal or humic acids beginning from week 6 (P<0.01 for week 6, P<0.001 for weeks 8-24, and P<0.05 for week 26.

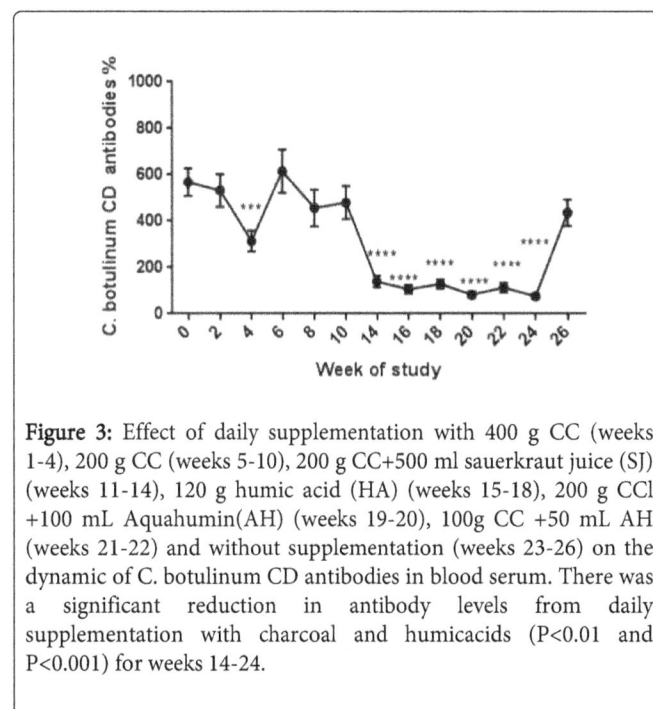

Figure 3: Effect of daily supplementation with 400 g CC (weeks 1-4), 200 g CC (weeks 5-10), 200 g CC+500 ml sauerkraut juice (SJ) (weeks 11-14), 120 g humic acid (HA) (weeks 15-18), 200 g CCl +100 mL Aquahumin(AH) (weeks 19-20), 100g CC +50 mL AH (weeks 21-22) and without supplementation (weeks 23-26) on the dynamic of C. botulinum CD antibodies in blood serum. There was a significant reduction in antibody levels from daily supplementation with charcoal and humicacids (P<0.01 and P<0.001) for weeks 14-24.

Detection of haptoglobin

Haptoglobin levels in blood serum were not significantly different with any of the supplements except for week 24 after they were taken off Aquahumin (Figure 4).

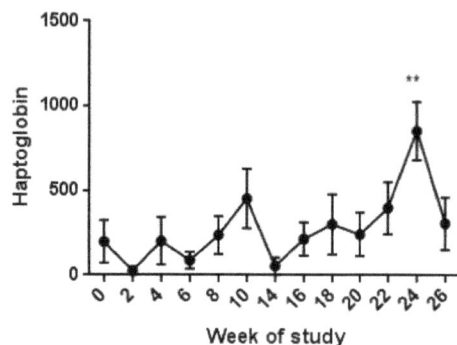

Figure 4: Haptoglobin in blood serum after the daily application of 440 g CC (weeks 1-4), 200 g CC (weeks 5-10), 200 g CC+500 ml sauerkraut juice (SJ) (weeks 11-14), 120 g humic acid (HA) (weeks 15-18), 200 g CCl+100 mL Aquahumin (AH) (weeks 19-20), 100 g CC +50 mL AH (weeks 21-22) and without supplementation (weeks 23-26). A significant (P<0.05) difference was only detected at week 24.

LBP results

There was a significant increase in LBP in blood serum on week 20 (P<0.001) (Figure 5).

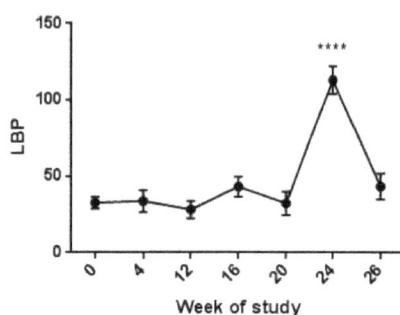

Figure 5: LBP in blood serum in relation to daily oral application of 400 g charcoal (CC) (weeks 1-4), 200 g CC (weeks 5-10), 200 g CC +500 ml sauerkraut juice (SJ) (weeks 11-14), 120 g humic acid (HA) (weeks 15-18), 200 g CCl+100 mL Aquahumin(AH) (weeks 19-20), 100 g CC +50 mL (AH) (weeks 21-22) and without supplementation (weeks 23-26). A significant (P<0.001) increase inLBP level was seen only at week 24.

Paraoxanase (PON) in blood serum

PON activity increased significantly only at 24-26 weeks (P<0.001) (Figure 6).

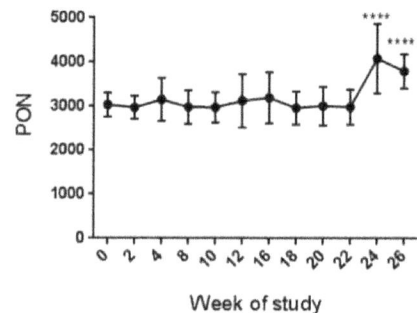

Figure 6: Paraoxanaseactivity in blood serum in relation to daily supplementation with 400g charcoal (CC) (weeks 1-4), 200g CC (weeks 5-10), 200 g CC+500 ml sauerkraut juice (SJ) (weeks 11-14), 120 g humic acid (HA) (weeks 15-18), 200 g CC+100 mL Aquahumin(AH) (weeks 19-20), 100 g CC +50 mL AH (weeks 21-22) and without supplementation (weeks 23-26). Significant (P<0.05) differences were only detected at weeks 24-26.

Discussion

We investigated the effect of an oral application of CC and humic acids (HA) alone or in combination with SJ on blood serum *C. botulinum* ABE and CD antibody levels. Chronic botulism is characterized by the sub-lethal generation of *C. botulinum* progenitor toxins in the hind gut. The incorporation of the progenitor toxin and free BoNT from the gastrointestinal tract (GIT) into the body could happen via three different routes. Small concentrations of the progenitor toxin and BoNT bind with hemagglutinins (HA) or the HC part of the molecule can bind to receptors on the surface of epithelial cells and transcytosis can occur. Translocated HA disrupts the epithelial barrier. This is different with type A, B and C progenitor toxins. Type A and B HAs disrupt the epithelial cell line paracellular without causing cytotoxic effects in the epithelial cells of their susceptible hosts while type C HAs possibly evoke cytotoxic-barrier disrupting activity in the epithelial cells of susceptible animals. Damaged epithelial cells are not a barrier for progenitor toxins and BoNTs [20,23,24]. The damaged epithelial barrier permits the toxins to be distributed throughout the body by blood and lymph vessels. Based on this knowledge, it is very important to bind these toxins with CC. The very strong reduction of CD antibodies after the daily application of 400 g of CC shows this effect. These very high CD antibody levels without the application of a CD vaccine have not been reported previously. Such high antibody levels have only been observed in conjunction with vaccination [3]. Wang et al. showed good sorption of the hydrophobic herbicide terbuthylacin by CC [35]. Maybe the hydrophobic surfactant of the commercial herbicide Roundup also could be absorbed by CC [36]. Graber found that glyphosate can be absorbed by CC. Our results don't support these results in animals [37]. Four weeks daily application of 400 g CC reduced the CD antibody level dramatically (Figure 3) but did not affect the excretion of glyphosate in urine (Figure 1). In our own investigation, we only found neutralization or absorption of a maximum of 300 µg glyphosate to 1 mg CC (data not shown). The daily application of 200 g CC in weeks 5-10 failed to reduce glyphosate excretion or *C. botulinum* type CD antibody levels. The mixed application of 200 g CC and 500 mL SJ significantly reduced the amount of glyphosate excreted and *C. botulinum* CD antibodies also significantly (P<0.001) decreased (Figures 1 and 3). *C. botulinum* ABE antibodies were significantly reduced by all the treatments from week 4 on Figure 2. The application of HA (WH67) significantly ($P<0.001$) reduced glyphosate excretion and *C. botulinum* ABE and CD antibody levels. Krüger et al. demonstrated that glyphosate reduced the Enterococcus spp. bacteria that are antagonistic to *C. botulinum* [34]. Shehata et al. were able to neutralize the antibacterial activity of glyphosate with different humic acid preparations in vitro [38]. Results from the application of 200 g CC and 100 mL Aquahumin (liquid preparation) for 2 weeks compared with 100 g CC with 50 mL Aquahumin for two weeks showed that a definite amount of these substrates is necessary to absorb or neutralize glyphosate and/or *C. botulinum* toxins. Mazzei and Piccolo found that glyphosate may spontaneously and significantly bind to soluble humic matter by non-covalent interactions at slightly acidic pH [39]. Binding to matrices such as soluble fulvic and humic acids could be the reason. Glyphosate excretion was reduced with the soluble Aquahumin (Figure 1). It was not anticipated that the combination of 200 g CC and 500 mL SJ per day would be so very effective. Fermentation of cabbage to SJ is mostly done by Lactobacillus plantarum [40]. Lactobacilli produce exopolysaccharides (EPS), homopolysaccharides and heteropolysaccharides. These biopolymers are widely distributed in nature and can be the polymers of neutral (pentoses and hexoses) or anionic sugars (hexoses). They are released into the extracellular medium by Archebacteria and Eubacteria (both Gram positive and negative). Approximately 30 species of Lactobacilli are described as EPS producers. Among them, the best known are *L. casei*, *L. acidophilus*, *L. brevis*, *L. curvatus*, *L. delbrueckii*, *L. bulgaricus*, *L. helveticus*, *L. rhamnosus*, *L. plantarum*, and *L. johnsonii*. *L. plantarum* generates heteropolymers of glucose, galactose and rhamnose. Galactose and lactose inhibit the absorption of *C. botulinum* progenitor toxins to the sugar bearing receptors on epithelial cells of the GIT [41]. The sugar polymer concentrations in nutrient broth culture of Lactobacilli are in hundreds of mg per liter. EPS may also interact with proteins, mineral, ions and other compounds [42,43]. Zhang et al. (2013) identified antioxidant effects of *L. plantarum* that may involve scavenging reactive oxygen species (ROS), up-regulation of enzymatic and non-enzymatic antioxidant activities, and reduction of lipid peroxidation [44]. ROS and lipid peroxidation are induced by glyphosate [45,46]. The neutralization of glyphosate with humic acids from WH67 was reported by Shehata et al. [33]. The binding mechanism could be hydrogen bonding to phenolic groups of humic acid [47]. The positive acute phase proteins (haptoglobine, LBP) only significantly increased at week 24 and by week 26, both acute phase proteins (APP) were reduced but *C. botulinum* ABE and CD antibodies increased. Inflammation indicated by the significant increase of haptoglobin ($P< 0.01$) and LBP ($P<0.001$) may be induced by proliferation of *C. botulinum*. At week 26, when *C. botulinum* ABE and CD antibodies were high, the APPs were low. There is a negative correlation between LBP and *C. botulinum* ABE and CD antibodies ($R2= -0.41$ and -0.51, respectively). It is interesting that even though positive APPs increased, the negative APP paraoxanase also increased at week 24. This indicates that the anti-oxidative capacity of the cows increased, but the causes for this are unknown.

Conclusion

Daily oral application of 400 g CC) significantly reduced *C. botulinum* ABE and CD antibodies by absorption of *C. botulinum* toxins in the gastrointestinal tract but did not reduce glyphosate excretion in urine. This result was not repeatable with 200 g CC alone

but 200 g CC plus 500 ml SJ reduced both glyphosate excretion and *C. botulinum* ABE and CD antibodies. The same excellent result was obtained highly significantly with 120 g humic acids. A certain amount of CC and/or humic acids are necessary to absorb and/or neutralize glyphosate and *C. botulinum* toxins.

References

1. Böhnel H, Schwagerick B, Gessler F (2001) Visceral botulism--a new form of bovine Clostridium botulinumtoxication. J Vet Med A PhysiolPatholClin Med 48: 373-383.

2. Krüger M, Große-Herrenthey A, Schrödl W, Gerlach A, Rodloff A (2012) Visceral botulism at dairy farms in Schleswig Holstein, Germany: prevalence of Clostridium botulinum in feces of cows, in animal feeds, in feces of the farmers, and in house dust. Anaerobe 18: 221-223.

3. Krüger M, Skau M, Shehata AA, Schrödl W (2013) Efficacy of Clostridium botulinum types C and D toxoid vaccination in Danish cows. Anaerobe 23: 97-101.

4. http://www.botulismus.org/index_htm_files/Boehnel_Rinder.pdf

5. Steinman A, Millet N, Frenkel C, King R, Shpigel NY (2007) Presence of antibotulinum neurotoxin antibodies in selected wild canids in Israel. J Wildl Dis 43: 548-550.

6. Steinman A, Kachtan I, Levi O, Shpigel NY (2007) Seroprevalence of antibotulinum neurotoxin type C antibodies in horses in Israel. Equine Vet J 39: 232-235.

7. Williamson JL, Rocke TE, Aiken JM (1999) In situ detection of the Clostridium botulinum type C1 toxin gene in wetland sediments with a nested PCR assay. Appl Environ Microbiol 65: 3240-3243.

8. Böhnel H, Lube K (2000) Clostridium botulinum and bio-compost. A contribution to the analysis of potential health hazards caused by bio-waste recycling. J Vet Med B Infect Dis Vet Public Health 47: 785-795.

9. Long SC, Tauscher T (2006) Watershed issues associated with Clostridium botulinum: a literature review. J Water Health 4: 277-288.

10. Bagge E, Persson M, Johansson KE (2010) Diversity of spore-forming bacteria in cattle manure, slaughterhouse waste and samples from biogas plants. J ApplMicrobiol 109: 1549-1565.

11. Barash JR, Arnon SS (2014) A novel strain of Clostridium botulinum that produces type B and type H botulinum toxins. J Infect Dis 209: 183-191.

12. Dover N, Barash JR, Hill KK, Xie G, Arnon SS (2014) Molecular characterization of a novel botulinum neurotoxin type H gene. J Infect Dis 209: 192-202.

13. Foran PG, Mohammed N, Lisk GO, Nagwaney S, Lawrence GW, et al. (2003) Evaluation of the therapeutic usefulness of botulinum neurotoxin B, C1, E, and F compared with the long lasting type A. Basis for distinct durations of inhibition of exocytosis in central neurons. J Biol Chem 278: 1363-1371.

14. Popoff MR (2014) Botulinum neurotoxins: more and more diverse and fascinating toxic proteins. J Infect Dis 209: 168-169.

15. Rummel A, Karnath T, Henke T, Bigalke H, Binz T (2004) Synaptotagmins I and II act as nerve cell receptors for botulinum neurotoxin G. J Biol Chem 279: 30865-30870.

16. Cai S, Singh BR (2007) Strategies to design inhibitors of Clostridium botulinum neurotoxins. Infect Disord Drug Targets 7: 47-57.

17. Bonventre PF (1979) Absorption of botulinal toxin from the gastrointestinal tract. Rev Infect Dis 1: 663-667.

18. Sakaguchi G (1982) Clostridium botulinum toxins. PharmacolTher 19: 165-194.

19. Park JB, Simpson LL (2003) Inhalational poisoning by botulinum toxin and inhalation vaccination with its heavy-chain component. Infect Immun 71: 1147-1154.

20. Fujinaga Y (2010) Interaction of botulinum toxin with the epithelial barrier. J Biomed Biotechnol 2010: 974943.

21. Kouguchi H, Watanabe T, Sagane Y, Ohyama T (2001) Characterization and reconstitution of functional hemagglutinin of the Clostridium botulinum type C progenitor toxin. Eur J Biochem 268: 4019-4026.

22. Sugawara Y, Matsumura T, Takegahara Y, Jin Y, Tsukasaki Y, et al. (2010) Botulinumhemagglutinin disrupts the intercellular epithelial barrier by directly binding E-cadherin. J Cell Biol 189: 691-700.

23. Jin Y, Takegahara Y, Sugawara Y, Matsumura T, Fujinaga Y (2009) Disruption of the epithelial barrier by botulinumhaemagglutinin (HA) proteins - differences in cell tropism and the mechanism of action between HA proteins of types A or B, and HA proteins of type C. Microbiology 155: 35-45.

24. Matsumura T, Jin Y, Kabumoto Y, Takegahara Y, Oguma K, et al. (2008) The HA proteins of botulinum toxin disrupt intestinal epithelial intercellular junctions to increase toxin absorption. Cell Microbiol 10: 355-364.

25. Lee K, Gu S, Jin L, Le TT, Cheng LW, et al. (2013) Structure of a bimodularbotulinum neurotoxin complex provides insights into its oral toxicity. PLoSPathog 9: e1003690.

26. Simpson LL (2004) Identification of the major steps in botulinum toxin action. Annu Rev PharmacolToxicol 44: 167-193.

27. Nishiki T, Tokuyama Y, Kamata Y, Nemoto Y, Yoshida A, et al. (1996) Binding of botulinum type B neurotoxin to Chinese hamster ovary cells transfected with rat synaptotagmin II cDNA. NeurosciLett 208: 105-108.

28. Neuvonen PJ, Olkkola KT (1988) Oral activated charcoal in the treatment of intoxications. Role of single and repeated doses. Med Toxicol Adverse Drug Exp 3: 33-58.

29. Lai IH, Tsao JH, Lu YP, Lee JW, Zhao X, et al. (2009) Neutrophils as one of the major haptoglobin sources in mastitis affected milk. Vet Res 40: 17.

30. Bannerman DD, Paape MJ, Hare WR, Sohn EJ (2003) Increased levels of LPS-binding protein in bovine blood and milk following bacterial lipopolysaccharide challenge. J Dairy Sci 86: 3128-3137.

31. Bionaz M, Trevisi E, Calamari L, Librandi F, Ferrari A, et al. (2007) Plasma paraoxonase, health, inflammatory conditions, and liver function in transition dairy cows. J Dairy Sci 90: 1740-1750.

32. Turk R, JuretiÄ‡ D, Geres D, Svetina A, Turk N, et al. (2008) Influence of oxidative stress and metabolic adaptation on PON1 activity and MDA level in transition dairy cows. AnimReprodSci 108: 98-106.

33. Schroedl W, Jaekel L, Krueger M (2003) C-reactive protein and antibacterial activity in blood plasma of colostrum-fed calves and the effect of lactulose. J Dairy Sci 86: 3313-3320.

34. Krüger M, Shehata AA, Schrödl W, Rodloff A (2013) Glyphosate suppresses the antagonistic effect of Enterococcus spp. on Clostridium botulinum. Anaerobe 20: 74-78.

35. Wang JY, Lin KD, Hou ZN, Richardson B, Gan J (2010): Sorption of the herbicide terbuthylazine in two New Zealand forest soils amended with biosolids and biochards. J Soils Sediments 10: 283-289.

36. Kim YH, Hong JR, Gil HW, Song HY, Hong SY (2013) Mixtures of glyphosate and surfactant TN20 accelerate cell death via mitochondrial damage-induced apoptosis and necrosis. Toxicol In Vitro 27: 191-197.

37. Graber ES, Tsechansky L, Gerstl Z, Lew B (2012) High surface area biochar negatively impacts herbicide efficacy. Plant Soil 353: 95-106.

38. Shehata AA, Kühnert M, Haufe S, Krüger M (2014) Neutralization of the antimicrobial effect of glyphosate by humic acid in vitro. Chemosphere 104: 258-261.

39. Mazzei P, Piccolo A (2012) Quantitative evaluation of noncovalent interactions between glyphosate and dissolved humic substances by NMR spectroscopy. Environ SciTechnol 46: 5939-5946.

40. Yu Z, Zhang X, Li S, Li C, Li D, et al. (2013) Evaluation of probiotic properties of Lactobacillus plantarum strains isolated from Chinese sauerkraut. World J MicrobiolBiotechnol 29: 489-498.

41. Fujinaga Y, Inoue K, Nomura T, Sasaki J, Marvaud JC, et al. (2000) Identification and characterization of functional subunits of Clostridium botulinum type A progenitor toxin involved in binding to intestinal microvilli and erythrocytes. FEBS Lett 467: 179-183.

42. Yang Z, Li S, Zhang X, Zeng X, Li D, et al. (2010) Capsular and slime-polysaccharide production by Lactobacillus rhamnosus JAAS8 isolated from Chinese sauerkraut: potential application in fermented milk products. J BiosciBioeng 110: 53-57.

43. Badel S, Bernardi T, Michaud P (2011) New perspectives for Lactobacilli exopolysaccharides. BiotechnolAdv 29: 54-66.

44. Zhang L, Liu C, Li D, Zhao Y, Zhang X, et al. (2013) Antioxidant activity of an exopolysaccharide isolated from Lactobacillus plantarum C88. Int J Biol Macromol 54: 270-275.

45. El-Shenawy NS (2009) Oxidative stress responses of rats exposed to Roundup and its active ingredient glyphosate. Environ ToxicolPharmacol 28: 379-385.

46. Beuret CJ, Zirulnik F, Giménez MS (2005) Effect of the herbicide glyphosate on liver lipoperoxidation in pregnant rats and their fetuses. ReprodToxicol 19: 501-504.

47. Albers CN, Banta GT, Hansen PE, Jacobsen OS (2009) The influence of organic matter on sorption and fate of glyphosate in soil--comparing different soils and humic substances. Environ Pollut 157: 2865-2870.

19

Comparing Heat-Treated Silica Particle with Silica Particles for the Ability to Induce Superoxide Release from Rat Alveolar Macrophages

Masayuki Ohyama[1*], Hideki Tachi[2], Chika Minejima[3] and Takayuki Kameda[4]

[1]*Department of Environmental Health, Osaka Prefectural Institute of Public Health, Japan*

[2]*Department of Textile & Polymer Section, Technology Research Institute of Osaka Prefecture, Japan*

[3]*Department of Material Science, College of Liberal Arts, International Christian University, Japan*

[4]*Department of Socio-Environmental Energy Science, Kyoto University, Japan*

*Corresponding author: Ohyama Masayuki, Osaka Prefectural Institute of Public Health, 1-3-69, Nakamichi, Higashinari-ku, Osaka 537-0025, Japan, E-mail: ohyama@iph.pref.osaka.jp

Abstract

Crystalline silica can devitrify with the formation of cristobalite and other crystalline silica species when exposed to prolonged high temperatures, which is of potential concern because crystalline silica is classified as carcinogenic. Silica particles activate macrophages to release oxidants, which contribute to inflammation and injury in the lower respiratory tract. Our aim was to compare silica particles with heat-treated silica particles for their ability to induce superoxide release from rat alveolar macrophages. We estimated the ability of four types of silica particle samples and heat-treated silica particles with different number average particle diameter to induce lucigenin-dependent chemiluminescence (CL) from macrophages based on the number of silica particles. A strong positive correlation was observed between particle diameter and the ability to induce CL in both the silica and heat-treated silica samples. Moreover, the ability of heat-treated silica samples to induce CL was approximately 43% of that of the silica samples. These results suggest that heat-treated silica reduces superoxide release from macrophages, and that the heat-treated reduces the biological effects of silica.

Keywords: Silica; Quartz; Heat-treated; Superoxide; Reactive oxygen species; Macrophage

Introduction

In 1987 the International Agency for Research on Cancer classified crystalline silica as a probable carcinogen [1] and in 1997 reclassified it as a Group 1 carcinogen [2]. Alveolar macrophages play a critical role in crystalline silica-induced cytotoxicity and genotoxicity [3,4].

Heating modifies the state of the silica surface and progressively decrease the membranolytic activity of silica dust toward erythrocytes [5-7], by eliminating from the surface the sites responsible for the interaction with cell membrane components. Fubini et al. demonstrated that cytotoxicity of crystalline silica to the rat lung alveolar epithelial cell line was greatly reduced for heat-treated silica at 800°C and eliminated for heat-treated silica at 1300°C [8].

We observed a close positive correlation between silica particle diameters and the ability to induce the release of superoxide from macrophages (in contributing). Therefore, it is possible to compare the ability to induce the release of superoxide with silica and heat-treated silica by the method.

The purpose of this study was to investigate the effect of heat-treated silica particles at 800°C in the ability to induce superoxide release from rat alveolar macrophages. Although the silica particles were heat-treated at 1300°C too, the samples could not be used for the experiment because of aggregating.

Materials and Methods

Silica samples

Silica (S-5631, Particle size: 0.5–10 μm) was obtained from Sigma Chemical Co. (St. Louis, MO, USA). We suspended silica particles in distilled water, and four samples (A, B, C and D) of different particle sizes were obtained depending on the sedimentation rate of the suspension. A part of each four sample (HA, HB, HC and HD) was heat-treated by an electric furnace (ks-1502, ADVANTEC, Tokyo, Japan). The electric furnace was programed as follows: 500°C for 1 h, 500°C for 10 min, 800°C for 4 h, 800°C for 1 h, and then turned off. The diameters of particles in the four samples were measured using a laser scattering particle size distribution analyzer (LA-700, Horiba Ltd., Kyoto, Japan). Silica particle numbers per unit weight were counted using a hemocytometer under an optical microscope (Microphot-FX, Nikon corp., Tokyo, Japan) (objective lens: (20; eyepiece: (10; intermediate magnifier: (2; resolving power of lens: λ/2N.A.=0.3667 μm, where λ=0.55 μm and numerical aperture (N.A.)=0.75).

All samples were dried and heat-sterilized at 80°C for 48 h and suspended in fetal bovine serum (FBS) at concentrations of 1 mg/ml. The suspensions were incubated for 15 min at 37°C, and spin-washed three times in Hanks' balanced salt solution (HBSS) at 900×g for 20 min. Pellets were resuspended at 0.77, 3.08, and 5.38 mg/ml. These suspensions were stored at 4°C.

Cell isolation

Bronchoalveolar lavage was performed on F344 rats (Japan Slc, Inc., Hamamatu, Japan) to isolate alveolar macrophages for in vitro experiments. Briefly, rats were injected peritoneally with 5% pentobarbital sodium at 25 mg/kg. The lungs were lavaged with cold (4°C) HBSS containing 100 U of penicillin and 100 μg of streptomycin per 1 ml with a 10 ml plastic syringe. This process was repeated until a total of 50 mL lavage fluid was collected. The lavage fluid was centrifuged at 250×g, for 10 min at 4°C. The pellet was resuspended in 5 mL of RPMI-1640 medium (HEPES modification, Sigma Chemical Co.) with 10% FBS and penicillin (100 U/mL) and streptomycin (100 μg/mL). In all experiments, the viability of cells was higher than 95 percent as measured by the trypan blue exclusion test. The suspension stored at 4°C until an assay. All procedures associated with this study were reviewed and approved by the Institutional Animal Care and Use Committee at Osaka Prefectural Institute of Public Health.

CL measurements

The method for measuring lucigenin-dependent CL from the macrophages exposed to various mineral samples has been described in previous reports [9-12].

The isolated cells (1.5×10^5) were transferred to a luminometer tube containing sample suspension (65 μl), 10% FBS, 0.1 mM lucigenin, and in some experiments 1,000 unit/ml superoxide dismutase (SOD). The final volume of each tube was 1 ml. The light emission of each sample was detected at 15-min intervals using a luminescence reader (ALOKA BLR-201, Mitaka, Tokyo, Japan). The CL response of all samples, including the negative control (no particle), was measured at constant rotation every 15 min using a stock suspension of cells. We performed all reactions at 37°C in RPMI 1640, and each measurement three times.

Statistical analysis

We estimated the ability to induce CL per sample particle for exclusion of sample dose effects, as described previously [10,11].

Briefly, we plotted the relationships between the administered numbers of samples and CL response. A slope (i.e., β_1) of linear regression of the administered numbers of samples and CL was estimated as the ability to induce CL per sample. As β_1 was a constant, it was possible to universally compare with each sample and to examine relationship between the ability to induce CL and sample geometries. In this study, we examined the relationship between β_1 and number average particle diameter of samples by linear regression in two groups of silica samples and heat-treated silica samples. Moreover, we compared the slopes (i.e., β_2) of linear regression of two groups to examine the reducibility of heat-treatment.

Results

Silica size per unit weight

Table 1 shows the results of silica samples from the laser scattering particle size distribution analyzer, and the results of particle number per unit weight of silica samples using a hemocytometer and an optical microscope. Each diameter of heat-treated silica was considerably similar with that of silica. We used the number average particle diameter as the particle size.

Time course of the ability to induce CL per dust particle (β_1)

We calculated β_1 to compare the CL response of each sample at a value not related to the number of sample particles. Table 2 shows β^1 and r^2 values of the regression line with CL and number of sample particles. All samples dose-dependently induced a CL response. Each response was almost completely inhibited by SOD, which is a superoxide scavenger (data not shown). Figure 1 shows a representative relationship between the number of sample particles and CL at 45 min. The ability to induce CL of heat-treated silica samples was reduced than silica samples.

Sample	A	HA	B	HB	C	HC	D	HD
median diameter (μm)	3.79	4.99	2.89	3.08	0.99	0.83	0.68	0.58
number average particle diameter (μm)	5.43	5.27	4.34	4.52	2.31	2.22	1.10	1.15
% diameter: 90.0% (μm)	8.09	8.95	6.71	6.92	2.95	2.84	1.39	1.08
number per unit weight (/μg)	6650	6780	9255	9285	55286	56143	340500	412500
ratio of number per unit weight	(1 : 1.020)		(1 : 1.003)		(1 : 1.016)		(1 : 1.211)	

Table 1: Particle diameter and number per unit weight of silica samples.

Timea	0		15		30		45		60		75		90		105		120	
	β_1[b]	r^2[c]	β_1	r^2	β_1	r^2	β_1	r^2	β_1	r^2	β_1	r^2	β_1	r^2	β_1	r^2	β_1	r^2
A	−0.6	0.59	25.2	0.73	40.5	0.99	66.2	0.95	104	0.97	151.3	0.99	174.7	0.98	166.4	0.95	145.6	0.95
HA	−0.3	0.40	5.5	0.49	15.9	0.85	27.6	0.98	48.3	0.99	66.4	1.00	87.0	0.98	92.1	0.99	88.9	0.97

B	-0.1	0.01	18.8	0.72	35.4	1.00	59.9	1.00	101.5	1.00	139.2	0.99	148.4	0.99	139.5	0.96	118.6	0.95
HB	-0.2	0.40	10.8	0.92	14.9	0.91	25.0	0.98	41.4	0.96	63.4	0.96	77.4	0.97	83.3	0.96	80.4	0.96
C	0.0	0.05	1.2	0.54	4.1	0.96	9.0	0.99	15.5	0.99	22.9	0.99	25.4	0.99	23.4	0.96	19.0	0.92
HC	0.0	0.02	4.0	0.94	5.3	0.93	7.3	0.98	10.3	0.98	15.1	0.97	17.9	0.97	19.6	0.97	19.1	0.96
D	0.0	0.86	0.1	0.14	1.2	0.99	1.8	0.99	2.5	1.00	3.2	0.99	3.7	0.99	3.8	0.97	3.5	0.96
HD	0.0	0.00	0.2	0.67	0.2	0.48	0.4	0.89	0.5	0.90	0.6	0.94	0.7	0.91	0.9	0.91	1.1	0.94

Table 2: Slope (β_1) and r^2 of the regression lines for CL and number of silica particles.

[a]Time after administration (min). [b]β_1 ($\times 10^{-8}$) is the slope of the regression line for the estimated number of silica particles administered and CL response with three concentrations and a duplicate negative control. The CL response is the mean value of the three measurements. [c]Square of the correlation coefficient of the regression line.

[a]Time after administration (min). [b]β_1 ($\times 10^{-8}$) is the slope of the regression line for the estimated number of silica particles administered and CL response with three concentrations and a duplicate negative control. The CL response is the mean value of the three measurements. [c]Square of the correlation coefficient of the regression line.

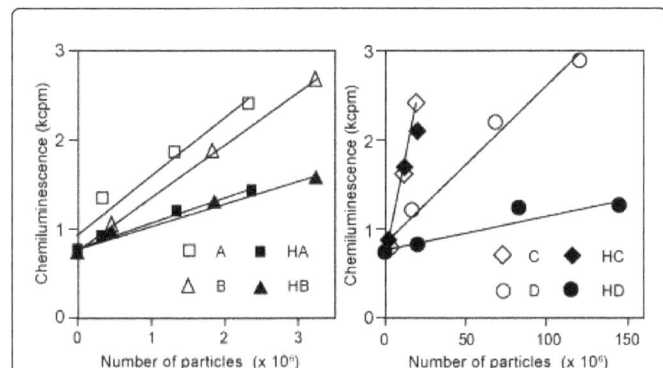

Figure 1: The relationship between number of dust particles and CL response at 45 min. The lines represent regression lines. The slope (β_1) of the line was taken as a measure of the ability to induce CL per silica particle.

Relationship between the ability to induce CL per dust particle (β_1) and silica diameter

Figure 2 shows a representative relationship between β_1 and number average particle diameter in the two groups (silica particles and heat-treated silica particles). A close correlation was found between β_1 and sample particle diameter in both the two groups. β_2 of regression lines of the heat-treated silica group was weaker than that of silica group.

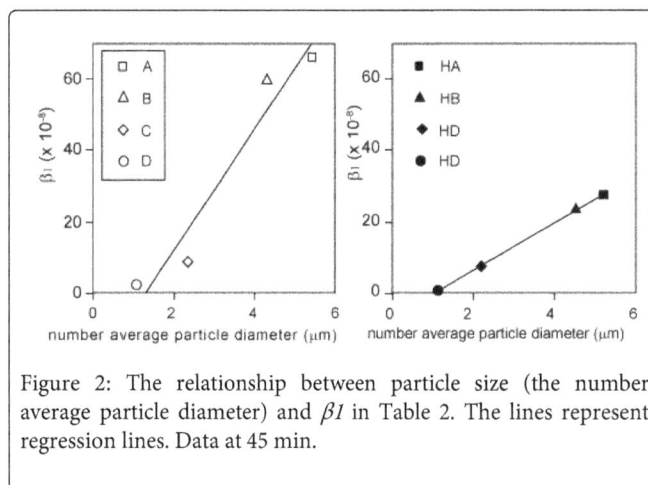

Figure 2: The relationship between particle size (the number average particle diameter) and $\beta1$ in Table 2. The lines represent regression lines. Data at 45 min.

Table 3 presents β_2 and r^2 of the regression lines with particle diameter and β_1. A close correlation was found between sample particle diameter and β_1 at each time-point in both the two groups. Silica group was more active than heat-treated silica group. β_2 of heat-treated silica group was 43 percent of silica group at the average measurement period.

Time[a]	15		30		45		60		75		90		105		120	
	β_2[b]	r^2[c]	β_2	r^2	β_2	r^2	β_2	r^2	β_2	r^2	β_2	r^2	β_2	r^2	β_2	r^2
Silica[d]	6.31	0.95	10.2	0.94	16.7	0.95	26.9	0.93	38.4	0.95	43.3	0.96	41.1	0.97	35.7	0.97
HS[e]	1.75	0.59	3.92	0.99	6.89	0.99	12.1	1.00	17.2	0.98	22.1	0.99	23.5	0.99	22.6	0.99
Ratio[f]	3.60		2.61		2.43		2.23		2.23		1.96		1.75		1.58	

Table 3: Slope (β_2) and r^2 of the regression lines for β_1 in Table 2 and particle size.

[a]Time after administration (min). [b]β_2 ($\times 10^{-8}$) is the slope of the regression line for $\beta1$ in Table 2 and particle size (the number average particle diameter). [c]Square of the correlation coefficient of the regression line for β_1 in Table 2 and particle size. [d]Group of four silica

samples. eGroup of heat-treated four silica samples (HS). $^f\beta_2$ of silic /β_2 of HS.

Discussion

We found the ability of heat-treated silica samples to induce CL from rat alveolar macrophages was weaker than that of silica samples. It was possible to universally compare the effect of particle diameter between the two groups when β_2 (Figure 2 and Table 3) was excluded.

These results suggest that the heat-treated of silica reduce the superoxide release from macrophages. Our results consist with oxidants from macrophages relate to carcinogenicity of silica particles.

Heating modifies the state of the silica surface and progressively decrease the membranolytic activity of silica dust toward erythrocytes [5-7], by eliminating from the surface the sites responsible for the interaction with cell membrane components. Although cytotoxicity of crystalline silica to the rat lung alveolar epithelial cell line was greatly reduced for heat-treated silica at 800°C and eliminated for heat-treated silica at 1300°C, heat-treated at 1300°C did not affect silica micromorphology and crystallinity. However, surface of silica, still showed some hydrophilic patches in heat-treated at 800°C, but heat-treated at 1300°C was fully hydrophobic [8]. Although we heat-treated the four types of silica particles at 800 and 1300°C, the samples of heat-treated silica at 1300°C were not examined by the particle aggregation. It was assumed that the surface of silica was made to change by the heat-treated at 1300°C very much.

We suggested previously that the induction superoxide release from macrophages occurs nonspecifically for various types of mineral fibers depending on fiber length, and that the kinetics of the induction superoxide release from macrophages is similar between silica particles and mineral fibers; moreover, this depends on silica particle size and mineral fiber geometry. However, present results show that the activity of the induction superoxide release from macrophages is different for two types of silica particles, may differ surface character. It seems that the present macrophage activity results are inconsistent with the nonspecific mineral fiber results. We considered to the inconsistency that the fiber length affects to release superoxide from macrophages further than the fiber surface characteristics. In fact, we previously demonstrated that the activity of mineral fiber to induce superoxide release from macrophages was approximately 8.3 times greater than that of silica [12].

In conclusion, our results suggest that the ability of heat-treated silica samples to release superoxide from macrophages reduced to approximately 43 percent of that of silica sample and that heat treatment reduces the biological effects of silica.

Acknowledgments

This study was supported by a Grant-in-Aid for Scientific Research from the Ministry of Education, Culture, Sports, Science and Technology.

References

1. IARC Monograph (1987) IARC Monograph on the Evaluation of the Carcinogenic Risk of Chemicals to Humans, Vol. 42: Silica and some silicates. IARC Press, Lyon.

2. [No authors listed] (1997) IARC Working Group on the Evaluation of Carcinogenic Risks to Humans: Silica, Some Silicates, Coal Dust and Para-Aramid Fibrils. Lyon, 15-22 October 1996. IARC Monogr Eval Carcinog Risks Hum 68: 1-475.

3. Fanizza C, Ursini CL, Paba E, Ciervo A, Di Francesco A, et al. (2007) Cytotoxicity and DNA-damage in human lung epithelial cells exposed to respirable alpha-quartz. Toxicol In Vitro 21: 586-594.

4. Zhang Z, Shen HM, Zhang QF, Ong CN (2000) Involvement of oxidative stress in crystalline silica-induced cytotoxicity and genotoxicity in rat alveolar macrophages. Environ Res 82: 245-252.

5. Pavan C, Tomatis M, Ghiazza M, Rabolli V, Bolis V, et al. (2013) In search of the chemical basis of the hemolytic potential of silicas. Chem Res Toxicol 26: 1188-1198.

6. Thomassen LC, Rabolli V, Masschaele K, Alberto G, Tomatis M, et al. (2011) Model system to study the influence of aggregation on the hemolytic potential of silica nanoparticles. Chem Res Toxicol 24: 1869-1875.

7. Sahai N (2002) Biomembrane phospholipid-oxide surface interactions: crystal chemical and thermodynamic basis. J Colloid Interface Sci. 252: 309-319.

8. Fubini B, Zanetti G, Altilia S, Tiozzo R, Lison D, et al. (1999) Relationship between surface properties and cellular responses to crystalline silica: studies with heat-treated cristobalite. Chem Res Toxicol 12: 737-745.

9. Ohyama M, Otake T, Morinaga K (2001) Effect of size of man-made and natural mineral fibers on chemiluminescent response in human monocyte-derived macrophages. Environ Health Perspect 109: 1033-1038.

10. Ohyama M, Otake T, Morinaga K (2000) The chemiluminescent response from human monocyte-derived macrophages exposed to various mineral fibers of different sizes. Ind Health 38: 289-293.

11. Nyberg P, Klockars M (1990) Measurement of reactive oxygen metabolites produced by human monocyte-derived macrophages exposed to mineral dusts. Int J Exp Pathol 71: 537-544.

12. Ohyama M, Tachi H, Minejima C, Kameda T (2014) Comparing the Role of Silica Particle Size with Mineral Fiber Geometry in the Release of Superoxide from Rat Alveolar Macrophages. J Toxicol Sci 39.

20

Improvement of QT Analysis for Evaluating the Proarrhythmic Risk of Drug: The Importance of Spatial and Temporal Dispersion of Repolarization

Gilles Hanton[*]

GH Toxconsulting, Brussels, Belgium

[*]**Corresponding author:** Dr. Gilles Hanton, 27 avenues Everard, B-1190, Bruxelles, E-mail: gilles.hanton@yahoo.fr

Abstract

Cardiac arrhythmias, in particular life-threatening Torsades de Pointes (TdP) are serious adverse effects associated with a number of pharmaceuticals belonging to different classes. It is therefore critical to have reliable biomarkers for assessing this risk during pre-clinical testing of new compounds. Prolongation of cardiac action potential and consequently of the QT interval of the ECG is generally considered as indicative of a risk of arrhythmia. Evaluation of drug effects on QT in preclinical studies is therefore requested by ICH (International Conference on Harmonization) guideline (S7B). However there is now growing evidence that the prolongation of mean QT interval is not an accurate indicator of the risk of arrhythmia and that other parameters of cardiac repolarization are more predictive. They include instability of action potential duration and increase in transmural heterogeneity of myocardial repolarization (spatial variability), which can be investigated in specific *in vitro* tests. We have conducted a number of experiments in dogs for evaluating the ECG correlates of both markers in studies testing the effects of isoproterenol, cisapride, astemizole and hypokaliemia, which are known to be associated with a proarrhythmic risk. Instability of action potential duration is associated with an increase in the beat-to-beat (temporal) variability of the QT interval that is evaluated by calculating the coefficient of variation of this parameter or by plotting QT from each beat versus QT of previous beat. Spatial variability of repolarization correlates with changes in the morphology of the T wave, in particular increase in the interval between the peak and the end of the T wave and notching of this wave. In these experiments, we have therefore established a simple method for *in vivo* assessment of spatial and temporal variability of cardiac repolarization, which may help in the evaluation the pro-arrhythmic risk of drugs.

Keywords: Cardiac arrhythmia; Cardiac repolarization; QT variability; T wave morphology

Introduction

Prolongation of the QT interval of the ECG corresponding to a delayed cardiac repolarization is produced by a number of drugs, in laboratory animals and humans and is generally considered as indicative of a risk of arrhythmia. Evaluation of drug effects on QT in preclinical studies is therefore requested by the ICH (International Conference on Harmonization) guideline S7B [1].

However there is now growing evidence that the prolongation of QT interval as such is not an accurate indicator of pro-arrhythmic risk and that other parameters of cardiac repolarization are more predictive [2-5]. They include time-related and spatial variability of cardiac action potential duration (CAPD) [6,7]. Time related variability of CAPD can be evaluated *in vitro* in isolated rabbit heart or *in vivo* as changes in beat-to-beat variability of the QT interval [8,9].

Spatial variability of CAPD, can be assessed *in vitro* in cardiac wedges preparation or *in vivo* by changes in the morphology of the T wave of the ECG [10].

We have established the methodology for these *in vivo* investigations in a few studies testing the effects of astemizole, cisapride, isoproterenol, and hypokaliemia, which are known to be associated with a proarrhythmic risk. Studies were conducted in dogs, which is the most frequent non-rodent species used in preclinical toxicity and safety pharmacology studies.

In vitro evaluation of time-related variability of CAPD associated instability of cardiac action potential

One of the best ways for this investigation is to use the Screenit model developed by Pr. Hondeghem [8]. Cardiac action potentials are recorded *in situ* in isolated rabbit heart. In addition to time-related variability (instability) of CAPD, two additional parameters, triangulation and reverse use dependency are recorded and constitute together a so called *TRIad*, which give critical information on the proarrhythmic risk.

Instability of action potential consists of increased beat-to-beat variability of CAPD. When it reaches a critical level it can lead to chaotic behavior of the myocardium and consequent arrhythmias [5]. Instability can be evaluated by plotting each action potential duration against the preceding one (Pointcaré plot). Proarrhythmic drugs produce instability as indicated by increased degree of scattering of the successive points [11]. Instability of the cardiac action potential is considered as one of the most sensitive predictors of proarrhythmia, since it frequently precedes the arrhythmic event and occurs at a much lower drug concentration than a prolongation of the action potential duration.

Triangulation of the action potential is a more oblique repolarization phase. It is considered to be proarrhythmic because it increases the duration of the vulnerable period of repolarization during which early after-depolarizations may occur and trigger Torsade de Pointes (TdP) [12].

Reverse-use dependence is characterized by more marked effects of compounds on the action potential at lower than at higher stimulation rates and therefore reflects the likelihood of TdP.

In vivo evaluation of time-related (beat-to-beat) variablility of CAPD

The variability of CAPD over time can be evaluated from the temporal variability QT intervals measured on ECG tracings. After recording individual QT intervals over 15 sec to 1 min, mean (mean $_{QT}$) and standard deviation (SD_{QT}) are calculated and the coefficient of variation $CV_{QT}=SD_{QT}/mean\ _{QT}$ is established as an evaluator of beat-to-beat variability of QT, especially in dog studies. The formula of QT temporal dispersion $QT_{td}=\log_{10}(CV_{QT}/CV_{RR})^2$, which is used in clinic, is not adapted to dogs because of the marked sinus arrhythmia in this species and consequently high value of CV_{RR} [13].

Another way for evaluating the temporal variability of QT is to establish the Poincaré plot in which the QT value from each beat is plotted against the following one. The spreading of the individual points gives the degree of variability of QT interval [9].

In vitro evaluation of spatial variability of CAPD

For evaluating the variability of CAPD in the different layers of the ventricle (transmural heterogeneity of myocardial repolarization), the arterially perfused cardiac wedge is one of the best models. Action potentials are recorded on the endocardium, epicardium and mid myocardium, in dogs.

This preparation allows evaluation of differences in CAPD across the ventricle wall. Indeed the different cardiomyocytes layers repolarize at different rates, the endocardium being the first and the mid-myocardium the latest to repolarize.

An increase in this transmural heterogeneity of repolarization has been assumed to be a key trigger of arrhythmias since it may result in reentry and subsequent TdP [14]. Notably, most pro-arrhythmic I_{Kr} blockers have a more marked effect on mid-myocardial cells in dogs (M cells) than on epicardial or subendocardial cells, and thus accentuate the heterogeneity of myocardial repolarization [6].

In vivo evaluation of spatial variability of cardiac repolarization

Transmural heterogeneity of repolarization times can be evaluated in dog toxicity studies from ECG tracings by assessing the changes in the morphology of the T wave. The T wave is the result of 2 opposing voltage gradients, between mid-myocardium M cell and epicardium. The full repolarization of epicardial cell corresponds to the peak of T wave whereas the full repolarization of M cells corresponds to end of T wave. An increased heterogeneity of repolarization of these different cell layers produced an increase in the interval between the peak and the end of the T wave interval (Tp –Te), which is considered in the clinic as a marker of the risk for ventricular arrhythmias [15]. When the transmural dispersion of repolarization is still more pronounced, it may lead to a notching of the T wave [16].

Experimental Assessment

Designs of studies

Effects on astemizole: Using a cross-over design, we treated 9 dogs/group with a single intravenous injection of astemizole at doses of 0, 1 or 3 mg/kg. ECGs were recorded before treatment, then 0.5 and 1 hour after treatment (100 beats).

Another group of 3 dogs received single intravenous injections of astemizole at increasing doses (6, 9 and 15 mg/kg.) over 3 successive days. ECGs were recorded before treatment, then 15 minutes, 30 minutes, 1 hour and 3 hours after treatment (40 beats).

Effects of cisapride: Using a cross-over design, we treated 9 dogs/group with a single intravenous injection of cisapride, at doses of 0, 1.5 or 6 mg/kg. ECGs were recorded before treatment, then 0.5 and 1 hour after treatment (100 beats).

Effects of hypokalemia: Hypokalemia was induced by oral treatment of 12 dogs with furosemide at increasing doses (5-60 mg/kg) over 12 days. ECGs were recorded before furosemide dosing, then 1.5 and 3.5 hours after each dosing (over 1 minute).

Effects of isoproterenol: A group of 3 dogs received increasing doses (2.5, 5 and 10 µg/kg) of isoproterenol by the subcutaneous route. ECGs were recorded before treatment, then 15 min, 30 min, 1 h, 3 h and 5 h after treatment (over 20 seconds).

ECG recording

Standard bipolar limb leads I, II, III, unipolar limb leads aVR, aVL, aVF and precordial leads CV6LL, CV5RL, CV6LU, V10 were recorded. T wave morphology and QT interval were assessed from CV5RL lead, since this lead gives the most accurate evaluation of end of T wave, which is monophasic and positive in untreated animals.

Evaluation of temporal variability of QT

QT values were recorded from individual beats and the coefficient of variation of QT: $CV_{QT}=SD_{QT}/mean\ _{QT}$ was calculated.

Evaluation of the morphology of the T wave

Modifications of the T wave were recorded from precordial lead CV5RL. In particular notching was noted. It consists in presence of 2 peaks on the wave. A grading system has been established as:

0: no notching.

1: minimal notching, mild rupture of continuity in ascending part of the T wave.

2: mild notching, plateau but single peak of the T wave.

3: moderate notching, second peak on the descending part of the wave, less than 0.1 mV between peak and trough, mild flattening

4: marked notching, second peak, with 0.1 to 0.3 mV between peak and trough, moderate flattening

5: severe notching, second peak with more than 0.3 mV between trough and peak, marked flattening and/or trough at the isoelectric line or slightly below.

Results

Detailed data have been provided in previous publications [13,17,18].

Effect of astemizole

In the cross over study, astemizole produced a dose-related increase in QT interval and in CV_{QT} at 30 and 60 min after dose (Table 1).

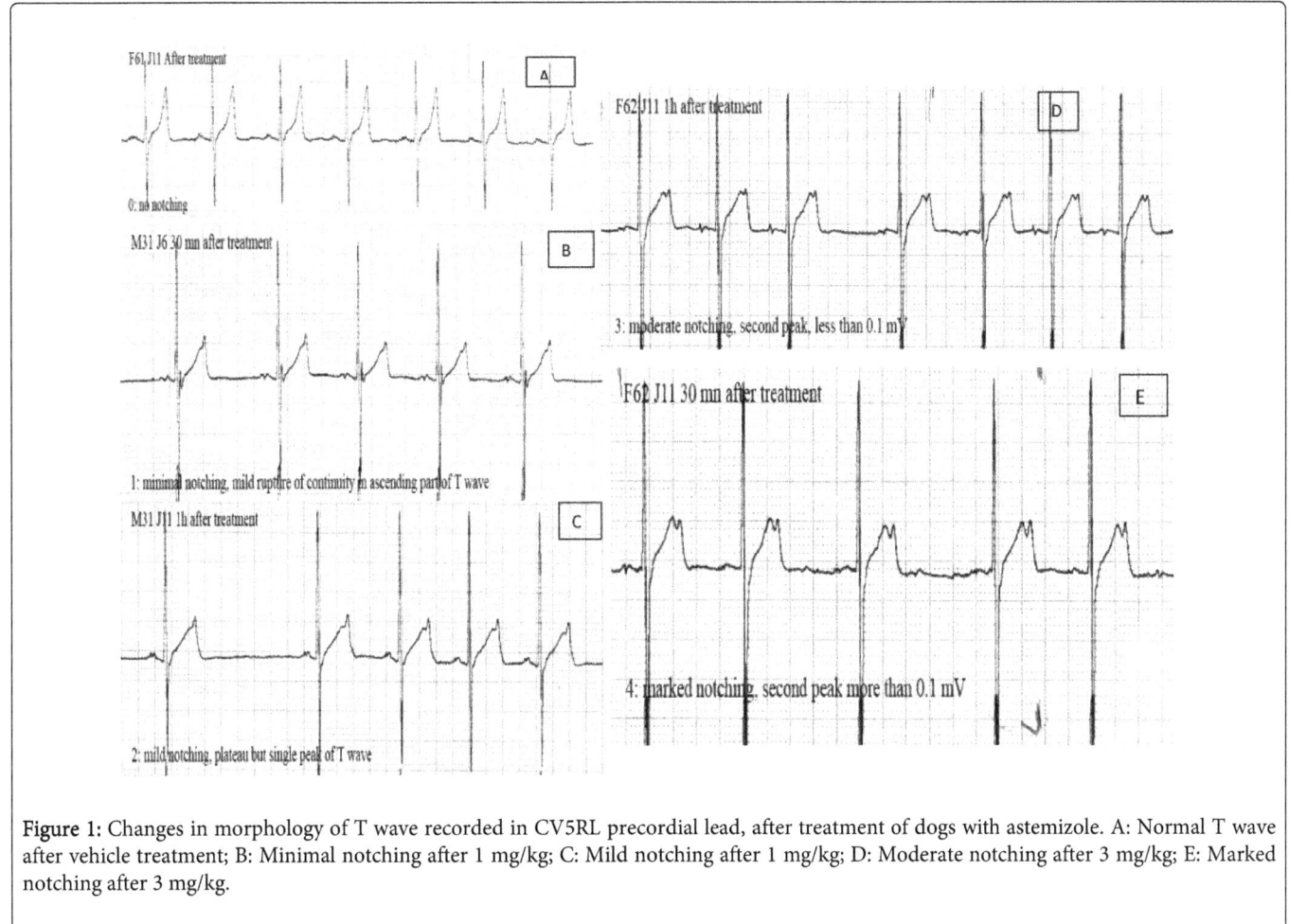

Figure 1: Changes in morphology of T wave recorded in CV5RL precordial lead, after treatment of dogs with astemizole. A: Normal T wave after vehicle treatment; B: Minimal notching after 1 mg/kg; C: Mild notching after 1 mg/kg; D: Moderate notching after 3 mg/kg; E: Marked notching after 3 mg/kg.

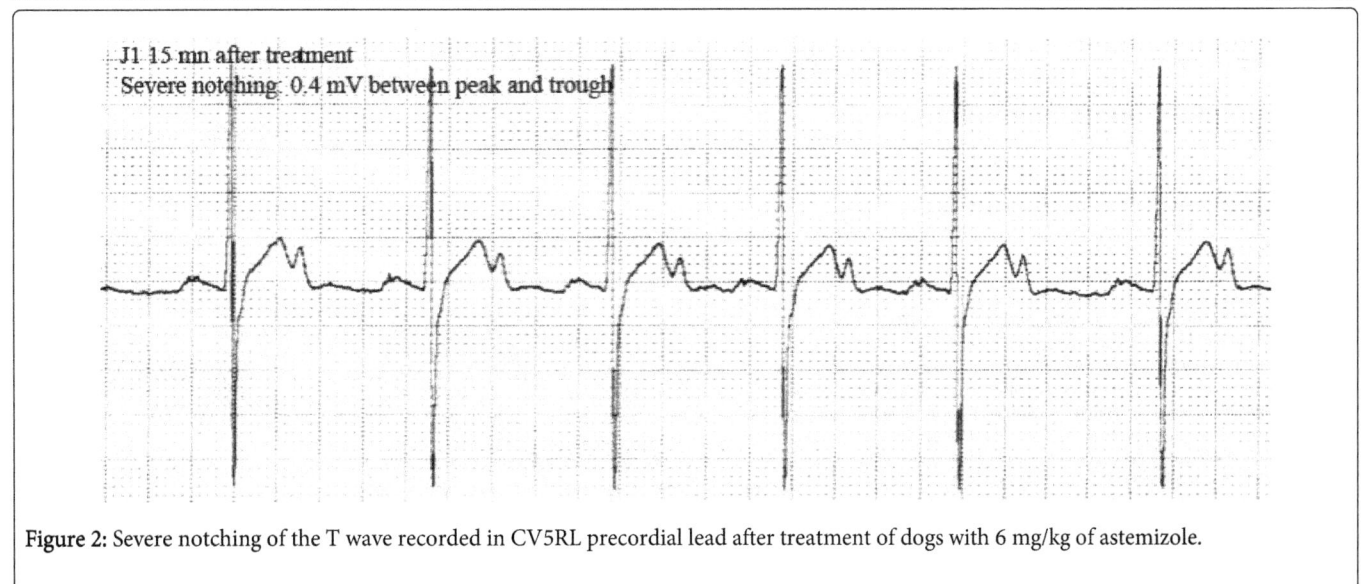

Figure 2: Severe notching of the T wave recorded in CV5RL precordial lead after treatment of dogs with 6 mg/kg of astemizole.

Notching of the T wave also occurred in both the cross over and the increased dose study and in some occasions was very pronounced and associated with a flattening of the wave (Table 2, Figure 1 and 2).

Effects of cisapride

The changes were similar to those produced by astemizole. The increase in CV_{QT} was slightly less pronounced for Cisapride than for astemizole (Table 3), but T wave notching was similar or even more marked in one animal (Table 2 and Figure 3).

Effects of hypokalemia

Hypokalemia produced an increase in QT interval and a number of changes in T wave morphology, in particular notching, flattening, inversion, biphasic of triphasic aspect (Figure 4).

	Mean values at 3 time points (n=9) Lead CV5RL			Difference compared to pre dose values	
	Pre-dose	30 min	60 min	30 min	60 min
Control	1.51 ± 0.33	1.47 ± 0.51	1.62 ± 0.37	-0.04	0.11
1 mg/kg	1.65 ± 0.41	2.48 ± 0.57	2.25 ± 0.74	0.84**	0.61
3 mg/kg	1.67 ± 0.35	2.89 ± 1.15	2.80 ± 1.22	1.22**	1.13**
Change compared to control at 1 mg/kg	0.13	1.01***	0.63*		
Change compared to control at 3 mg/kg	0.16	1.42***	1.18**		

*: $p<0.05$; **: $p<0.01$; ***: $p<0.001$ (data analyzed with a linear mixed model of analysis of variance with time, dose and the dosetime interaction as fixed effects and animal as a random effect).

Table 1: Effect of astemizole on coefficient of variation of QT in dogs.

		Mean score (n = 9) (range mini-max)		
		Before	30 minutes	60 minutes
Astemizole	Control	0.55 (0-2)	0.22 (0-1)	0.75 (0-2)
	1 mg/kg	0.55 (0-2)	2.11 (0-3)	2.22 (0-4)
	3 mg/kg	0.55 (0-1)	3.22 (1-4)	2.67 (0-4)
Cisapride	Control	0.4 (0-2)	0.7 (0-2)	0.6 (0-2)
	1.5 mg/kg	0.3 (0-2)	1.6 (0-3)	0.7 (0-2)
	6 mg/kg	0.2 (0-1)	2.6 (0-4)	2.3 (0-5)

Table 2: Notching of the T wave recorded in CV5RL precordial lead, after treatment of dogs with astemizole or cisapride.

	Mean values at 3 time points (n=9) Lead CV5RL			Difference compared to predose values	
	Pre-dose	30 min	60 min	30 min	60 min
Control	1.45 ± 0.42	1.41 ± 0.43	1.58 ± 0.25	-0.04	0.13
1.5 mg/kg	1.56 ± 0.41	2.06 ± 0.52	1.79 ± 0.39	0.5*	0.23
6 mg/kg	1.56 ± 0.33	2.16 ± 0.82	1.67 ± 0.58	0.6**	0.11
Change compared to control at 1 mg/kg	0.11	0.65*	0.21		
Change compared to control at 3 mg/kg	0.11	0.75*	0.09		

*: $p<0.05$; **: $p<0.01$; ***: $p<0.001$ (data analyzed with a linear mixed model of analysis of variance with time, dose and the dosetime interaction as fixed effects and animal as a random effect).

Table 3: Effect of cisapride on coefficient of variation of QT in dogs.

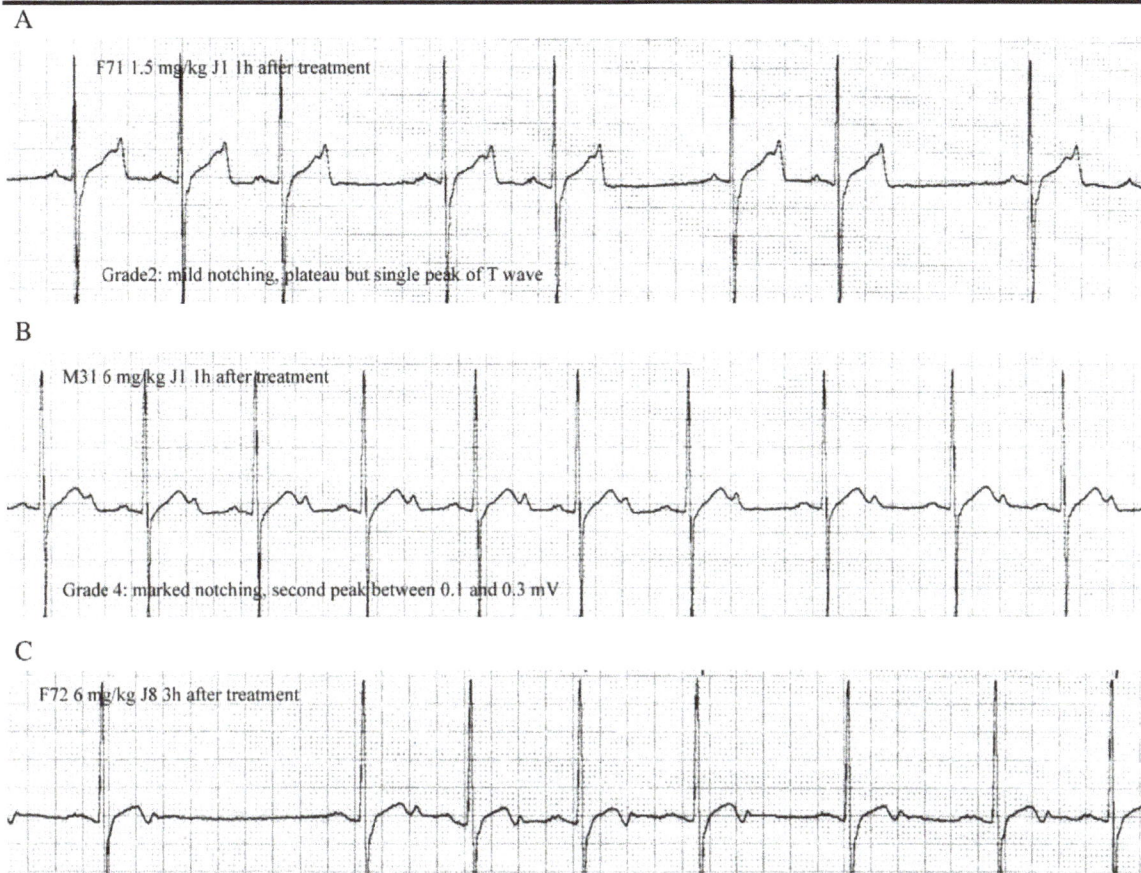

Figure 3: Changes in morphology of T wave recorded in CV5RL precordial lead, after treatment of dogs with cisapride. To be compared with normal monophasic T wave. **(A)** Mild notching 1 h after treatment with 1.5 mg/kg: (grade 2); **(B)** Marked notching with flattening of the T wave 1 h after treatment with 6 mg/kg (grade 4); **(C)** Severe notching of the T wave, 3 h after treatment with 6 mg/kg (grade 5).

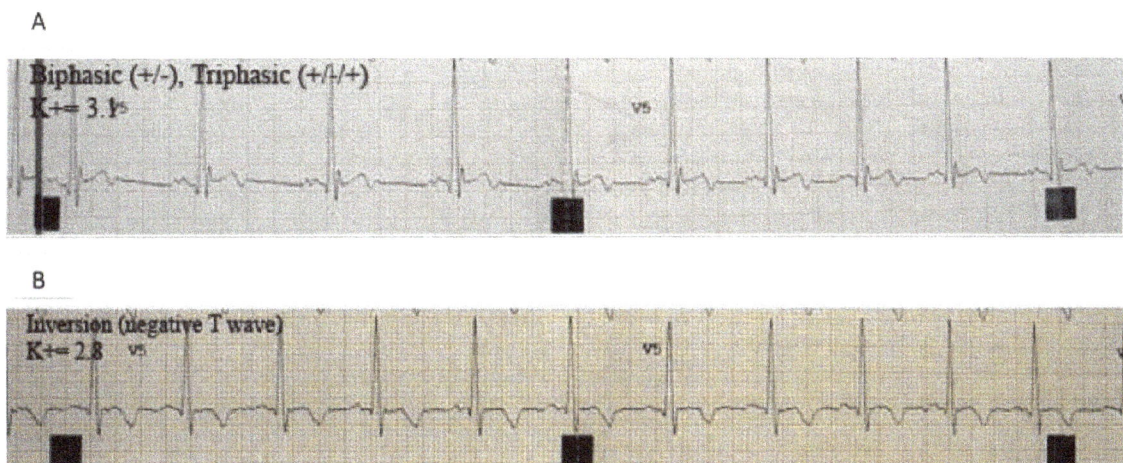

Figure 4: Severe changes inmorphology of T wave recorded in CV5RL precordial lead in hypokalemic dogs (treatment with furosemide). To be compared with normal T wave monophasic and positive. **(A)** Biphasic or triphasic T wave; **(B)** Inversion of T wave.

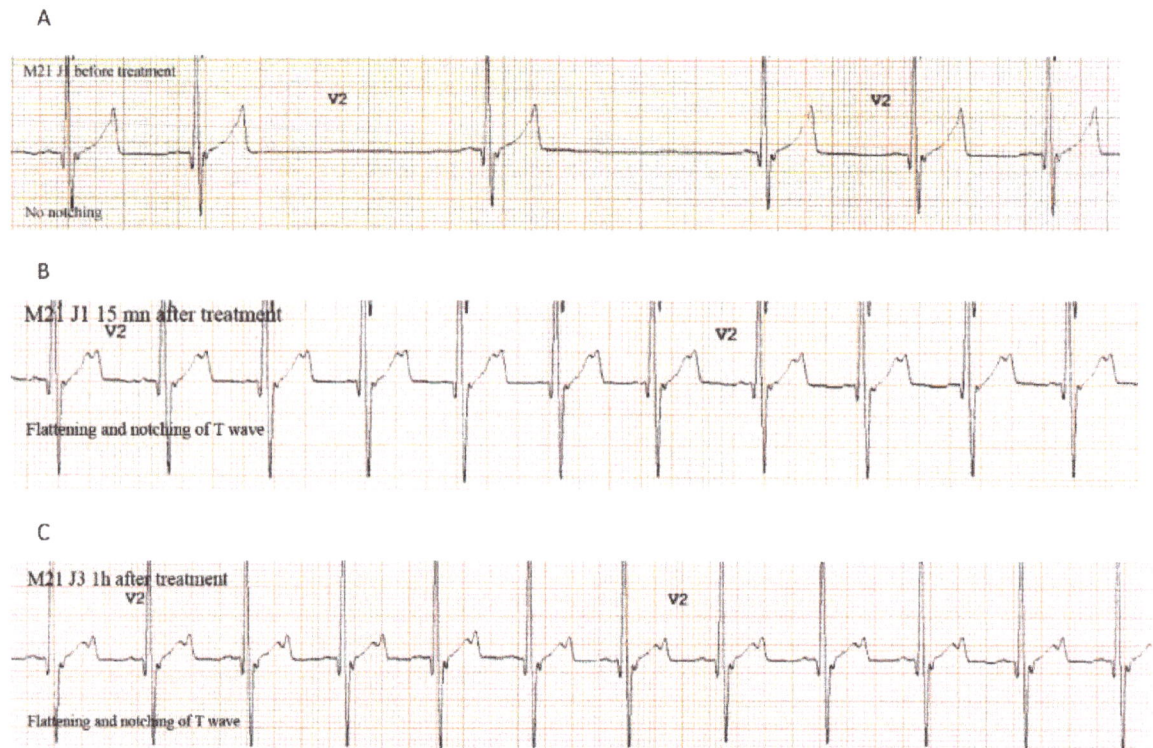

Figure 5: Changes in morphology of T wave recorded in CV5RL precordial lead, in a dog treated with 5 μg/kg of isoproterenol.

Effect of isoproterenol

Isoproterenol produced a marked increase in heart rate, a decrease in corrected QT interval (QTc) and a notching of T wave (Figure 5).

Discussion

The temporal variability of the QT interval of the ECG is the *in vivo* correlate of cardiac action potential instability, which has been shown to be markedly increased by arrhythmogenic drugs, in particular I_{Kr} blockers and is considered as a reliable and sensitive predictor for the risk of arrhythmia [12]. In the astemizole experiment, the CV of QT was markedly increased, indicating an effect on the temporal variability of cardiac repolarization. The CV of QT was also increased by cisapride but to a lesser extent as compared to astemizole. Results from both studies indicate that the CV of QT can assess the temporal variability of QT in dogs treated with pro-arrhythmic I_{Kr} blockers. These findings were consistent with those of previous authors [9].

Clinical investigations have shown that increased beat-to-beat QT variability is an indicator of temporal myocardial repolarization liability and predicts ventricular tachyarrhythmias, sudden cardiac death and cardiovascular mortality [19-21].

The second key observation after treatment with astemizole and cisapride was a clear notching of the T wave, consisting of presence of 2 peaks of the T wave, with the intermediate trough sometimes reaching the isoelectric line, giving an impression of U wave. Notching of the T wave indicates an increase in the heterogeneity of repolarization of the different layers of cardiomyocytes across the ventricular wall and consequent modification of the transmural voltage gradient [22-24]. The change is considered to be due to differences in the action of the compounds on different cardiac cells. I_{Kr} blockers like astemizole or cisapride act predominantly on the M cells, which are more sensitive to I_{Kr} blocking than epicardial or endocardial cells [25,26]. Notching of the T wave has been previously observed in dogs and humans after treatment with I_{Kr} blockers [26-28].

Notching of the T wave in dogs was therefore found to be a predictive biomarker for the evaluation of potential proarrhythmic risk of I_{Kr} blockers and the aim of further studies was to verify this finding in situations potentially producing arrhythmia by other ways than I_{Kr} blocking. These experiments indicated that diuresis-induced hypokalemia and isoproterenol, an adrenergic β-agonist both produce T wave abnormalities.

Notching and/or flattening of the T wave in CV5RL in dogs treated with isoproterenol is also probably related to an increase in heterogeneity of the repolarisation of the different cardiomyocytes layers across the ventricular wall. *In vitro* studies on canine cardiac tissues have shown that isoproterenol produced a greater shortening of the action potential in epicardial than in endocardial cardiomyocytes and prolonged the action potential of M cells [29,30]. These changes resulted from a large augmentation in I_{Ks} current in epicardial and endocardial cells but not in M cells in which I_{Ks} is weak.

The changes in T wave morphology in hypokalemic dogs is consistent with *in vivo* and *in vitro* data and find a similar explanation as the changes produced by astemizole, cisapride and isoproterenol. In isolated cardiac tissues, a decrease in extracellular potassium prolongs the duration of cardiac action potential to a greater extent in the epicardium than in other myocardial layers, which is attributed to a predominant I_{to} current (responsible for transient early outflow of potassium) in the epicardium [14]. Electrophysiological studies in isolated cardiac cells also showed that when extracellular potassium decreases, the slope of phase 2 of the action potential becomes steeper and phase 3 slower, resulting in an increased duration of the action potential. The period of incomplete repolarization tends to be longer in Purkinje fibres than in ventricular cells, resulting in an increased dispersion of repolarization [31]. In humans, hypokalemia is known to produce typical changes in the ECG, in particular a decrease in T wave amplitude and the appearance of a U wave [32]. Similar changes have been observed in hypokalemic dogs [33].

Notching of the T wave thus occurred in different conditions known to be associated with arrhythmic events. Notably this indication of proarrhythmic risk was found in association with QT prolongation (astemizole, cisapride and hypokaliemia) but also with QT shortening (isoproterenol). The findings of the current experiments are therefore consistent with clinical investigations showing that changes in the morphology of the T wave, in particular T wave notching and increase in Tp-Te, are reliable markers of the proarrhythmic risk [34-36].

In conclusion, we have established a simple method for *in vivo* assessment of spatial and temporal variability of cardiac repolarization, which may help in the evaluation the pro-arrhythmic risk of drugs. The precordial lead CV5RL was found to be the best lead for these investigations. This methodology could help in the interpretation of findings in pre-clinical studies.

References

1. Guth BD, Germeyer S, Kolb W, Markert M (2004) Developing a strategy for the nonclinical assessment of proarrhythmic risk of pharmaceuticals due to prolonged ventricular repolarization. J Pharmacol Toxicol Methods 49: 159-169.

2. Hoffmann P, Warner B (2006) Are hERG channel inhibition and QT interval prolongation all there is in drug-induced torsadogenesis? A review of emerging trends. J Pharmacol Toxicol Methods 53: 87-105.

3. Belardinelli L, Antzelevitch C, Vos MA (2003) Assessing predictors of drug-induced torsade de pointes. Trends Pharmacol Sci 24: 619-625.

4. Redfern WS, Carlsson L, Davis AS, Lynch WG, MacKenzie I, et al. (2003) Relationships between preclinical cardiac electrophysiology, clinical QT interval prolongation and torsade de pointes for a broad range of drugs: Evidence for a provisional safetymargin in drug development. Cardiovasc Res 58: 32-45.

5. Shah RR, Hondeghem LM (2005) Refining detection of drug-induced proarrhythmia: QT interval and TRIaD. Heart Rhythm 2: 758-772.

6. Shimizu W, Antzelevitch C (1999) Cellular basis for long QT, transmural dispersion of repolarization, and torsade de pointes in the long QT syndrome. J Electrocardiol 32 Suppl: 177-184.

7. De Clerk F, Van de Water A, D'Aubioul J, Lu HR, Van Rossem K, et al. (2002) In vivo measurement of QT prolongation, dispersion and arrhythmogenesis: application to the preclinical cardiovascular safety pharmacology of a new chemical entity. Fundam Clinical Pharmacol 16: 125-140.

8. Hondeghem LM, Lu HR, van Rossem K, De Clerck F (2003) Detection of proarrhythmia in the female rabbit heart: blinded validation. J Cardiovasc Electrophysiol 14: 287-294.

9. Van der Linde H, Van de Water A, Loots W, Van Deuren B, Lu HR, et al. (2005) A new method to calculate the beat-to-beat instability of QT duration in drug-induced long QT in anesthetized dogs. J Pharmacol and Toxicol Meth 52: 168-177.

10. Antzelevitch C, Shimizu W (2002) Cellular mechanisms underlying the long QT syndrome. Curr Opin Cardiol 17: 43-51.

11. Valentin JP, Hoffmann P, De Clerck F, Hammond TG, Hondeghem L (2004) Review of the predictive value of the Langendorff heart model (Screenit system) in assessing the proarrhythmic potential of drugs. J Pharmacol Toxicol Methods 49: 171-181.

12. Hondeghem LM, Carlsson L, Duker G (2001) Instability and triangulation of the action potential predict serious proarrhythmia, but action potential duration prolongation is antiarrhythmic. Circulation 103: 2004-2013.

13. Hanton G, Yvon A, Racaud A (2008) Temporal variability of QT interval and changes in T wave morphology in dogs as markers of the clinical risk of drug-induced proarrhythmia. J Pharmacol Toxicol Methods 57: 194-201.

14. Antzelevitch C, Sicouri S, Litovsky SH, Lukas A, Krishnan SC, et al. (1991) Heterogeneity within the ventricular wall. Electrophysiology and pharmacology of epicardial, endocardial, and M cells. Circ Res 69: 1427-1449.

15. Ravensbergen HJ, Walsh ML, Krassioukov AV, Claydon VE (2012) Electrocardiogram-based predictors for arrhythmia after spinal cord injury. Clin Auton Res 22: 265-273.

16. Xue J, Chen Y, Han X, Gao W (2010) Electrocardiographic morphology changes with different type of repolarization dispersions. J Electrocardiol 43: 553-559.

17. Hanton G, Bonnet P, Loiret C (2007) In vivo assessment of temporal and transmural variability of cardiac repolarization as a tool for evaluating pro-arrhythmic risk. The Toxicologist 96: 76.

18. Hanton G, Yvon A, Provost JP, Racaud A, Doubovetzky M (2007) Quantitative relationship between plasma potassium levels and QT interval in beagle dogs. Lab Anim 41: 204-217.

19. Berger RD, Kasper EK, Baughman KL, Marban E, Calkins H, et al. (1997) Beat-to-beat QT interval variability: novel evidence for repolarization lability in ischemic and nonischemic dilated cardiomyopathy. Circulation 96: 1557-1565.

20. Piccirillo G, Rossi P, Mitra M, Quaglione R, Dell'Armi A, et al. (2013) Indexes of temporal myocardial repolarization dispersion and sudden cardiac death in heart failure: any difference? Ann Noninvasive Electrocardiol 18: 130-139.

21. Tereshchenko LG, Cygankiewicz I, McNitt S, Vazquez R, Bayes-Genis A, et al. (2012) Predictive value of beat-to-beat QT variability index across the continuum of left ventricular dysfunction: competing risks of noncardiac or cardiovascular death and sudden or nonsudden cardiac death. Circ Arrhythm Electrophysiol 5: 719-727.

22. Yan GX, Antzelevitch C (1998) Cellular basis for the normal T wave and the electrocardiographic manifestations of the long-QT syndrome. Circulation 98: 1928-1936.

23. Fei L, Statters DJ, Camm AJ (1994) QT-interval dispersion on 12-lead electrocardiogram in normal subjects: its reproducibility and relation to the T wave. Am Heart J 127: 1654-1655.

24. Wolk R, Mazurek T, Lusawa T, Wasek W, Rezler J (2001) Left ventricular hypertrophy increases transepicardial dispersion of repolarisation in hypertensive patients: a differential effect on QTpeak and QTend dispersion. Eur J Clin Invest 31: 563-569.

25. Shimizu W, Antzelevitch C (1998) Cellular basis for the ECG features of the LQT1 form of the long-QT syndrome: effects of beta-adrenergic agonists and antagonists and sodium channel blockers on transmural dispersion of repolarization and torsade de pointes. Circulation 98: 2314-2322.

26. Lupoglazoff JM, Denjoy I, Berthet M, Neyroud N, Demay L, et al. (2001) Notched T waves on Holter recordings enhance detection of patients with LQt2 (HERG) mutations. Circulation 103: 1095-1101.

27. Jackman WM, Friday KJ, Anderson JL, Aliot EM, Clark M, et al. (1988) The long QT syndromes: a critical review, new clinical observations and a unifying hypothesis. Prog Cardiovasc Dis 31: 115-172.

28. Weissenburger J, Nesterensko VV, Antzelevitch C (2000) Transmural heterogeneity of ventricular repolarization under baseline and long QT conditions in the canine heart in vivo: torsades de pointes develops with

halothane but not pentobarbital anesthesia. J CardiovasElectrophysiol 11, 290-304.

29. Litovsky SH, Antzelevitch C (1990) Differences in the electrophysiological response of canine ventricular subendocardium and subepicardium to acetylcholine and isoproterenol. A direct effect of acetylcholine in ventricular myocardium. Circ Res 67: 615-627.

30. Shimizu W, Antzelevitch C (2000) Differential effects of beta-adrenergic agonists and antagonists in LQT1, LQT2 and LQT3 models of the long QT syndrome. J Am Coll Cardiol 35: 778-786.

31. Vera Z, Janzen D, Desai J (1991) Acute hypokalemia and inducibility of ventricular tachyarrhythmia in a nonischemic canine model. Chest 100: 1414-1420.

32. Surawicz B, Braun HA, Crum WB, Kemp RL, Wagner S, et al. (1957) Quantitative analysis of the electrocardiographic pattern of hypopotassemia. Circulation 16: 750-763.

33. Felkai F (1985) Electrocardiographic signs in ventricular repolarization of experimentally induced hypokalaemia and appearance of the U-wave in dogs. Acta Vet Hung 33: 221-228.

34. Lin YH, Lin LY, Chen YS, Huang HC, Lee JK, et al. (2009) The association between T-wave morphology and life-threatening ventricular tachyarrhythmias in patients with congestive heart failure. Pacing Clin Electrophysiol 32: 1173-1177.

35. Xue J, Gao W, Chen Y, Han X (2009) Identify drug-induced T wave morphology changes by a cell-to-electrocardiogram model and validation with clinical trial data. J Electrocardiol 42: 534-542.

36. Zhou Y, Sedransk N (2013) A new functional data-based biomarker for monitoring cardiovascular behavior. Stat Med 32: 153-164.

21

Protective and Anti-Oxidant Activity of the *Euryops arabicus* against Paracetamol Induced Hepatorenal Toxicity in Rats

Essam Mahmoud Hafez[1*], **Milad Gad Paulis**[1], **Mostafa Abotaleb Ahmed**[1], **Marian NagyFathy**[2], **Ahmed Abdel-Lateff** [3,4] and **Mardi M. Algandaby**[5]

[1]*Department of Forensic Medicine and Clinical Toxicology, Faculty of Medicine, Minia University, Minia 61519, Egypt*

[2]*Department of Pathology, Faculty of Medicine, Minia University, Minia 61519, Egypt*

[3]*Department of Natural Products and Alternative Medicine, Faculty of Pharmacy, King Abdulaziz University, Jeddah, Saudi Arabia*

[4]*Department of Pharmacognosy, Faculty of Pharmacy, Minia University, Minia 61519, Egypt*

[5]*Department of Biological Sciences, Faculty of Science, King Abdulaziz University, Jeddah, Saudi Arabia*

*Correspondence author: Essam M. Hafez, Department of forensic medicine and clinical toxicology, Faculty of Medicine, Minia University, Minia, Egypt, E-mail: essamtox@yahoo.com

Abstract

Paracetamol overdose is a predominant cause of hepatorenal toxicity in both humans and experimental animals. The extract of *Euryops arabicus* was evaluated for its protective and anti-oxidant effect against paracetamol-induced hepatic and renal injuries in rats. The extract of *Euryops arabicus* was administered at100 mg/kg and 200 mg/kg followed by paracetamol at 1g/kg for seven days. The animals were sacrificed after 24 hrs of paracetamol challenge .Indices of liver such as aspartate aminotransferase (AST), alanine aminotransferase (ALT), alkaline phosphatase (ALP), total bilirubin (TB), serum albumin (SA) and renal indices blood urea (BU) and serum creatinine (SC) were measured. Liver and kidney homogenates were analyzed for oxidative stress biomarkers namely Thiobarbituric acid reactive substances TBARS. Finally, histopathological examinations of both previous organs were examined. The significantly disturbed liver and kidney functions by paracetamol toxicity were restored to almost normal values by administration of *Euryops arabicus*. Also, the elevated TBARS in groups received paracetamol alone decreased in groups given paracetamol and *Euryops arabicus*. Histological effect of paracetamol on liver and kidney was also markedly abolished by co-administration of *Euryops arabicus*. These results suggest that *Euryops arabicus* may protect from paracetamol-induced liver and kidney toxicity.

Keywords: *Euryops arabicus*; paracetamol; Thiobarbituric acid reactive substances; hepatorenal histopathology; protective and anti-oxidant

Introduction

Asteraceae is a large family of herbaceous plants contains about 1100 genera and 25,000 species, widely distributed in the tropical and subtropical regions. It is economically important as a source of food, such as lettuce and artichokes, cooking oils, sweetening agents, and tea infusions [1]. Among 100 species of the genus *Euryops,* only *Euryops arabicus* (*E. arabicus*) is known in Saudi Arabia [2].

E. arabicus (Jabur) is dome shaped shrub ranged from three to five feet tall with interesting two inches long narrow lobed leathery leaves which are clustered at the tips of the branches. The fall appears in summer and the composite heads of spaced out yellow ray flowers and orange-yellow disk flowers are appeared. It is attractive plant that it has been described as a dwarf pine tree because of its elongated and narrow leaves. It is native to the Arabian Peninsula south to Somalia where the heated leaves and stems were once used in the treatment of wounds. The first description had been done by Ernst Gottlieb von Steudel, a German physician in 1852. The name for the genus comes from the Greek words 'eury' (or 'eurys') meaning "large" or "broad" and 'ops' (or 'opos') meaning "resemblance", "sight" or "the eye" probably in reference to the large eye-like flowers [1-3]. Metabolites from *E. arabicus* were studied for their anti-oxidant, antimicrobial and antiproliferative effects. For instances, flavonoids,

secofuroermophilanes, furoermophilanes and eremophilanolides were identified from the genus Euryops [3-6].

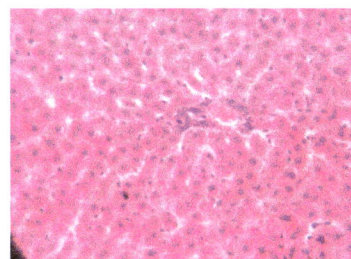

Figure 1: Group I rat liver served as normal negative control and they received normal saline 1 mL/kg bw, orally, normal architecture (H and E x 200).

Drug-induced liver injury is a potential complication of virtually every prescribed medication, because the liver occupies the main role in the metabolic disposition of all drugs and foreign substances. Most of the hepatotoxic chemicals damage liver cells mainly by lipid peroxidation and other oxidative damages and this applies also to paracetamol which is a widely used analgesic and antipyretic which is safe when used at therapeutic levels [4]. Paracetamol is representing the drug of choice in children. However, paracetamol hepatotoxicity is the leading cause of drug induced liver failure and an acute or cumulative overdose can cause severe liver injury with the potential to progress to liver failure [5].

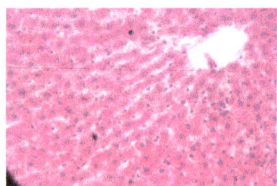

Figure 2: Group II rat liver served as normal positive control and they received 1%.carboxy methyl cellulose 1 mL/kg bw orally, normal architecture (H and E x 200).

Paracetamol induced toxicity in rats is one of the widely used experimental model to evaluate the hepatoprotective nature of herbal extracts [6]. A computer survey including different databases, especially, Scifinder, indicated no publication had been reported about in-vivo anti-oxidant activity of *E. arabicus*.

The main goal of the current study is to evaluate whether the extract of *E. arabicus* has in-vivo antioxidant and protective effect against hepatorenal toxicity induced by paracetamol. The in-vitro antioxidant effect was studied employing the volatile oil which obtained from the areal part of *E. rabicus* and showed moderate activity [7]. Interesting is the chemical composition of *E. arabicus*, is mainly polyphenolic compounds. Thus the current study is interesting in the in-vivo study its antioxidant effect. A combination of biochemical and histological parameters were used to investigate the protective potential of *E. arabicus* extract on paracetamol induced hepatorenal toxicity.

Materials and Methods

Chemicals

All the materials used for this experiment were of analytical grade. Paracetamol (EPICO Company), thiobarbituric acid and potassium phosphate buffer used for determination of Thiobarbituric acid reactive substances (TBARS) level, carboxy methyl cellulose (CMC) were purchased from Sigma and Merck Chemical Companies. Diagnostic kits for the estimation of aspartate aminotransferase (AST) and alanine aminotransferase (ALT), alkaline phosphatase (ALP), serum albumin (SA), total bilirubin (TB), blood urea (BU), and serum creatinine (SC) were manufactured by Ranbaxy Diagnostics Ltd. (UK).

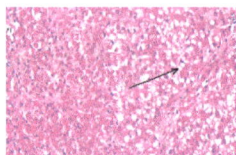

Figure 3: Group III rat liver received paracetamol at dose of 1 g/kg bw p.o. (paracetamol) showing extensive areas of hepatocellular necrosis and inflammatory cell infiltration. Most of the centrilobular hepatocytes were swollen with marked cytoplasmic vacuolation and pyknotic nuclei with obliterated intervening hepatic sinusoids (H and E x 100).

Plant material

The aerial parts *E. arabicus* (Family Asteraceae) were collected from Al-Taeif, 200 Km south Jeddah, Saudi Arabia. The powdered air-dried *E. arabicus* was extracted and prepared according to Walied et al. [7]. The extract was dissolved in 1% CMC just before administration.

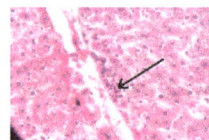

Figure 4: Group IV rat liver received paracetamol and 100 mg/kg bw, p.o. of *E. arabicus* leaves extract. H and E staining of liver showing scattered inflammatory cells (H and E x 200).

Animals

Healthy adult male albino rats weighting about 150-170 grams were obtained from the animal house in Faculty of Science Minia University. All animals were allowed free access to distilled water and laboratory chow ad libitum. To avoid stress of isolation or overcrowdings, 6 rats were housed per cage. They were left freely wandering in their cage for two weeks with 12 hour dark: light cycle for acclimatization before starting the experiment. They were fasted 12h before administration of paracetamol. All protocols used in this study were approved by the Committee of Minia University.

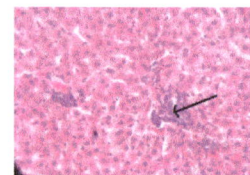

Figure 5: Group V rat liver received paracetamol and 200 mg/kg bw, p.o. of *E. arabicus* leaves extract. H and E staining of liver showing few scattered inflammatory cells (H and E x 200).

Acute toxicity of the extract

The acute toxicity of the extract was performed as per OECD-425 guidelines. Five rats of similar weight were chosen. One animal was fasted overnight with access to drinking water. They were given 2000 mg/kg of the extract and observed for 24h for mortality. The animal survived and then four additional animals were tested sequentially so that a total of five animals were tested. All the animals were observed closely for 24 h and daily for 14 days, no mortality was observed. Hence, we selected 200 mg/kg (1/10th of 2000 mg/kg) as maximum safety dose with descending dose levels with 2 fold interval i.e., 100 mg/kg and 200 mg/kg body weight of the test animal.

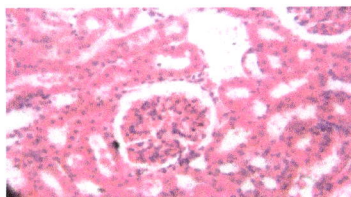

Figure 6: Group I rat renal tissue served as normal negative control and they received normal saline 1 mL/kg bw, orally normal architecture (H and E x 200).

Rats were divided into five groups of 6 animals each and were given orally the following treatment for seven days.

Group I: served as normal negative control and they received normal saline 1 ml/kg body weight, orally (bw, p.o).

Group II: served as normal positive control and they received 1%.carboxy methyl cellulose 1 mL/kg bw, p.o.

Group III: received paracetamol at dose of 1 g/kg bw, p.o.

Group IV: received 100 mg/kg E. arabicus leaves extract followed by 1g /kg paracetamol bw, p.o.

Group V: received 200 mg/kg E. arabicus leaves extract followed by 1g /kg paracetamol bw, p.o.

After 24 h of the last treatment, blood was collected from retro-orbital plexus, allowed to clot for 1 h at room temperature and serum was separated by centrifugation at 2500 rpm for 15 min. The serum was then collected and analyzed for various biochemical parameters.

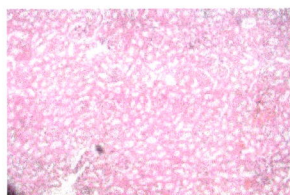

Figure 7: Group II rat renal tissue served as normal positive control and they received 1%.carboxy methyl cellulose 1 mL/kg bw orally (H and E x 200).

Serum biochemical assays

The following tests were done to assess the hepatoxicity of paracetamol AST, ALT, TB, and SA. Kidney functions were looked for by measuring BU and SC. Tests were used according to the standard procedures using commercially available diagnostic kits.

Oxidative stress

Twenty four hour after the last treatment; rat were decapitated. The liver and kidney tissues were dissected from the surrounding fat and connective tissue. Left lobe of liver and left kidney specimens were longitudinally sectioned, kept at -20°C and subsequently homogenized in cold potassium phosphate buffer (0.05 M, pH 7.4). The ratio of tissue weight to homogenization buffer was 1:10. The tissue specimens'

homogenates were centrifuged at 5000 r.p.m for 10 minutes at 4°C. The resulting supernatant was used for determination of TBARS level according to the method of Ohkawa et al. [8].

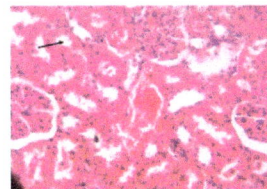

Figure 8: Group III rat renal tissue received paracetamol. H and E staining of kidney showing many tubules with cloudy swelling manifested as enlarged tubules with conical shaped cells, abundant eosinophilic cytoplasm, satellite shaped lumen and luminal cast (H and E x 200).

Histological studies

The right lobe of the liver and right kidney was fixed in 10% buffered formalin and was processed for paraffin sectioning. Sections of about 5 ml thickness were stained with haematoxylin and eosin to be examined and photographed [9].

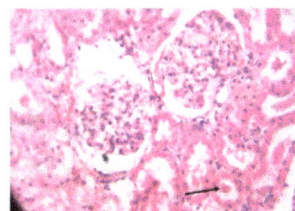

Figure 9: Group IV rat renal tissue, received paracetamol and 100 mg/kg bw, p.o. of E. arabicus leaves extract. . H and E staining of kidney showing few tubules with cloudy swelling, less luminal cast (H and E x 200).

Statistical analysis

All data were represented as mean ± standard deviation (M ± SD). For comparison between groups one-way analysis of variance was used. P value was considered significant if it was less than 0.05.

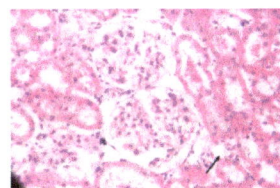

Figure 10: Group V rat renal tissue received paracetamol and 200 mg/kg bw, p.o. of E. arabicus leaves extract. H and E staining of kidney showing very few tubules with cloudy swelling with no luminal cast (H and E x 200).

Results

As shown in table 1 there is significant difference in hepatic and renal biochemistry parameters between the two control groups and paracetamol group indicating toxicity induced by paracetamol. There was significant elevation of AST, ALT, ALP, TB, BU, and SC in group that received paracetamol. Also, there was significant decrease in SA in paracetamol group compared with control ones.

In pretreatment groups with *E. Arabicus* there is significant lowering of the hepatic and renal injury indicators as there is a decrease of the increased level of AST, ALT, ALP, bilirubin, and increase albumin; also, decrease blood urea and serum creatinine.

There is also, much improvement in hepatic and renal function in group pretreated with 200 mg/kg *E. Arabicus* than in that treated with 100 mg/kg.

Table 2 demonstrates thiobarbituric acid reactive substances levels in liver and kidney tissues, there are statistically significant difference between TBARS level between different groups. It much increase in paracetamol group indicating oxidative damage produced by paracetamol but it decrease in rats pretreated with *E. Arabicus*, although it did not reach normal level. There are also little changes between 100 mg/kg pretreated group and 200 mg/kg one.

Groups/ parameters	Liver Function tests					Kidney function tests	
	AST (IU/L)	ALT (IU/L)	ALP (IU/L)	TB (mg/dl)	SA (gm/dl)	SC (mg/dl)	BU (mg/dl)
Group I (-ve control)	64.2 ± 1.23	39.8 ± 2.4	120.1 ± 4.3	0.4 ± 0.04	3.3 ± 0.60	0.2 ± 0.85	23.6 ± 3.12
Group II (+veControl)	61.4 ± 2.02	37.7 ± 2.34	115.3 ± 3.81	0.6 ± 0.05	4.1 ± 0.23	0.3 ± 0.39	28.3 ± 4.68
Group III (Paracetamol group)	160.3 ± 3.42***	89.7 ± 0.32***	389.8 ± 16.51***	0.9 ± 0.04***	1.9 ± 0.34***	1.3 ± 0.62***	55.7 ± 5.12***
Group IV (Paracetamol +100EA)	110.7 ± 2.3**	64.2 ± 2.81**	310.2 ± 17.17**	0.7 ± 0.03**	2.6 ± 0.43**	1.0 ± 0.23**	40.2 ± 5.90**
Group V (Paracetamol +200EA)	98.7 ± 1.24*	54.8 ± 1.91*	212.1 ± 14.50*	0.6 ± 0.04*	2.9 ± 0.67*	0.8 ± 0.42*	39.3 ± 4.70*
Data represent Mean ± SD of the each group. *P <0.05, **P < 0.01, ***P < 0.001							

Table 1: Biochemistry levels of the groups.

Histopathological examination also provided supportive evidence for the results obtained from the enzyme analysis. Microscopically, liver slices from control animals stained with haematoxylin and eosin showed normal parenchymal architecture with cords of hepatocytes, portal tracts and terminal veins without noticeable alterations (Figures 1 and 2).

Liver section of paracetamol treated rats showing extensive areas of hepatocellular necrosis and inflammatory cell infiltration. Most of the centrilobular hepatocytes were swollen with marked cytoplasmic vacuolation and pyknotic nuclei with obliterated intervening hepatic sinusoids (Figure 3).

Liver section of rats treated with paracetamol and 100 mg/kg bw of *E. Arabicus* showed less inflammatory cells around central vein and absence of necrosis (Figure 4). Liver section of rats treated paracetamol and 200 mg/kg bw of *E. Arabicus* showed minimal inflammatory cellular infiltration, regeneration of hepatocytes around central veinwas also observed and almost near normal liver architecture (Figure 5) , indicating the hepatoprotective activity of *E. Arabicus*.

Regarding to the renal histology, group I and II show normal kidney architecture (Figures 6 and 7). In group III; rats received toxic dose of paracetamol, there are many tubules with cloudy swelling manifested as enlarged tubules with conical shaped cells, abundant eosinophilic cytoplasm, satellite shaped lumen and luminal cast (Figure 8). In group IV and V; there was much decrease in the inflammation and cast than paracetamol group with more improvement in group V comparing with group IV (Figures 9 and 10).

Discussion

Paracetamol induced hepatic injury is considered as one of the most commonly used model for hepatoprotectivity drug screening through estimation of serum cytoplasmic enzymes; aspartate aminotransferase (AST), alanine aminotransferase (ALT), alkaline phosphatase (ALP), serum albumin (SA), total bilirubin (TB), blood urea (BU) and serum creatinine (SC) activities is a useful as quantitative markers of the extent, type of hepatocellular and renal affection by paracetamol [10,11]. In the current study, the significant elevation of the enzymes levels, particularly, serum aspartate aminotransferase, alanine aminotransferase, alkaline phosphatase, total bilirubin blood urea, and serum creatinine in the rats which treated with paracetamol, indicate the deterioration of the hepatic functions due to the toxic effects of the drug and consequently, they have been attributed to the damage of structural integrity of the liver, because these enzymes released into the circulation after autolytic breakdown or cellular necrosis [12].

The reduction in the level of hepatic markers by the *E. arabicus* is an indicator of stabilization of the plasma membrane as well as repair of hepatic tissue damage caused by paracetamol. This effect is in agreement with the commonly accepted view that serum levels of transaminases return to normal with the healing of hepatic parenchyma and the regeneration of hepatocytes [13].

There is statistically significant TBARS level difference as it increases in paracetamol group indicating oxidative damage produced by paracetamol but it decreases in rats pretreated with *E. Arabicus* although it did not reach normal level. There are also little changes between 100 mg/kg pretreated group and 200 mg/kg one. All these results are in agreement with published data [14-16], that indicated the elevation in TBARS level in paracetamol group is an indicator of lipid peroxidation which is due to paracetamol induced tissue damage.

Groups/parameters	Hepatic TBARS	Renal TBARS
Group I (-ve control)	35.2 ± 5.20	22.9 ± 3.65
Group II (+veControl)	28.8 ± 6.78	21.2 ± 5.34
Group III (Paracetamol group)	93.1 ± 7.41***	37.2 ± 2.12***
Group IV (Paracetamol +100EA)	65.9 ± 7.97**	32.6 ± 1.3**
Group V (Paracetamol +200EA)	60.8 ±8.11*	28.7 ± 4.3*
TBARS is measured in μmol of malondialdehyde/mg of tissue proteins. *P < 0.05, **P < 0.01, ***P < 0.001		

Table 2: Thiobarbituric acid reactive substances in liver and kidney tissues.

Histological findings of tissue damage induced by paracetamol in the liver confirmed previous laboratory results that showing extensive areas of hepatocellular necrosis and inflammatory cell infiltration and this coincides with Roomi et al. [17] who found mild and significant lobular focal hepatitis in paracetamol studied group.

Rregarding renal histological finding there are many tubules with cloudy swelling manifested as enlarged tubules with conical shaped cells, abundant eosinophilic cytoplasm, satellite shaped lumen and luminal cast. These results are in agreement with Madhukiran et al. [18] who reported that kidneys of paracetamol treated rats, the inflammatory cell infiltration in the interstitium and significant tubular damage were detected. In contrast, Ahmed et al. [19] who observed that the ingestion of paracetamol (500 mg/kg/day) did not produce papillary necrosis nor interstitial nephritis.

Flavonoids isolated from *E. arabicus* had been proved to increase the expression of the rate limiting enzyme in the synthesis of c-glutamylcysteine synthetase with a concomitant increase in the intracellular glutathione concentrations [20-21].

The reactive species mediated hepatotoxicity can be effectively managed upon administration of agents possessing anti-oxidant [22], free radical scavenger [23] and anti-lipid per oxidant activities [24]

A potential of hepatoprotective property underlying *E. arabicus* may be attributed to the polyphenolic principles, particularly, flavonoids. This finding could be explained by the comparing results with those plants that mainly used for treatment of liver disorders. For instance, *Curcuma longa* (turmeric), *Glycyrrhiza glabra* (licorice), and *Camellia sinensis* (Green tea), are reported to be hepatoprotective due to the powerful anti-oxidative properties [25-28]. In addition, the antioxidant properties of *Trichosanthes cucumerina* are attributed to flavonoids, carotenoids, lycopene, phenolics, and β-carotene [29].

Conclusion

E. arabicus has the ability to protect the liver and kidneys from the damaging effects of paracetamol in acute toxic doses and stimulation of endogenous anti-oxidant defense system.

References

1. Underberg AA, Baldwin BG, Bayer RG, Compositae (2007) The Families and Genera of Vascular Plants, In: Kadereit JW, Jeffrey C (eds.), Flowering Plants, Dicots, Asterales, VIII, Springer, Berlin, Heidelberg, New York 61.

2. Özçelik B, Orhan I, Toker G (2006) Antiviral and antimicrobial assessment of some selected flavonoids. Z Naturforsch C 61: 632-638.

3. Mothana RA, Alsaid MS, Al-Musayeib NM (2011) Phytochemical analysis and in vitro antimicrobial and free-radical-scavenging activities of the essential oils from Euryops arabicus and Laggera decurrens. Molecules 16: 5149-5158.

4. Rumack BH (2004) Acetaminophen misconceptions. Hepatology 40: 10-15.

5. Lee WM (2004) Acetaminophen and the U.S. Acute Liver Failure Study Group: lowering the risks of hepatic failure. Hepatology 40: 6-9.

6. Nirmala M, Girija K, Lakshman K, Divya T (2012) Hepatoprotective activity of Musa paradisiaca on experimental animal models. Asian Pac J Trop Biomed 2: 11-15.

7. Walied M Alarif, Ahmed Abdel-Lateff, Ahmed M Al-Abd (2013) Selective cytotoxic effects on human breast carcinoma of new methoxylated flavonoids from Euryops arabicus grown in Saudi Arabia. European Journal of Medicinal Chemistry 66: 204-210.

8. Ohkawa H, Ohishi N, Yagi K (1979) Assay for lipid peroxides in animal tissues by thiobarbituric acid reaction. Anal Biochem 95: 351:8.

9. Romero-Sarmiento Y, Soto-Rodrguez I, Arzaba-Villalba A, Garca HS, Alexander-Aguilera A (2012) Effects of conjugated linoleic acid on oxidative stress in rats with sucrose-induced non-alcoholic fatty liver disease. J. Funct. Food 4: 450–458.

10. Dash Deepak K, Yeligar Veerendra C, Nayak Siva S, Tirtha Ghosh, Rajalingam D (2007) Evaluation of hepatoprotective and antioxidant activity of Ichnocarpus frutescens (Linn.) R.Br. on paracetamol - induced hepatotoxicity in rats. Trop J Pharm Res 6: 755–765.

11. Ehsan Kheradpezhouh, Mohammad-Reza Panjehshahin, Ramin Miri , Katayoun Javidnia et al. (2010) Curcumin protects rats against acetaminophen-induced hepatorenal damages and shows synergistic activity with N-acetyl cysteine . European Journal of Pharmacology 628: 274–281.

12. Zhang R, Hu Y, Yuan J, Wu D (2009) Effects of Puerariae radix extract on the increasing intestinal permeability in rat with alcohol-induced liver injury. J Ethnopharmacol 126: 207-214.

13. Thabrew MI, Joice PD, Rajatissa W (1987) A comparative study of the efficacy of Pavetta indica and Osbeckia octandra in the treatment of liver dysfunction. Planta Med 53: 239-241.

14. Knight TR, Kurtz A, Bajt ML, Hinson JA, Jaeschke H (2001) Vascular and hepatocellular peroxynitrite formation during paracetamol-induced liver injury: Role of mitochondrial oxidant stress. Toxicol. Sci 62: 212–220.

15. Sener G, Sehirli AO, Ayan DG (2003) Protective effects of melatonin, vitamin E and N-acetylcysteine against acetaminophen toxicity in mice: a comparative study. J Pineal Res 35: 61-68.

16. Khan RA, Khan MR, Sahreen S, Shah NA (2000) Hepatoprotective activity of Sonchus asper against carbon tetrachloride-induced injuries in male rats: a randomized controlled trial. BMC Complem. Altern. Med 201: 1-90.

17. Roomi MW, Kalinovsky T, Ivanov V, Rath M, Niedzwiecki A (2008) A nutrient mixture prevents acetaminophen hepatic and renal toxicity in ICR mice. Hum Exp Toxicol 27: 223-230.

18. Madhukiran P, Ganga Rao B (2011) Invitro evaluation for free radical scavenging activity of methanolic leaf extract of Cyathea gigantean (wall Ex.hook). Int J Pharm Res Dev 3: 2.

19. Ahmed MH, Ashton N, Balment RJ (2003) Renal function in a rat model of analgesic nephropathy: effect of chloroquine. J Pharmacol Exp Ther 305: 123-130.

20. Myhrstad MC, Carlsen H, Nordstrom O, Blomhoff R, Moskaug JJ (2002) Flavonoids increase the intracellular glutathione level by transactivation

of the gamma-glutamylcysteine synthetase catalytical subunit promoter. Free Radic. Biol. Med 32: 386–393.

21. Moskaug JØ, Carlsen H, Myhrstad MC, Blomhoff R (2005) Polyphenols and glutathione synthesis regulation. Am J Clin Nutr 81: 277S-283S.

22. Attri S, Rana SV, Vaiphei K, Sodhi CP, Katyal R, et al. (2000) Isoniazid- and rifampicin-induced oxidative hepatic injury--protection by N-acetylcysteine. Hum Exp Toxicol 19: 517-522.

23. Sadanobu S, Watanabe M, Nakamura C, Tezuka M (1999) In vitro tests of 3-dithia-2-thioxo-cyclopent-4-ene to evaluate the mechanisms of its hepatoprotective action. J Toxicol Sci 24: 375-381.

24. Lim HK, Kim HS, Choi HS, Oh S, Jang CG, et al. (2000) Effects of acetylbergenin against D -galactosamine-induced hepatotoxicity in rats. Pharmacol Res 42: 471-474.

25. Donatus IA, Sardjoko, Vermeulen NP (1990) Cytotoxic and cytoprotective activities of curcumin. Effects on paracetamol induced cytotoxicity, lipid peroxidation and glutathione depletion in rat hepatocytes.Biochem Pharmacol 39: 1869–1875.

26. Soni KB, Lahiri M, Chackradeo P, Bhide SV, Kuttan R (1997) Protective effect of food additives on aflatoxin-induced mutagenicity and hepatocarcinogenicity. Cancer Lett 115: 129-133.

27. Wang GS, Han ZW (1993) The protective action of glycyrrhiza flavonoids against carbon tetrachloride hepatotoxicity in mice. Yao Xue Xue Bao 28: 572-576.

28. Miyagawa C, Wu C, Kennedy DO, Nakatani T, Ohtani K, et al. (1997) Protective effect of green tea extract and tea polyphenols against the cytotoxicity of ,4-naphthoquinone in isolated rat hepatocytes. Biosci Biotechnol Biochem 61: 1901-1905.

29. Lavelli V, Peri C, Rizzolo A (2000) Antioxidant activity of tomato products as studied by model reactions using xanthine oxidase, myeloperoxidase, and copper induced lipid peroxidation. J Agric Food Chem 48: 1442–1448.

22

Effects of Selected Inhibitors of Protein Kinases and Phosphatases on Cellular Respiration: An *In Vitro* Study

Saeeda Almarzooqi[1], Alia Albawardi[1], Ali S. Alfazari[2], Dhanya Saraswathiamma[1], Hidaya Mohammed Abdul-Kader[2], Sami Shaban[3], Robert Mallon[4] and Abdul-Kader Souid [5,*]

[1]Departments of Pathology, UAE University, Al-Ain, Abu Dhabi, United Arab Emirates
[2]Medicine, UAE University, Al-Ain, Abu Dhabi, United Arab Emirates
[3]Medical Education, UAE University, Al-Ain, Abu Dhabi, United Arab Emirates
[4]RHP Associates, Caldwell NJ
[5]Pediatrics, UAE University, Al-Ain, Abu Dhabi, United Arab Emirates

*Corresponding author: Abdul-Kader Souid, Departments of Pediatrics, UAE University, Al-Ain, Abu Dhabi, United Arab Emirates, E-mail: asouid@uaeu.ac.ae

Abstract

Inhibitors of protein kinases/phosphatases are known to alter cellular metabolism. Effects of these rapidly identified small molecules on cellular respiration (mitochondrial O_2 consumption) have not been adequately investigated, especially in healthy organs. This in vitro study measured cellular respiration in tissues from C57BL/6 mice with and without GSK2126458 (PI3K/mTOR inhibitor), BEZ235 (PI3K/mTOR inhibitor), GDC0980 (PI3K/mTOR inhibitor), GSK1120212 (trametinib, MEK inhibitor), sorafenib, regorafenib (multikinase inhibitors), and cyclosporine (calcineurin inhibitor). Cellular respiration was measured by the phosphorescence oxygen analyzer, aided by the O_2 probe Pd(II)-meso-tetra-(4-sulfonatophenyl)-tetrabenzoporphyrin. Cyanide inhibited O_2 consumption, confirming the oxidation occurred in the respiratory chain. Renal cellular respiration decreased 26-34% in the presence of 10 µM GSK2126458 ($p < 0.001$), 10 µM BEZ235 ($p < 0.001$), or 1.0 µM GDC0980 ($p < 0.001$). Liver cellular respiration decreased 20-32% with 10 µM GSK2126458 ($p = 0.048$), 0.1 µM BEZ235 ($p = 0.028$), or 0.1 µM GDC0980 ($p = 0.016$). Heart cellular respiration decreased 19-27% with 10 µM GSK2126458 ($p = 0.078$), 10 µM BEZ235 ($p = 0.040$), or 10 µM GDC0980 ($p = 0.036$). GSK1120212, sorafenib, regorafenib, and cyclosporine had no effects on cellular respiration. Thus, cellular bioenergetics (the biochemical processes involved in energy conversion) is interconnected with PI3K/PTEN/Akt/mTOR; and inhibitors of this cascade impair cellular respiration. This biomarker (cellular respiration) senses the activity/toxicity of this class of molecularly targeted agents.

Keywords: Cellular respiration; PI3K inhibitor; mTOR inhibitor; MEK-1/2 inhibitor; Multikinase inhibitor; Calcineurin inhibitor

Abbreviations

PI3K: Phosphoinositide 3-kinase; Mtor: Mammalian Ttarget of Rapamycin; MEK: Mitogen-activated Protein/extracellular Signal-regulated Kinase; PBS: Phosphate-buffered Saline; Pd phosphor: Pd(II) Complex of Meso-tetra-(4-sulfonatophenyl)-tetrabenzoporphyrin; $1/\tau$: Phosphorescence Decay Rate; k: Rate of Cellular Respiration (in µM O_2 min^{-1}); kc: Corrected Rate of Cellular Respiration (in µM O_2 min^{-1} mg^{-1}).

Introduction

Intracellular kinase-dependent signals regulate vital cellular functions including nutrient transport, metabolic reactions, proliferation, and response to toxins [1]. Inhibitors of some of these enzymes (protein kinases and phosphatases) have been developed for treatment of various human diseases (e.g., cancer and aberrant immune responses) [2,3]. Many of these small molecules are in clinical use as monotherapy or with conventional cytotoxic agents. This therapeutic approach promotes apoptosis by targeting critical reactions involving cellular respiration and production of adenosine triphosphate (ATP)) [4,5].

processes, such as survival pathways (e.g., PI3K/PTEN/Akt/mTOR and Ras/Raf/MEK/ERK) and cellular bioenergetics (metabolic

Studies addressing the effects of these agents targeting biomolecules on organ functions are limited, as drug development studies focus on derangements involving target organs. Agents that target regulators of the metabolic pathways are in clinical development and many (e.g., inhibitors of MEK, PI3K, mTOR, and Akt) are in phase 3 clinical trials [4] and one is recently approved (the PI3K inhibitor idelalisib). Inhibiting these signals is expected to disturb the metabolic processes of normal tissue. Blocking PI3K, for example, causes multifaceted alternations in glucose transport/ metabolism including feedback activation of insulin signals. Inhibition of mTOR activates AMP-activated protein kinase, resulting in improved cellular bioenergetics, including increased substrate-level phosphorylation and ↑oxidative phosphorylation [4].

This study investigated the effects of selected inhibitors of PI3K, mTOR, MEK, sorafenib family multikinases, and calcineurin (a calcium-dependent serine-threonine phosphatase) on renal, cardiac, and hepatic cellular respiration.

Methods

Reagents and solutions

GSK2126458 (PI3K inhibitor, cat. #HY-10297), BEZ235 (PI3K/mTOR inhibitor, cat. #HY-15174), GDC0980 (PI3K/mTOR inhibitor, cat. #HY-13246), and GSK1120212 (MEK inhibitor, cat. #HY-10999) were purchased from MedChem Express, LLC (Princeton, NJ). Sorafenib (multikinase inhibitor) and regorafenib (multikinase inhibitor) were purchased from Selleck Chemicals (Houston, TX, USA). All compounds were dissolved in DMSO (5 mg/mL) and stored at -20°C. The immunosuppressant cyclosporine (calcineurin inhibitor, m.w. 1202.61; dissolved in DMSO at 50 mg/dL and stored at -20°C) was purchased from MedChem Express, LLC (Princeton, NJ). Pd(II) complex of meso-tetra-(4-sulfonatophenyl)-tetrabenzoporphyrin (Pd phosphor) was purchased from Porphyrin Products (Logan, UT). Pd phosphor (2.5 mg/mL=2 mM) and Na cyanide (1.0 M) were stored at -20°C. Roswell Park Memorial Institute medium (RPMI) 1640 and remaining reagents were purchased from Sigma-Aldrich (St. Louis, MO).

Mice

C57BL/6 (9-10 weeks old) mice were housed at the animal facility in rooms maintained at 22°C, 60% humidity and 12-h light-dark cycles. The mice had ad libitum access to standard rodent chow and filtered water. The study received approval from the Animal Ethics Committee-College of Medicine and Health Sciences (A29-13; in vitro assessment of the effects of nephrotoxic drugs and toxins on renal cellular respiration in mice).

Tissue collection and processing

Urethane (25% w/v, 100 μL per 10 g) was used to anesthetize the mice. Tissue fragments (10 to 20 mg each) were cut manually with sterile scalpels (Swann-Morton, Sheffield, England) and immediately processed for measuring cellular respiration in the presence and absence of designated concentrations of the drugs [6,7]. Alternately, specimens were incubated at 37°C in 50 mL RPMI or phosphate-buffered saline (gassed with 95% O_2: 5% CO_2) with and without the drugs for up to 6 h; at designated times, samples were removed from the incubation solution and processed for measuring cellular respiration [6,7].

Cellular respiration

The phosphorescence O_2 analyzer was used to measure O_2 consumption [6-9]. Briefly, samples were exposed to 600 per min pulsed flashes. O_2 concentration was measured with the Pd phosphor, 625 nm absorption/800 nm emission. The phosphorescence was detected by the Hamamatsu photomultiplier tube (#928). The phosphorescence decay rate ($1/\tau$) was exponential; $1/\tau$ was linear with O_2 concentration: $1/\tau=1/\tau_o + k_q[O_2]$, $1/\tau$=phosphorescence decay rate with O_2, $1/\tau_o$=phosphorescence decay rate without O_2, and k_q=second-order O_2 quenching rate constant ($s^{-1} \cdot \mu M^{-1}$) [8]. Rate of respiration (k, μM O_2 min^{-1}) was the negative of the slope $d[O_2]/dt$. The value of k was divided by specimen weight (k_c, μM O_2 min^{-1} mg^{-1}). A program was developed using Microsoft Visual Basic 6, Microsoft Access Database 2007, and Universal Library components (Universal Library for Measurements Computing Devices), which allowed direct reading from the PCI-DAS 4020/12 I/O Board (PCI-DAS 4020/12 I/O Board) [9]. O_2 measurements were performed at 37°C in sealed glass vials. Respiratory substrates were endogenous metabolic fuels and nutrients (e.g., glucose) in RPMI. [O_2] decreased linearly with time. This zero-order process was inhibited by cyanide, confirming O_2 consumption occurring due to the process of respiration [6,7].

Statistical analysis

Data were analyzed on SPSS statistical package (version 19), using the nonparametric (2 independent samples) Mann-Whitney test.

Results

Figure 1A shows representative runs of renal cellular O_2 consumption in RPMI with and without the PI3K/mTOR inhibitor GSK2126458. Each run represented a specimen that was collected from a mouse and processed for measuring cellular respiration immediately after collection. A summary of the results is shown in Figure 1C. The rate of respiration (k_c in μM O_2 min^{-1} mg^- mean ± SD) without addition (control) was 0.99 ± 0.24 (n=11 mice) and with the addition of 10 μM GSK2126458 was 0.74 ± 0.18 (n=11 mice, p=0.023), Figure 1C. Thus, GSK2126458 significantly decreased renal cellular respiration by 25%.

The same experiments were repeated in phosphate-buffered saline (PBS). Representative runs are shown in Figure 1B and a summary of the results in Figure 1D. The value of k_c without addition was 0.90 ± 0.06 μM O_2 min^{-1} mg^{-1} (n=7 mice) and with the addition of 10 μM GSK2126458 was 0.68 ± 0.11 μM O_2 min^{-1} mg^{-1} (24% lower, n=6 mice, p=0.004), Figure 1D. Thus, the inhibition of renal cellular respiration by GSK2126458 was independent of nutrients (e.g., glucose) present in RPMI.

Figure 2A shows representative runs of renal cellular mitochondrial O_2 consumption in samples incubated in vitro with and without GSK2126458 (PI3K/mTOR inhibitor), GSK1120212 (MEK inhibitor), or both agents. Briefly, several renal specimens were collected from one mouse and incubated at 37°C in RPMI with and without the compounds. At designated times; specimens were removed from incubation solutions, rinsed with RPMI, and processed for measuring O_2 consumption at 37°C. A summary of the results is shown in figure 2B (five separate experiments, five mice, 8-15 runs per condition). The rate of respiration (k_c in μM O_2 min^{-1} mg^{-1}) without addition was 0.53 ± 0.14 (n=15 mice), with 10 μM GSK2126458 was 0.39 ± 0.09 (26% lower, p=0.031), with 10 μM GSK1120212 was 0.47 ± 0.08 (11% lower, p=0.397), and with 10 μM of both compounds was 0.35 ± 0.07 (34% lower, p=0.004). Thus, renal cellular respiration was significantly decreased in the presence of the PI3K/mTOR inhibitor GSK2126458, but not the MEK inhibitor GSK1120212. The degree of inhibition was similar to that observed over the shorter incubation discussed above.

It is worth noting, however, that the values of kc in untreated specimens incubated for ≤6 h (Figure 2B) were significantly lower than untreated specimens without incubation (Figure 1C), p<0.001. This finding reflects deterioration of the renal tissue in vitro. More pronounced deteriorations were observed in heart and liver specimens (data not shown). Therefore, the remaining experiments were performed as described for Figures 1B and 1C).

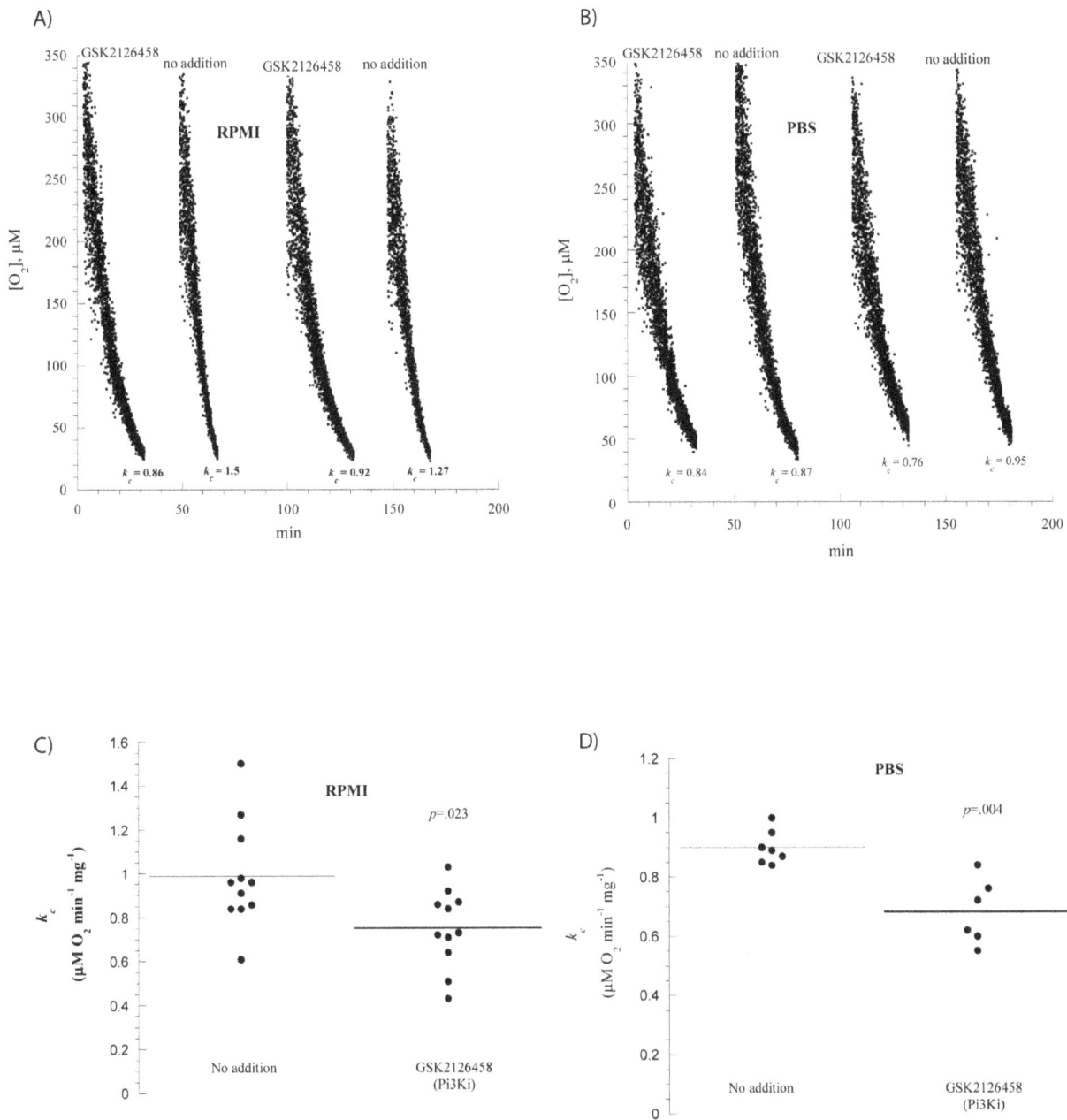

Figure 1: Effects of the PI3K inhibitor GSK2126458 on renal cellular respiration. Panels A-B: Each run represented a renal specimen that was collected from a C57BL/6 mouse and processed immediately for measuring cellular respiration in RPMI (A) or PBS (B) with and without the addition of 10 μM GSK2126458. Rate of respiration (k, μM O_2 min^{-1}) was the negative of the slope of $[O_2]$ vs. t. The values of kc (μM O_2 min^{-1} mg^{-1}) are shown at the bottom of each run. Panels C-D are summaries of all measurements in RPMI (C; 11 separate experiments, 11 mice per condition) and PBS (D; six separate experiments, 7 mice for untreated condition and 6 mice for treated condition). The lines are means.

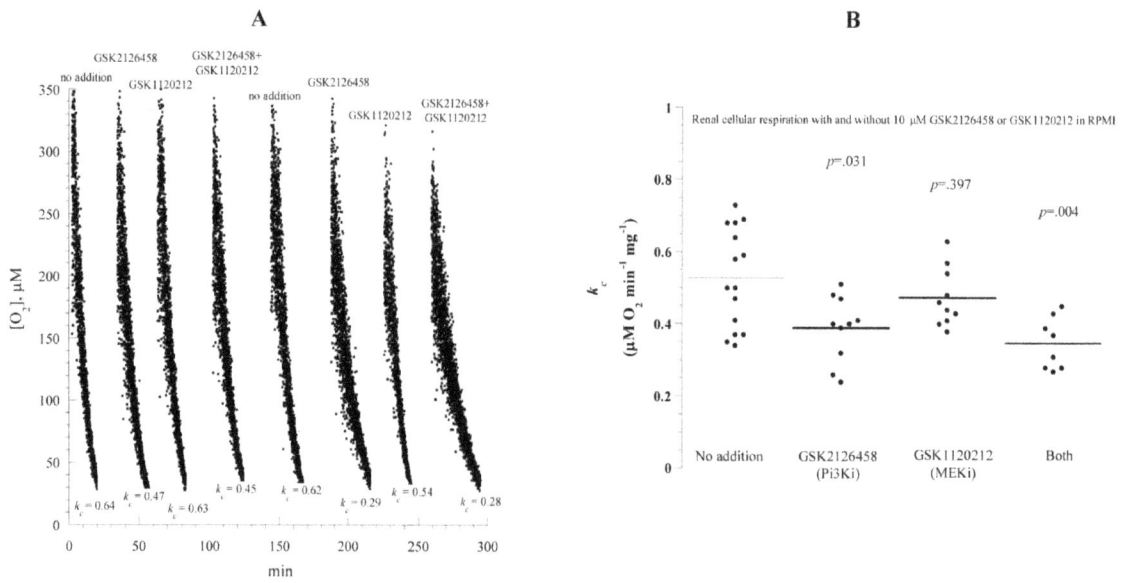

Figure 2: Effects of GSK2126458 (PI3K inhibitor) and GSK1120212 (MEK inhibitor) on renal cellular respiration. Panel A: Representative runs of renal cellular respiration. Multiple renal specimens were collected from a C57BL/6 mouse and incubated at 37°C in RMPI with and without the addition of 10 μM GSK2126458 alone, 10 μM GSK1120212 alone or combination of both compounds. At designated periods, specimens were removed from the incubation solution, rinsed with RPMI, and then placed in the O_2 vial for measuring cellular respiration. Rate of respiration (k, μM O_2 min^{-1}) was the negative of the slope of $[O_2]$ vs. t. The values of k_c (μM O_2 min^{-1} mg^{-1}) are shown at the bottom of each run. Panel B is a summary of all measurements in RPMI (five separate experiments, one mouse per experiment, 8-15 runs per condition); the lines are means.

	Drug Concentration	kc (μM O_2 min^{-1} mg^{-1})	Inhibition (%)	P
GSK2126458 (PI3K/mTOR inhibitor)	0	1.12 ± 0.27 (22)	-	-
	0.1 μM	1.36 ± 0.23 (4)	0	0.150
	1.0 μM	1.02 ± 0.19 (9)	9	0.453
	10 μM	0.74 ± 0.18 (11)	34	<0.001
BEZ235 (PI3K/mTOR inhibitor)	0	0.72 ± 0.18 (18)	-	-
	0.1 μM	0.75 ± 0.20 (8)	0	0.724
	1.0 μM	0.62 ± 0.15 (16)	16	0.126
	10 μM	0.40 ± 0.13 (10)	31	<0.001
GDC0980 (PI3K/mTOR inhibitor)	0	0.93 ± 0.20 (12)	-	-
	0.1 μM	0.98 ± 0.21 (7)	0	0.400
	1.0 μM	0.62 ± 0.07 (8)	27	<0.001
	10 μM	0.64 ± 0.10 (12)	26	0.003
GSK1120212 (MEK inhibitor)	0	1.30 ± 0.32 (4)	-	-
	10 μM	1.03 ± 0.18 (7)	21	0.164
Cyclosporine (calcineurin inhibitor)	0	1.07 ± 0.17 (4)	-	-

			10 µM	1.00 ± 0.23 (8)	7	0.461
Sorafenib (multikinase inhibitor)			0	0.96 ± 0.18 (6)	-	-
			10 µM	0.90 ± 0.22 (12)	6	0.494
Regorafenib (multikinase inhibitor)			0	1.02 ± 0.28 (4)	-	-
			10 µM	1.01 ± 0.20 (8)	0	1.00

Table 1: Effects of selected inhibitors of protein kinases and phosphatases on renal cellular respiration. For each measurement, a renal fragment was collected from C57BL/6 mouse and processed immediately for measuring cellular respiration in RPMI with and without designated concentrations of the drugs. The values of k_c are mean ± SD (n); n=number of animals. Each measurement is a separate experiment.

Tables 1 and 2 summarize the results of the studied compounds in renal, cardiac, and hepatic tissues. All measurements were determined in RPMI with and without designated drugs exactly as described for Figures 1B and 1C.

As shown, the PI3K/mTOR inhibitors GSK2126458, BEZ235, and GDC0980 significantly inhibited cellular respiration in the three studied organs (Tables 1 and 2). The inhibition was concentration-dependent; 100 nM BEZ235 or GDC0980 significantly inhibited hepatic cellular respiration (Table 2). GSK1120212 (MEK inhibitor), cyclosporine (calcineurin inhibitor), sorafenib (multikinase inhibitor), and regorafenib (multikinase inhibitor), on the other hand, had no significant effect on cellular respiration (Table 1).

		Drug Concentration	k_c (µM O_2 min^{-1} mg^{-1})	Inhibition (%)	P
Heart	GSK2126458	0	0.48 ± 0.09 (6)	-	-
		10 µM	0.39 ± 0.12 (11)	19	0.078
	BEZ235	0	0.33 ± 0.08 (8)	-	-
		0.1 µM	0.26 ± 0.07 (6)	21	0.142
		10 µM	0.24 ± 0.12 (7)	27	0.040
	GDC0980	0	0.37 ± 0.11 (8)	-	-
		10 µM	0.29 ± 0.08 (16)	22	0.038
Liver	GSK2126458	0	0.93 ± 0.20 (6)	-	-
		10 µM	0.73 ± 0.18 (11)	22	0.048
	BEZ235	0	0.87 ± 0.16 (4)	-	-
		0.1 µM	0.60 ± 0.12 (8)	20	0.028
	GDC0980	0	1.06 ± 0.24 (4)	-	-
		0.1 µM	0.72 ± 0.16 (8)	32	0.016

Table 2: Effects of the PI3K/mTOR inhibitors on heart and liver cellular respiration. For each measurement, a tissue fragment was collected from C57BL/6 mouse and processed immediately for measuring cellular respiration in RPMI with and without designated concentrations of the drugs. The values of k_c are mean ± SD (n); n=number of animals. Each measurement is a separate experiment.

Discussion

The adverse impact of disrupting PI3K signaling on cellular respiration is demonstrated here using highly selective PI3K/mTOR inhibitors (GSK2126458, BEZ235, and GDC0980) with three vital organs (the heart, liver, and kidney), Tables 1 and 2. These results are consistent with the well-known roles of PI3K/PTEN/Akt/mTOR pathway in cell metabolism, including insulin and insulin signaling [4].

GSK1120212 (trametinib, an oral MEK1/2 inhibitor) has no effect on renal cellular respiration (Table 1), even when the incubation is extended to about 6 h (Figures 2A and 2B). The combination of GSK1120212 and GSK2126458, however, is more potent than GSK2126458 alone (apparently additive, Figure 2B). GSK1120212 is effective in melanoma and colorectal cancer (inducing cell cycle arrest). The drug is typically given with other targeted therapies [10,11].

The sorafenib family multikinase inhibitors (sorafenib and regorafenib) and cyclosporine have no effect on cellular respiration (Table 1). The results are consistent with a recent finding that the multikinase inhibitors are much more effective when combined with

PI3K inhibitors [12]. The results are also consistent with a previous study showing cyclosporine has no effect on cell line respiration [13].

It is important to explain the rational for using relatively high drug concentrations (≥100 nM, Tables 1 and 2) to elicit the cellular response to blocking the PI3K signals. First, drug exposure time is relatively brief (≤1 h). Second, distribution of the drug in *ex vivo* tissue fragments is relatively slow. Due to these experimental limitations, it is unclear whether concentrations <100 nM are inhibitory over a longer incubation time.

Signal transduction controls vital cellular processes including: metabolism, growth, and survival [1-5]. Consistently, derangements in cellular bioenergetics are expected in therapies that alter cell signaling [14]. The PI3K/PTEN/Akt/mTOR pathway regulates cell glucose uptake [15]. Consistently, insulin resistant hyperglycemia is a common dose-limiting toxicity of PI3K inhibitors [16]. This adverse bioenergetic event, however, has not been adequately investigated in off-target organs, such as the heart, liver, and kidney. The results in Tables 1 and 2 show the studied PI3K/ mTOR inhibitors impair cellular respiration in these vital body organs. This finding suggests monitoring therapies that block PI3K/mTOR signaling should include biomarkers of cellular bioenergetics.

The activities of BEZ235 and GSK2126458 were compared in tamoxifen-resistant breast cancer cell lines. Both drugs inhibited AKT signaling, but BEZ235 was a more potent inhibitor of p70S6K and rpS6 [17].

The rapamycin derivatives temsirolimus and everolimus (mTOR-targeted therapies) are approved treatments for renal cell carcinoma [18]. Exposure to these drugs leads to feedback activation of PI3K-PTEN-AKT, which overcomes the effects of inhibiting mTOR [19]. BEZ235, on the other hand, targets both mTOR and PI3K, preventing the undesirable feedback activation of PI3K [20].

Signals through PI3K/PTEN/Akt/mTOR integrate critical processes between the plasma membrane and cellular compartments. Aberrant pathways have been implicated in numerous cancers [2,3]. Consistently, increased phosphatidylinositol 3,4,5-trisphosphate, generated by the activity of PI3K, has been associated with tumor survival; and agents that block PI3K have been shown to induce rapid apoptosis [4,5]. Activities of these rapidly identified small molecules have been linked to suppressing cellular metabolism [21]. Some of these drugs (sirolimus, cyclosporine, and tacrolimus) are potent immunosuppressants, and monitoring their cytotoxicities requires novel systems, such as the one described here.

Mitochondria use energy derived from oxidations in the respiratory chain to generate adenosine 5'-triphoshate (oxidative phosphorylation). These vital organelles respond to apoptotic signals by releasing pro-apoptotic molecules that trigger the caspase (*cys*teine-dependent *asp*artate-directed prote*ase*) cascade. Caspase activation leads to mitochondrial perturbation, which involves opening mitochondrial permeability transition and collapsing the electrochemical potential. Thus, induction of apoptosis and mitochondrial dysfunction are coupled processes. These facts emphasize the need for using mitochondrial biomarkers for monitoring adverse events of molecularly targeted therapies.

Caspase activation is more likely to result in cell death in the presence of mitochondrial dysfunction (impaired cellular bioenergetics). This cellular dependency on aerobic metabolism does not necessarily apply to cancer cells, which are more capable of surviving on anaerobic metabolism ("aerobic glycolysis" or Warburg effect) [22]. It is worth noting that other biomarkers of mitochondrial function include modulators of thioredoxin/thioredoxin-interacting protein [23] and death-associated protein kinase interactome [24]. These important reactions are involved in mitochondria respiration, permeability, and electrochemical potential, generation of reactive O_2 species, induction of caspases, and regulation of calcium homeostasis. O_2 consumption, however, is the easiest method of monitoring drug-induced cellular toxicities.

In summary, inhibitors of PI3K/ mTOR invoke potent inhibitory effects on the cellular respiration of vital organs (Figures 1 and 2, Tables 1 and 2). Inhibitors of MEK, sorafenib family multikinases, and calcium-dependent serine-threonine phosphatase have no effects on cellular respiration (Table 1). Cellular respiration is a useful tool for assessing compounds that inhibit PI3K/mTOR signaling.

Author Contribution

Saeeda Almarzooqi, Alia Albawardi, Ali Alfazari, Robert Mallon, and Abdul-Kader Souid designed the study, carried out the analysis, interpreted the data, and drafted the manuscript. Sami Shaban programed the oxygen analyzer and performed the data analysis. Dhanya Saraswathiamma and Hidaya Mohammed Abdul-Kader performed the oxygen measurements. All authors read, edited, and approved the final manuscript.

Funding

This research was supported by a grant from the UAE University, NRF (31M096).

References

1. Cantley LC (2002) The phosphoinositide 3-kinase pathway. Science 296: 1655-1657.

2. Berridge MJ (2009) Signaling defects and disease. Cell Signalling Biology 12.1-12.66.

3. Osaki M Oshimura M, Ito H (2004) PI3K-Akt pathway: its functions and alterations in human cancer. Apoptosis 9: 667-676.

4. Tennant DA Durán RV, Gottlieb E (2010) Targeting metabolic transformation for cancer therapy. Nat Rev Cancer 10: 267-277.

5. Markman B Dienstmann R, Tabernero J (2010) Targeting the PI3K/Akt/mTOR pathway--beyond rapalogs. Oncotarget 1: 530-543.

6. Alfazari AS Al-Dabbagh B, Almarzooqi S, Albawardi A, Souid AK (2013) A preparation of murine liver fragments for in vitro studies: liver preparation for toxicological studies. BMC Res Notes 6: 70.

7. Alfazari AS Al-Dabbagh B, Almarzooqi S, Albawardi A, Souid AK (2013) Bioenergetic study of murine hepatic tissue treated in vitro with atorvastatin. BMC Pharmacol Toxicol 14: 15.

8. Lo LW Koch CJ, Wilson DF (1996) Calibration of oxygen-dependent quenching of the phosphorescence of Pd-meso-tetra (4-carboxyphenyl) porphine: a phosphor with general application for measuring oxygen concentration in biological systems. Anal Biochem 236: 153-160.

9. Shaban S Marzouqi F, Al Mansouri A, Penefsky HS, Souid AK (2010) Oxygen measurements via phosphorescence. Comput Methods Programs Biomed 100: 265-268.

10. Zeiser R (2014) Trametinib. Recent Results Cancer Res 201: 241-248.

11. Akinleye A, Avvaru P, Furqan M, Song Y, Liu D (2013) Phosphatidylinositol 3-kinase (PI3K) inhibitors as cancer therapeutics. J Hematol Oncol 6: 88.

12. Sajithlal GB Hamed HA, Cruickshanks N, Booth L, Tavallai S, et al. (2013) Sorafenib/regorafenib and phosphatidyl inositol 3 kinase/

thymoma viral proto-oncogene inhibition interact to kill tumor cells. Mol Pharmacol 84: 562-571.

13. Tao Z Jones E, Goodisman J, Souid AK (2008) Quantitative measure of cytotoxicity of anticancer drugs and other agents. Anal Biochem 381: 43-52.

14. Kroemer G Pouyssegur J (2008) Tumor cell metabolism: cancer's Achilles' heel. Cancer Cell 13: 472-482.

15. Fleming IN Andriu A, Smith TA (2014) Early changes in [18F]FDG incorporation by breast cancer cells treated with trastuzumab in normoxic conditions: role of the Akt-pathway, glucose transport and HIF-1α. Breast Cancer Res Treat 144: 241-248.

16. Bendell JC Rodon J, Burris HA, de Jonge M, Verweij J, et al. (2012) Phase I, dose-escalation study of BKM120, an oral pan-Class I PI3K inhibitor, in patients with advanced solid tumors. J Clin Oncol 30: 282-290.

17. Leung E Kim JE, Rewcastle GW, Finlay GJ, Baguley BC (2011) Comparison of the effects of the PI3K/mTOR inhibitors NVP-BEZ235 and GSK2126458 on tamoxifen-resistant breast cancer cells. Cancer Biol Ther 11: 938-946.

18. Ravaud A Bernhard JC, Gross-Goupil M, Digue L, Ferriere JM (2010) [mTOR inhibitors: temsirolimus and everolimus in the treatment of renal cell carcinoma]. Bull Cancer 97: 45-51.

19. Chen J, Zhao KN, Li R, Shao R, Chen C (2014) Activation of PI3K/Akt/MTOR pathway and dual Inhibitors of PI3K and MTOR in endometrial cancer. Curr Med Chem 26:3070-3080.

20. Kuger S Cörek E Polat B, Kämmerer U, Flentje M et al. (2014) Novel PI3K and mTOR Inhibitor NVP-BEZ235 Radiosensitizes Breast Cancer Cell Lines under Normoxic and Hypoxic Conditions. Breast Cancer (Auckl) 8: 39-49.

21. Dehnhardt CM Venkatesan AM, Chen Z, Delos-Santos E, Ayral-Kaloustian S, et al. (2011) Identification of 2-oxatriazines as highly potent pan-PI3K/mTOR dual inhibitors. Bioorg Med Chem Lett 21: 4773-4778.

22. Dang CV (2012) Links between metabolism and cancer. Genes Dev 26: 877-890.

23. Yoshihara E Masaki S Matsuo Y Chen Z Tian H, et al. (2014) Thioredoxin/Txnip: redoxisome, as a redox switch for the pathogenesis of diseases. Front Immunol 4: 514.

24. Bialik S Kimchi A (2014) The DAP-kinase interactome. Apoptosis 19: 316-328.

23

Serum Proteomic Analysis for the Identification of Biomarkers by Two-Dimensional Differential Gel Electrophoresis (2D-DIGE) after Exposure to the Food-Processed Contaminant Furan

Santokh Gill[*1], Meghan Kavanagh[1], Christine Poirier[2], Dorcas Weber[2], and Terry Koerner[2]

[1]Regulatory Toxicology Research Division, Health Canada

[2]Food Research Division, Bureau of Chemical Safety, Food Directorate, Health, Canada

[*]**Corresponding author:** Dr. Santokh Gill, Health Canada, Regulatory Toxicology Research Division, Health Products and Food Branch, Tunney's Pasture, Health, 251 Sir Frederick Banting Driveway, Ottawa, ON, K1A 0K9, Canada, E-mail: Santokh.gill@hc-sc.gc.ca

Abstract

Background: Furan is a compound known to be present in cooked or thermally-processed foods by formation through traditional heat treatment processes and also known to be a potent hepatotoxin. To identify potential biomarkers of furan exposure, two-dimensional differential gel electrophoresis (2D-DIGE) was performed on individual serum samples to identify proteomic profiles that were differentially expressed in rats exposed to furan at 0, 0.03, 0.5 and 8.0 mg/kg bw/day.

Results: There were no differences in protein expression between control and the 0.03 and 0.5 mg/kg bw/day dose groups (one-way ANOVA $P<0.05$, avg ratio +1.5). At the 8.0 mg/kg bw/day of furan exposure, there were 22 protein spots that showed a difference in expression when compared to the control animals (one-way ANOVA $P<0.05$, avg ratio +1.5). After manual spot picking, four proteins were identified by standard in-gel tryptic digestion followed by mass spectrometry and bioinformatics.

Conclusions: Of these four proteins apolipoprotein C-III (isoform CRA_b) and fetuin-B (precursor) were up-regulated, whereas α-1-macroglobulin and pre-proapolipoprotein A-1 were down-regulated. These biomarkers could be of diagnostic relevance to identify furan exposure.

Keywords: Furan; Biomarkers; Serum protein profiling

Introduction

Furan is a colorless, volatile, lipophilic compound that is formed during traditional heat treatment processes such as cooking, canning, and baking [1]. A recent survey performed by the United States Food and Drug Administration [2] on approximately 300 food samples showed that furan is present in a wide range of foods up to levels greater than 100 ng/g. For example, it is found in cooked and canned meats, roasted coffee, beer and wheat breads [1,3-5]. These data have been supported by similar findings by the European Food Safety Authority [6] and the Swiss Office of Public Health [7]. In humans, furan has been observed in breast milk samples and in the breath of both smokers and non-smokers [8-10]. Hence, based on the widespread industrial use and potential exposure to furan, the toxic properties of this compound are a public health concern. Furan had been previously found to be a potent hepatotoxin [11,12] although little toxicological information was available until recently [13]. Recent proteomic studies of human body fluids have resulted in identifying potential biomarker candidates for many conditions [14,15]. Of particular interest in preclinical and clinical safety assessments are biomarkers in the peripheral blood or serum that are quantitatively altered functionally or morphologically as an indication of the early exposure to chemicals or in the progression of diseases. This is particularly true for diseases that are either asymptomic or where a late diagnosis generally results in a poor outcome. Early detection of hazardous exposures of humans may significantly reduce adverse health effects through appropriate reductions [16]. Plasma or serum is a preferred specimen for the early diagnosis of malignant tumors or chemical exposure because samples are readily accessible by non-invasive methods. Protein profiling of serum offers opportunities to discover potentially new biomarkers for the early detection of chemical exposure or diseases and could also facilitate their prognosis [14,15].

Recent advances in proteomic technologies by two-dimensional differential gel electrophoresis (2D-DIGE) and improved mass spectrometry have provided new opportunities for identifying biomarkers and therapeutic targets [17]. 2D-DIGE is effective in separating and quantifying complex protein samples. A pool of all the samples within an experiment is used as a common internal standard on each gel with a dedicated fluorescent dye (Cy2TM). This allows all proteins to be included within the experiment to ultimately match and normalize protein patterns within the same gel and across different gels thus reducing the problems of intra- and inter-gel variations. Quantitative comparisons of proteins from individual samples randomized through additional fluorescent dyes (Cy3TM/ Cy5TM) are analysed by the relative changes between the protein spots and the internal standard (Cy2TM) thus allowing accurate quantification of induced biological change between samples with an associated statistical significance (Ettan DIGE System User Manual, 18-1173-17, Edition AB). Proteins of interest (POIs) can then be selected, excised and identified by tandem mass spectrometry (LC-MS/MS) and bioinformatics.

The object of this study was to use proteomic approaches (2D-DIGE/LC-MS/MS) to assess possible biomarkers of exposure in male rats that were administered furan at 0.0, 0.03, 0.5 and 8.0 mg/kg bw/day. Significant differences in protein expression (one-way ANOVA P<0.05, avg ratio+1.5) between control and various dose groups was used to establish protein profiles that could be relevant for early discrimination between these groups. In addition, our objectives were to identify serum proteins in rats that might serve as sensitive indicators of hepatomegaly, hepatocellular necrosis or hepatobiliary injury as these were the histological observations from our previous study [13].

Method and Material

Test compound and dosing solutions

Furan doses were prepared by mixing the appropriate quantity of furan with Mazola* corn oil to deliver final concentrations at 0, 0.03, 0.12, 0.5, 2.0 and 8.0 mg/ml. Each dose was prepared separately on a volume-to-weight (v:w) ratio. Chilled corn oil was weighed to the nearest milligram in a conical flask. Chilled furan solution was drawn up in a Hamilton syringe, measured to the nearest microliter, injected into corn oil and mixed using a magnetic stir bar. Dosing solutions were dispensed into brown glass vials and capped with plastic closures adapted with silicon septa ensuring no remaining air space. Dosing solutions were stored at 4°C with fresh solutions were prepared every 14 days [18].

Animal studies

Fischer-344 male and female rats were obtained from Charles River Laboratories Inc. (St.-Constant, QC) at 5-6 weeks of age and were acclimatized for a period of twelve days before studies began. Animals were handled and treated according to the Guidelines of the Canadia Council of Animal Care (Ottawa, ON). Animals received treatment by gavage over a 90-day period, dosing 5 days a week final furan concentrations at 0, 0.03, 0.12, 0.5, 2.0 and 8.0 mg/kg bw/day. These animals were weighed daily on weekdays prior to gavage. Food consumption was measured on a weekly basis [13].

Sample collection

At the end of the study, animals were sacrificed by exsanguination under isofluorane anaesthesia. Blood from the abdominal aorta was collected in SST Vacutainer* tubes (Becton-Dickinson, Franklin Lakes, NJ) and allowed to clot at room temperature. Serum was separated by centrifugation at 3,000x g, aliquoted and stored at -80°C for two-dimensional differential gel electrophoresis (2D-DIGE) and clinical chemistry analysis. Each sample was limited to a maximum of 3 freeze/thaws cycles [13].

Immunodepletion of serum

Randomly selected male serum samples (n=5) at doses of 0, 0.03, 0.5 and 8.0 mg/kg bw/day were processed using the Albumin and IgG Depletion Spintrap Kit (GE Healthcare) following the manufacturer's instructions. This allowed the removal of high abundant proteins (Albumin/IgG) allowing a larger quantity of less abundant proteins to be analyzed by 2D-DIGE. In brief, each column was depleted of storage solution by centrifugation for 30 seconds at 100 xg. Columns were then equilibrated several times with 400 l binding buffer (20 mM sodium phosphate, 0.15 M sodium chloride pH 7.4) followed by centrifugation

for 30 sec at 800 xg and discarding the flow through. Each diluted serum sample (50 l serum: 50l binding buffer) was added to a column in a new tube and incubated at room temperature for 5 min. The depleted sample was collected by centrifugation for 30 seconds at 800x g. Binding buffer (100 l) was added twice to each column and centrifuged for 30 seconds at 800x g to give a final volume of 300 l of depleted serum. Immunodepleted serum was diluted (1:2) in binding buffer to determine protein concentrations by the Bradford assay (BioRad). Samples were stored at -80°C until further proteomic analysis.

Preparation of samples for two-dimensional gel electrophoresis

Samples were additionally precipitated while removing interfering substances to improve the labelling efficiency by using the 2D Clean-up Kit (GE Healthcare) following the manufacturer's instructions. All other reagents were purchased from GE Healthcare unless otherwise specified. Pellets were resuspended in Standard Cell Lysis Buffer (pH 9.0) containing 7 M urea, 2 M thioruea, 30 mM Tris-HCl, 4% (w/v) 3-[3-cholamidopropyl) dimethylammonio]-1-propanesulfonate (CHAPS) to a final concentration of [10 g/l]. All samples were adjusted to a final pH of 9.0. Stock solution of CyDye DIGE Fluor Cy2TM, Cy3 TM and Cy5 TM minimal dyes were made by adding 5 l of fresh dimethylformamide (Sigma-Aldrich) to each vial containing 5nmol of dye. To take advantage of the multiplexing capabilities of 2D-DIGE, an internal standard representing a pool of all samples (n=20) was labelled with Cy2TM to be included on each gel to facilitate gel-to-gel matching and statistical analysis. The internal standard protein (Cy2TM) was labelled in a single tube for all gels in the study for improved consistency. For analytical gels, each sample containing 50 g of protein was labelled with 400 pmol of the appropriate dye. Each individual protein sample was labelled with either Cy3 TM or Cy5 TM alternating dyes between doses in a random fashion. Labelling was conducted in the dark for 30 minutes and the reaction was stopped with 0.2 μl of 10 mM Lysine as outlined for 2D-DIGE minimal labelling in the EttanTM DIGE Imager user manual (GE Healthcare).

Two-dimensional gel electrophoresis

First dimensional separation was completed using 18 cm Immobiline Drystrips pH 4-7 (GE Healthcare) with the Ettan IPGphor3 Isoelectric Focusing System. The Cy2 TM , Cy3 TM and Cy5TM labelled samples for each analytical gel were combined and the total volume adjusted to 340 l by the addition of rehydration buffer containing 7 M Urea, 2 M Thioruea, 2% (w/v) 3-[3-cholamidopropyl) dimethylammonio]-1-propanesulfonate (CHAPS), 0.5% IPG Buffer pH 4-7, 0.2% (w/v) Dithiothreitol (DTT) and bromophenol blue. Proteins were separated in 18 cm ceramic strip holders (GE Healthcare) by active rehydration following the manufacturer's instructions (GE Healthcare). In brief, each labelled sample in rehydration buffer was placed into an 18 cm ceramic strip holder between the electrodes. Immobiline DryStrips 18 cm pH 4-7 were placed gel side down into the stripholder using forceps. DryStrip Cover Fluid was added to the top of each strip to prevent the evaporation of sample or urea crystallization. Ceramic strip holders were added to the Ettan IPGphor3 unit for first dimensional separation of proteins by isoelectric focusing (IEF) at 20°C and 75 A/strip using the outlined running protocol: 14 hrs at 30 V; 1 hr at 500 V; 1 hr gradient up to 1,000 V; 3 hr gradient up to 8,000 V and a final step of 8,000 V to a total of 33217 V hrs. The focused Immobiline Drystrips had the excess cover fluid removed and were stored at -80°C for several hours until the equilibration of strips and second dimensional separation was performed.

Second dimensional separation (SDS-PAGE) was completed by casting 15% polyacrylamide gels using the Ettan DALT Gel Caster and low fluorescent Ettan DALT plates (GE Healthcare). Gels were overlaid with water-saturated butanol for one hour followed by 1x SDS DALT electrophoresis running buffer and allowed to polymerize overnight. Focused Immobline Drystrips were removed from -80°C and left in a solution containing Equilibration Buffer (6 M Urea, 30% glycerol, 2% (w/v) SDS, 50 mM Tris-HCl (1.5 M, pH 8.8) and 0.02% bromophenol blue) with the addition of 0.5% (w/v) of DTT for 15 minutes. This was followed by a second incubation of Equilibration Buffer but with the addition of 4.5% (w/v) Iodoacetamide for 15 minutes. The strip was added to the top of each gel and covered with 0.5% (w/v) agarose overlay solution containing 0.02% bromophenol blue. Electrophoresis was performed using the Ettan DALT six electrophoresis system with a Multitemp III cooling unit and the EPS601 Electrophoresis Power Supply (GE Healthcare) by applying 0.5 W/gel overnight followed by 17 W/gel until the bromophenol blue dye front reached the bottom of the gels.

Image acquisition and statistical analysis

Analytical gels were scanned using the EttanTM DIGE Imager (GE Healthcare) at 100 μm resolution using excitation/emission wavelengths specified by selecting the DIGE File Naming Format: Cy2 TM at 480 nm/530 nm, Cy3 TM at 540 nm/595 nm and Cy5 TM at 635 nm/680 nm which enabled the fluorescence proteins to be visualized. The exposure was set for each channel in that the maximum pixel value was achieved without saturation as outlined in the EttanTM DIGE Imager user manual (GE Healthcare). Images were analysed using the Decyder 2D software v7.0 (GE Healthcare) according to the manufacturer's recommendation. In brief, all gel images were viewed and cropped in the Image Loader. This allowed the images to be the same size and exclude areas (i.e., vertical streaks at extreme pH, Immobline Drystrip, dye front) to achieve relevant areas of interest and optimize spot matching across the individual gels. A single cropped "master" gel containing an internal standard (Cy2 TM) and two individual samples (Cy3 TM, Cy5 TM) was analyzed in the DIA (Differential In-Gel Analysis) module. Spot detection was performed using an estimation of 10, 000 spots with an exclusion of background by selecting the volume of the first true spot. Cropped images (n=30) representing each channel (Cy2 TM, Cy3 TM and Cy5 TM) of all gels were processed using the Batch Processor module which performs automated matching of spot boundaries from all gels to the " master" gel using the parameters selected in the DIA module. Samples were specified into dose groups or as internal standards with the master gel identified. Individual samples (Cy3 TM, Cy5 TM) were compared to the corresponding protein spot of the internal standard (Cy2 TM) on the same gel to provide spot protein abundance ratios (i.e., Cy2: Cy3, Cy2: Cy5) used for normalization. In addition, the identical pooled internal standard (Cy2 TM) from each gel was matched and spot protein abundance ratios were compared from each gel to reduce the amount of gel-to-gel variability. Overall, the intra- and inter-gel variation is reduced allowing only the biological variation to be compared in future analysis. Images were then viewed in the BVA (Biological Variation Analysis) module to verify that all spots on the gel images were matched.

Statistical analysis was conducted using the EDA (Decyder Extended Data Analysis) module. A base set was created to filter both proteins and spot maps by selecting proteins spots present in 90% of the gel images and removing unassigned proteins. Differential Expression Analysis calculations for one-way ANOVA (P<0.05) with a multi-comparison test between all doses as well as the t-test and average ratio between each dose and the control were performed. An additional set was created by filtering only those proteins which had a one-way ANOVA (P<0.05) and a change in avg ratio expression of +1.5 to be used for future analysis. Principle Component Analysis (PCA) was conducted to analyse the protein distribution patterns for dose related changes and identify differentially expressed proteins. Pattern Analysis was completed by Hierarchical Clustering, Kmeans and Self-Organizing Maps to visualize the data and group similar data into subsets or clusters. Points of interest (POIs) for further analysis were identified based on results of the Differential Expression Analysis (one-way ANOVA P<0.05, avg ratio +1.5) compared to the control dose. All the POIs identified as significant, were exported as a pick list into BVA where all spots were manually confirmed before proceeding with the preparative gels for spot picking.

Preparative gels and spot picking

Preparative gels were conducted in duplicate using the same protocol as analytical gels with the following exceptions. A single sample containing 500 g of pooled unlabelled protein was used which represented all dose groups. This enabled more protein to be selected for mass spectrometry analysis. First dimensional separation was completed on the unlabelled sample and the total volume was adjusted to 340 l by the addition of rehydration buffer. For second dimensional separation, the glass plates were first washed in 1% Decon (v/v) overnight, 1% HCL for one hour and then treated with Bind Saline working solution (GE Healthcare) and left to dry for a minimum of 1.5 hours before casting the gels. Upon completion of the electrophoresis, the glass plates were separated with the gel remaining on the bind saline treated plate. Gels were notched for identification and placed in a tray covered with fixing solution (50% Methanol, 7% Acetic acid) for 30 minutes on an orbital shaker twice. Fixed gels were placed in a new tray covered with SYPRO Ruby staining solution in the dark until optimal staining was achieved. In order to minimize background, gels were transferred to a tray with wash solution (10% Methanol, 7% Acetic acid) for 30 minutes on an orbital shaker. This was followed by two washes in ultrapure water before imaging. Preparative gels were scanned using the EttanTM DIGE Imager (GE Healthcare) at 480 nm/595 nm (SR1-filter setting) which enabled the fluorescence proteins to be visualized. The exposure was set in that the maximum pixel value was achieved without saturation. Gels were scanned to identify POIs and improve manual spot picking. Gels were placed on a Dark Reader* Transilluminator (Clare Chemical Research, Dolores, CO, USA) and POI's were manually picked using the OneTouch Plus spot-picker pipette with disposable tips (Gel Company Inc., San Francisco, CA, USA). Selected gel plugs containing POIs were placed in a microcentrifuge tube containing 1% acetic acid and then stored at -20°C until identification. Gels were scanned a second time to confirm spot picking.

Tryptic digestion

Excised spots were placed in low-binding tubes (LoBind, Eppendorf) and washed with 200 μl of water (Milli-Q 18 Ω). The gel pieces were dehydrated with 200 μl of 50% acetonitrile (ACN)/buffer

(50 mM NH_4HCO_3) followed by another 200 µl of 100% ACN. The ACN was removed and the gel pieces were dried in a vacuum centrifuge (Thermo Electron Corporation, Savant, DNA 120 SpeedVac Concentrator) to remove residual solvent. The gel pieces were rehydrated with 50 µl DTT (500 mM in buffer) and the protein cysteine residues were allowed to reduce for 30 minutes at 37°C. The proteins were alkylated in the dark at room temperature for 30 minutes by the addition of 50 µl of a freshly prepared iodoacetamide (1 M in buffer). The gel pieces were washed with 400 µl Milli-Q water to remove any residual iodoacetamide and the digestion was initiated by the addition of trypsin (10 µl of 20 ng/µl Promega Sequence Grade Modified in buffer) and a minimal amount of buffer (30 µl) to cover the gel pieces. The samples were incubated overnight at 37°C. The digested peptides were extracted from the gel plugs with 50 l of 1% formic acid (FA) and mixed for 10 minutes (max speed on bench top centrifuge) and the supernatant was removed and put into a new low binding tube. The gel pieces were then extracted with 80 µl of 70% ACN/5% FA and mixed for 10 minute, adding the supernatant to the previous supernatant. The peptide solution was dried in a vacuum centrifuge and reconstituted in mass spectrometry buffer (30 l of 0.1% FA).

LC-MS/MS analysis and protein identification

Liquid chromatography (LC) and mass spectrometry (MS) was performed on a hybrid MALDI Q-TOF Premier (Waters, Milford, MA) fitted with a nanolockspray source, which was coupled to a nanoAcquity UPLC system (Waters, Milford, MA). An auxiliary solvent manager was used to deliver a reference mass calibration standard [Glu1]-Fibrinopeptide B in 50% aqueous methanol (0.5 µM)). The LC system consisted of a trap column (Symmetry C18, 5 µm 180 µm x 20 mm, Waters) and an analytical column (BEH 130 C18, 1.7 µm 100 µm x 100 mm, Waters). Solvent A consisted of H_2O with 0.1% FA and solvent B consisted of ACN with 0.1% FA. In a typical experiment, digests were injected (4 µL) onto the trap column for 3 minute at a flow rate of 3.0 µL/min using 99% solvent A. The samples were then diverted to the analytical column and eluted at 300 nL/min. The elution program started with 99% A for 1 minute followed by a gradient to 50% B in 35 minutes.

The mass spectrometer was operated in positive ion mode in a V configuration (resolution >10000 FWHH) and the acquired data collected using MassLynx v4.1 software package. Data was collected in both MS full scan survey mode and an automated data directed analysis (DDA) mode. MS survey scan data was acquired in continuum mode from m/z 100 to 1500 and the collection of MS/MS information (m/z 100 to 1500) was triggered when the threshold rose above a minimum (5 counts/sec). Data was collected on up to three simultaneous masses and the system was returned to MS survey scan mode when the counts for each triggered mass returned to a minimum (10 counts/sec) or a time constraint was reached (4.8 sec). Data collection continued with mass- and charge-dependent collision energies for charge states of 2+, 3+ or 4+ until of the above set of specifications was reached.

Peak lists were developed from the data collected in the LC-MS/MS analysis of each gel sample using MassLynx 4.1 and submitted directly to an in-house Mascot server with distiller software version 2.4.3.1. The tandem MS information was then searched against the NCBI database (version 20130503) with specific taxonomy (Rattus, 68, 381 sequences), 1 missed cleavage site, a fixed carbamidomethylation modification at cysteine, variable modifications deamidation (NQ), oxidation (M),

phosphorylation (ST), phosphorylation (Y), peptide tolerance ± 0.1 Da, and MS/MS fragment tolerance ± 0.1 Da. Proteins were identified and included if detected in all samples, a protein score above the confidence threshold and sequence coverage of at least 10% based on at least 2 identified peptides [19].

Results

Proteome differential expression in serum between treated and control animals

Statistical analysis was conducted using the EDA (Decyder Extended Data Analysis) module. The differential expression analysis (DEA) module was used to established the base set of proteins (n=238) by the filtering criteria by selecting proteins spots present in 90% of the gel images and removing unassigned proteins. Of these proteins, those with a one-way ANOVA with multiple comparison test (P<0.05) were further reduced (n=92). Comparisons between control and each dose group by the t-test and average ratio allowed the further filtering of a differential protein average ratio expression of +1.5 as a parameter. At both the 0.03 or 0.5 mg/kg bw/day dose groups, no proteins were identified as significantly changed (one-way ANOVA P<0.05, avg ratio of +1.5). In comparison, there were 22 protein spots differentially expressed at the 8.0 mg/kg bw/day dose group. A gel image illustrating the proteins identified (one-way ANOVA P<0.05, avg ratio +1.5) and the randomization of samples between dyes is shown (Figure 1).

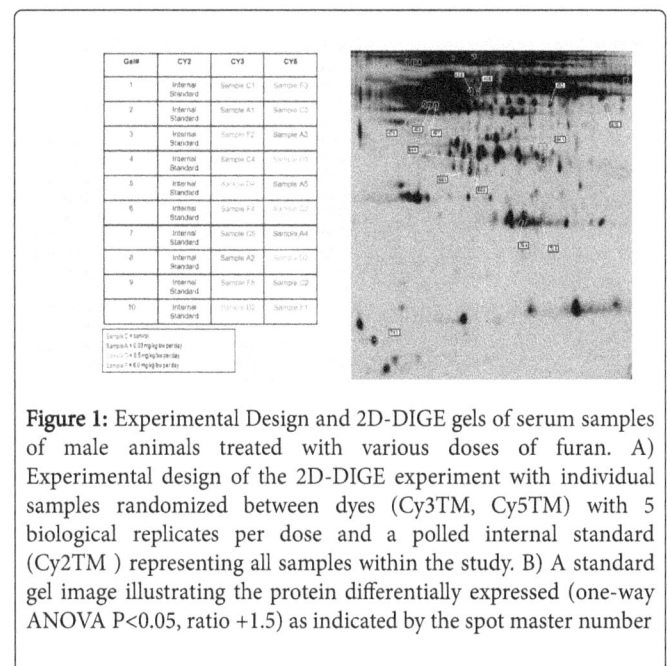

Figure 1: Experimental Design and 2D-DIGE gels of serum samples of male animals treated with various doses of furan. A) Experimental design of the 2D-DIGE experiment with individual samples randomized between dyes (Cy3TM, Cy5TM) with 5 biological replicates per dose and a polled internal standard (Cy2TM) representing all samples within the study. B) A standard gel image illustrating the protein differentially expressed (one-way ANOVA P<0.05, ratio +1.5) as indicated by the spot master number

Principle Component Analysis was conducted to analyse the protein distribution patterns for dose related changes and identify those differentially expressed. The experimental groups are represented by each of the four dose groups of furan (0, 0.03, 0.5 and 8.0 mg/kg bw/ day). The samples within each dose group (n=5) are grouped together thus illustrating that the biological replicates are responding in a similar way. The 8.0 mg/kg bw/day group are clearly separated from the remaining dose groups on the spot maps thus they are responding differently (Figure 2). The PCA analysis also displays several proteins which are found outside of the ellipse representing a 95% significance level (Figure 2). This represents proteins that have a strong differential expression.

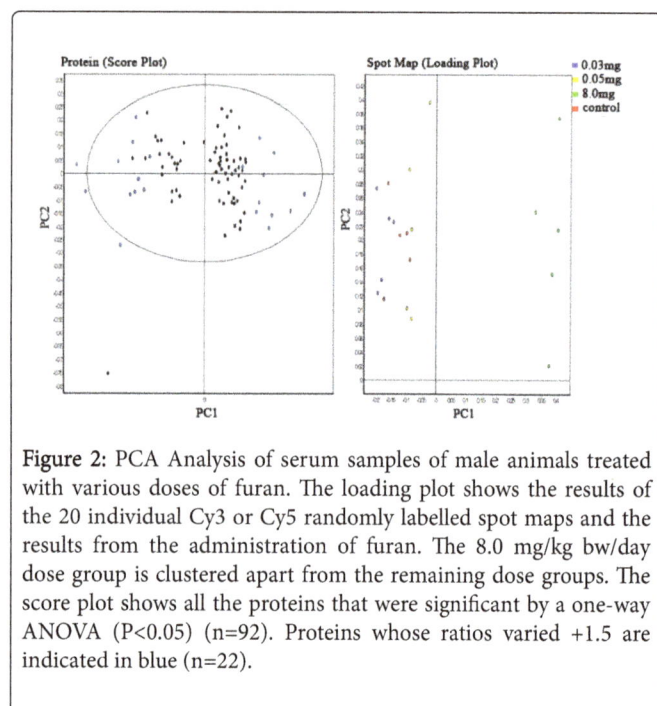

Figure 2: PCA Analysis of serum samples of male animals treated with various doses of furan. The loading plot shows the results of the 20 individual Cy3 or Cy5 randomly labelled spot maps and the results from the administration of furan. The 8.0 mg/kg bw/day dose group is clustered apart from the remaining dose groups. The score plot shows all the proteins that were significant by a one-way ANOVA (P<0.05) (n=92). Proteins whose ratios varied +1.5 are indicated in blue (n=22).

Pattern Analysis was completed by Hierarchical Clustering, Kmeans and SOM analyses to visualize the data and group similar data (proteins and treatment groups) into subsets or clusters (Figure 3). Hierarchical Clustering analysis of proteins (one-way ANOVA P<0.05, avg ratio +1.5) resulted in separating the 8.0 mg/kg bw/day dose group from all other dose groups. This also was confirmed by Kmeans2 analysis where Cluster #1 (q=92.9) (n=5) represents the highest dose group and further supports the previous results from the PCA analysis. Kmeans1 analysis of proteins (one-way ANOVA P<0.05, avg ratio +1.5) results in four clusters which were significant. Cluster #1

(q=81.2) (n=9) and Cluster #4 (q=81.3) (n=3) were the results of proteins that were down-regulated as a result of an increase in furan exposure. Cluster #2 (q=81.3) (n=6) and Cluster #3 (q=78.5) (n=4) represented proteins that were up-regulated under the same conditions. At the 8.0 mg/kg bw/day dose group, 22 protein spots were significantly altered (one-way ANOVA P<0.05, avg ratio +1.5) but only 4 of these spots were able to be manually picked and identified with high confidence with the previously mentioned parameters [19]. Fetuin B (precursor) and apolipoprotein C-III, isoform CRA_b, were up-regulated and α-1-macroglobulin and pre-proapolipoprotein A-1 were down-regulated (Table 1).

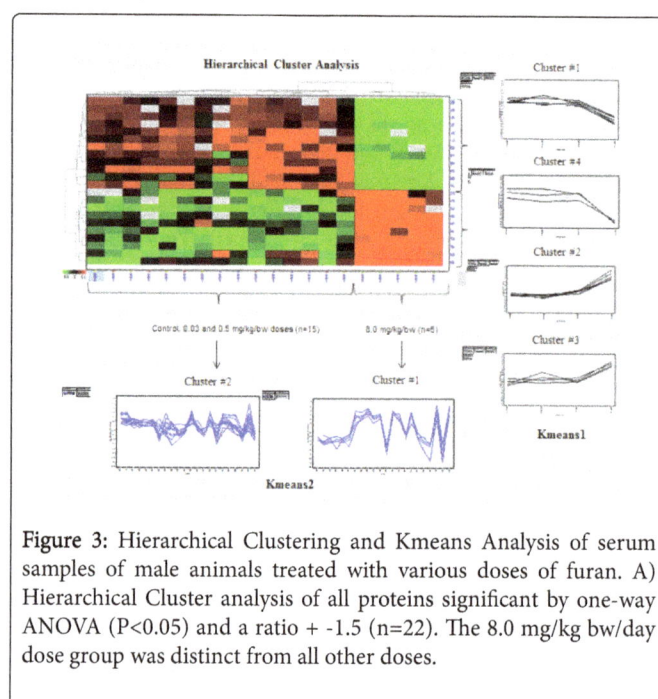

Figure 3: Hierarchical Clustering and Kmeans Analysis of serum samples of male animals treated with various doses of furan. A) Hierarchical Cluster analysis of all proteins significant by one-way ANOVA (P<0.05) and a ratio + -1.5 (n=22). The 8.0 mg/kg bw/day dose group was distinct from all other doses.

Proteins	gi |	Mass	pI	score	% coverage	#peptides	Biological Function	Fold change
Fetuin-B (precursor)	gi|17865327	42361	6.71	465	49	23	Immune system regulation and inflammation	-2.4
Apolipoprotein C-III, isoform CRA_b	gi|149041555	7847	4.65	150	27	3	Lipid metabolism	-2.2
Pre-proapolipoprotein A-1	gi|55747	30126	5.52	439	42	18	Anti-inflammatory and anti-oxidant	2.1
α-1-macroglobulin	gi|205384	168422	6.46	223	4	10	Immune system regulation and inflammation	1.6

Table 1: Identification of proteins that were differentially expressed in animals exposed to 8.0 mg/kg bw/day of furan. Expression levels were determined using 2 DIGE and proteins were identified by in-gel digestion, mass spectrometry (q-TOF MS/MS) and bioinformatics (MASCOT).

Discussion

Serum and other body fluids are non-invasive resources to gain access to information for the clinical diagnosis and identification of novel biomarkers. Serum provides a rich sample for diagnostic analyses because of the expression and release of potential protein biomarkers into the bloodstream via various tissues or organs in response to specific physiological states. Potential protein biomarkers may be present at low concentrations and could be masked by high abundant proteins if not depleted since they possess similar biophysical characteristics [20]. In this study, a serum proteomic profiles were used for the exposure assessment of furan which is found through food processing. Principle Component Analysis, Hierarchical Clustering and the Kmeans Analysis of identified proteins (one-way ANOVA P<0.05, avg ratio +1.5) confirm that the 8.0 mg/kg bw/day dose group of furan is distinct from all other doses as no proteins were identified as significant at the 0.03 or 0.5 mg/kg bw/day dose groups. At the the 8.0 mg/kg bw/day dose group, four proteins were identified having a significant differential expression and were identified by bioinformatic analysis of mass spectrometry data. Pre-proapolipoprotein A-1 (+2.1) and α-1-macroglobulin (+1.6) were upregulated whereas apolipoprotein C-III- isoform CRA_b (-2.2) and fetuin-B precursor (-2.4) were down-regulated. These proteins belong to the class of acute-phase protein (APPs) which are a large group of biochemically and functionally unrelated proteins whose plasma concentrations can decrease and/or increase following exposure to inflammatory conditions such as external trauma, hemorrhage/tissue injury, acute infections, burns and chronic inflammation [21]. The changes in APP plasma levels correlate with changes in the rate of hepatic synthesis and in the hepatic levels of the corresponding mRNA [22-24]. The serum concentrations of macroglobulins have been shown to more than double after injury [22]. This glycoprotein serves as the principal circulatory proteinase binder. Proteinases released in response to tissue injury, necrosis or inflammation would be bound and inactivated by α-1-macroglobulin, and in turn the protein complex would stimulate the liver to synthesize a number of acute-phase proteins. Fetuin is a transporter protein in the serum and is an anti-inflammatory mediator that is critical to regulating the innate immune response following tissue injury in response to pro-inflammatory cytokines early in the inflammatory response. During inflammation, circulating fetuin levels substantially decrease as fetuin becomes associated with the membranes of macrophages. It is thought to mediate serum calcium homeostasis and mineralization and to potentially participate in the transport of bioactive molecules. The calcium levels were not altered in clinical biochemistry [13]. Pre-proapolipoprotein, in addition to being a marker of inflammation, is also a major precursor or component of plasma HDL which mediates the reverse transport of cholesterol from the tissues into the liver. The increased synthesis of pre-proapolipoprotein A-1 suggests an up-regulation of HDL synthesis and the subsequent increase in cholesterol catabolism in the liver. Apolipoprotein C-III, isoform CRA_b is involved in lipid metabolism. A decrease of approximately two-fold in the amount of apolipoprotein C-III-containing HDL particles was found in rats 24hr after the induction of inflammation [24]. Its production rate is strongly correlated with plasma triglyceride levels [25-27]. Triglycerides were significantly reduced at the same dose [13] supporting the down- regulation of the apolipoprotein C-III, isoform CRA_b by 2D-DIGE analysis.

The APPs results in a complex systemic reaction with the goal of re-establishing homeostasis and promoting healing. These proteins are generally referred to as the 'molecular thermometer' whereby

quantitation of individual APPs can provide an assessment of the response to the triggering event [28,29]. These APPs can be of diagnostic relevance and also of prognostic value. Within a few hours after exposure to toxicants, the pattern of protein synthesis by the liver is drastically altered resulting in an increase of some of these APPs [30,31]. The changes in the concentrations of APPs are due largely to changes in their production by hepatocytes. The magnitude of the increases varies from about 50 percent in the case of ceruloplasmin to as much as 1000-fold in the case of C-reactive protein and serum amyloid A, the plasma precursor of amyloid A. The maximal level could be seen after 8-10 days and it is maintained during each stage of disease [30]. Although, the acute phase response typically lasts only a few days, in cases of chronic or recurring inflammation, an aberrant continuation of some aspects of the acute phase response may contribute to the underlying tissue damage that accompanies the disease and may also lead to further complications. This was seen in the case of the subchronic study of furan for both the clinical biochemistry and histology [13] as well as being documented in other conditions such as cardiovascular or protein deposition diseases such as reactive amyloidosis.

Serum proteomic profiling as a tool to determine chemical exposure is still in its infancy stages. Humans are unavoidably exposed to a variety of environmental toxicants and combinations potentially contributing to an increased risk for a number of diseases. Detection of novel biomarkers could aid in the identification of an early-stage of chemical exposure and/or stages of disease. Biomarkers in accessible body fluids could greatly enhance the ability to identify exposures and could provide a warning sign prior to being symptomatic [17]. This is particularly important for asymptomatic conditions where a late diagnosis generally results in a poor outcome.

Conclusions

In the present study, we used 2D-DIGE, mass spectrometry and bioinformatics for a translational approach using serum proteomic profiling for the identification of novel biomarkers related to the subchronic exposure to furan. Proteomic profiling may expand the repertoire of identified predictive biomarkers of toxicant exposures to not only provide critical tools in the evaluation of their safety for future health risk assessment but also the appropriate measures to minimize adverse effects. All the identified serum proteins were involved in the acute phase response pathway and lipid metabolism which also corroborates the histological and clinical biochemistry results of our earlier publication.

Acknowledgements

We thank Andrea Kocmarek and Paul Rowsell for reviewing the manuscript.

References

1. Morehouse KM, Nyman PJ, McNeal TP, Dinovi MJ, Perfetti GA (2008) Survey of furan in heat processed foods by headspace gas chromatography/mass spectrometry and estimated adult exposure. Food Addit Contam Part A Chem Anal Control Expo Risk Assess 25: 259-264.

2. US FDA (US Food and Drug Administration) (2004) Exploratory data on furan in food.

3. Bolger PM, Tao SS, Dinovi M (2008) Hazards of dietary furan. In Process-induced Toxicants: Occurrence Formation, Mitigation and Health Risks, R. H. Stadler and D, R, Lineback (2nd eds.) John Wiley, Hoboken, NJ pp. 111-32.

4.   Crews C, Castle L (2007) A review of the occurrence, formation and analysis of furan in heat processed foods. Trends Food Sci Tech 18: 365-72.

5.   Maga JA (1979) Furans in foods. CRC Crit Rev Food Sci Nutr 11: 355-400.

6.   EFSA (European Food Safety Authority) (2004) Report on the scientific panel on contaminants in the food chain on provisional findings on furan in food. EFSA J 137: 1-20.

7.   Reinhard H, Sager F, Zimmermann H, Zoller O (2004) Furan in foods on the Swiss markets method and results. Mitt Lebensmittelunters Hyg 95: 532-35.

8.   Butterworth BE, Sprankle CS, Goldsworthy SM, Wilson DM, Goldsworthy TL (1994) Expression of myc, fos, and Ha-ras in the livers of furan-treated F344 rats and B6C3F1 mice. Mol Carcinog 9: 24-32.

9.   International Agency for Research on Cancer (1995) IARC Monographs on the Evaluation of Carcinogenic Risks to Humans 63: 3194-407.

10. Mugford CA, Carfagna MA, Kedderis GL (1997) Furan-mediated uncoupling of hepatic oxidative phosphorylation in Fischer-344 rats: an early event in cell death. Toxicol Appl Pharmacol 144: 1-11.

11. Wiley RA, Traiger GJ, Baraban S, Gammal LM (1984) Toxicity-distribution relationships among 3-alkylfurans in mouse liver and kidney. Toxicol Appl Pharmacol 74: 1-9.

12. Ravindranath V, McMenamin MG, Dees JH, Boyd MR (1986) 2-Methylfuran toxicity in rats--role of metabolic activation in vivo. Toxicol Appl Pharmacol 85: 78-91.

13. Gill S, Bondy G, Lefebvre DE, Becalski A, Kavanagh M, et al. (2010) Subchronic oral toxicity study of furan in Fischer-344 rats. Toxicol Pathol 38: 619-630.

14. Hu S, Loo JA, Wong DT (2006) Human body fluid proteome analysis. Proteomics 6: 6326-6353.

15. Gianazza E, Wait R, Eberini I, Sensi C, Sironi L, et al. (2012) Proteomics of rat biological fluids--the tenth anniversary update. J Proteomics 75: 3113-3128.

16. Maurya P, Meleady P, Dowling P, Clynes M (2007) Proteomic approaches for serum biomarker discovery in cancer. Anticancer Res 27: 1247-1255.

17. Ritorto, MS, Borlak J (2008) A simple and reliable protocol for mouse serum proteome profiling studies by use of two-dimensional electrophoresis and MALDI TOF/TOF mass spectrometry. Proteome Sci 6: 25.

18. NTP (National Toxicology Program) (1993) Toxicology and Carcinogenesis Studies of Furan (CAS No. 110-00-9) in F344/N rats and B6C3F1 Mice (Gavage Studies). Natl Toxicol Program Tech Rep Ser 402: 1-286.

19. Mally A, Graff C, Schmal O, Moro S, Hamberger C, et al. (2010) Functional and proliferative effects of repeated low-dose oral administration of furan in rat liver. Mol Nutr Food Res 54: 1556-1567.

20. Liu B, Qiu FH, Voss C, Xu Y, Zhao MZ, et al. (2011) Evaluation of three high abundance protein depletion kits for umbilical cord serum proteomics. Proteome Sci 9: 24.

21. Ruminy P, Gangneux C, Claeyssens S, Scotte M, Daveau M, et al. (2001) Gene transcription in hepatocytes during the acute phase of a systemic inflammation: from transcription factors to target genes. Inflamm Res 50: 383-390.

22. Zorin NA, Zhabin SG, Belogorlova TI, Chirikova TS, Krayushkina NA, et al. (1994) Changes in tissue distribution of rat alpha 1-macroglobulin and pregnancy-associated alpha 1-glycoprotein after inflammatory injury. Int J Exp Pathol 75: 425-431.

23. Ho AS, Cheng CC, Lee SC, Liu ML, Lee JY, et al. (2010) Novel biomarkers predict liver fibrosis in hepatitis C patients: alpha 2 macroglobulin, vitamin D binding protein and apolipoprotein AI. J Biomed Sci 17: 58.

24. Shen P, Howlett G (1993) Alteration in rat apolipoprotein C-III gene expression and lipoprotein composition during inflammation. Inflammation 17: 153-166.

25. Rahman SM, Choudhury M, Janssen RC, Baquero KC, Miyazaki M, et al. (2013) CCAAT/enhancer binding protein ß deletion increases mitochondrial function and protects mice from LXR-induced hepatic steatosis. Biochem Biophys Res Commun 430: 336-339.

26. Mauger JF, Couture P, Bergeron N, Lamarche B (2006) Apolipoprotein C-III isoforms: kinetics and relative implication in lipid metabolism. J Lipid Res 47: 1212-1218.

27. Lee HY, Birkenfeld AL, Jornayvaz FR, Jurczak MJ, Kanda S, et al. (2011) Apolipoprotein CIII overexpressing mice are predisposed to diet-induced hepatic steatosis and hepatic insulin resistance. Hepatology 54:1650-1660.

28. Feingold KR, Grunfeld C (2010) The acute phase response inhibits reverse cholesterol transport. J Lipid Res 51: 682-684.

29. Cray C, Zaias J, Altman NH (2009) Acute phase response in animals: a review. Comp Med 59: 517-526.

30. Gabay C, Kushner I (1999) Acute-phase proteins and other systemic responses to inflammation. N Engl J Med 340: 448-454.

31. Tirziu E (2009) Acute-Phase Proteins in Immune Response. Lucrari Stiiniifice MedicinaVeterinara p 42.

24

Biochemical Characterization of a PLA$_2$ Btae TX-I Isolated from *Bothriopsis taeniata* Snake Venom: A Pharmacological and Morphological Study

Frey Francisco Romero-Vargas[1], Thalita Rocha[2,3], Maria Alice Cruz-Höfling[3*], Lea Rodrigues-Simioni[4], Luis Alberto Ponce-Soto[1] and Sergio Marangoni[1]

[1]*Department of Biochemistry, Institute of Biology, State University of Campinas (UNICAMP), Campinas, SP, Brazil*

[2]*Multidisciplinary Research Laboratory, San Francisco University (USF), Bragança Paulista, SP, Brazil*

[3]*Department of Histology and Embryology, Institute of Biology, State University of Campinas (UNICAMP), Campinas, SP, Brazil*

[4]*Department of Pharmacology, Faculty of Medical Sciences, State University of Campinas (UNICAMP), Campinas, SP, Brazil*

*Corresponding author: Dr. Maria Alice da Cruz-Höfling, Department of Histology and Embryology, Institute of Biology, State University of Campinas (UNICAMP), P.O. Box 6109, Zip Code 13083-865, Campinas, SP, Brazil, E-mail: **hofling@unicamp.br**

Abstract

In this research a preliminary identification and biochemical and biological characterization of a PLA$_2$ (Btae TX-I) from the venom of a viperid snake, *Bothriopsis taeniata* (Speckled forest pit viper) were obtained. Btae TX-I was purified by two chromatographic steps, molecular exclusion chromatography followed by analytical chromatography reverse phase HPLC. Molecular mass behaved as a homogeneous single chain protein on SDS–PAGE, confirmed by MALDI-TOF spectrometry, indicating a molecular mass of 13889.98 Da. Tryptic peptides were determined *in tandem* mass spectrometry and showed similarity with other myotoxic PLA$_2$s. Btae TX-I belongs to the Asp49 PLA$_2$ class, is enzymatically active in presence of a synthetic substrate and shows a minimum sigmoidal behavior, reaching its maximal activity at pH 8.0 and 35–45°C. PLA$_2$ activity in presence of Mn^{2+}, Mg^{2+}, Cd^{2+} and Zn^{2+} was reduced either in presence or absence of Ca^{2+}, suggesting that the arrangement of the catalytic site presents an exclusive structure for Ca^{2+}. Crotalic crotapotins from rattlesnake venom has significantly inhibited (p<0.05) the enzymatic activity of Btae TX-I. In ex vivo experiment, Btae TX-I caused partial blockade of the neuromuscular transmission in chick biventer cervicis preparations in a similar way to other *Bothrops* species. Btae TX-I also inhibited contractures in the upper concentration (50 μg) to exogenous KCl (20 mM). Histological analysis of the biventer cervicis incubated with Btae TX-I showed that just the highest Btae TX-I PLA$_2$ dose (50 μg) caused almost 27.4 ± 0.3% damaged fibers. The results give evidence that the main effect of type Asp49 Btae TX-I PLA$_2$ from *Bothriopsis taeniata* is at the post-synaptic site.

Keywords: Speckled forest pit viper; *Bothriopsis taeniata* venom; Phospholipase A$_2$; Histopathological analysis; Neurotoxic activity

Introduction

Phospholipase A$_2$s (PLA$_2$s, EC 3.1.1.4) represent a superfamily of lipolytic esterases that hydrolyze the *sn*-2 ester bond of phospholipids releasing free fatty acid and lysophospholipid. Initially, PLA$_2$ family members were included according with their biochemical characteristics and cellular origin in three main classes, secretory (sPLA$_2$), cytosolic (cPLA$_2$) and intracellular (iPLA$_2$) [1]. At present with the discovery of additional PLA$_2$s and based on amino acid sequences, 16 distinct groups of PLA$_2$s were now reported [2,3]. The sPLA$_2$ are the oldest class of PLA2, being also found in prokaryotes [4]. sPLA$_2$ molecular mass ranges from 13 to 19 kDa and typically requires Ca^{2+} at millimolar concentrations for their catalytic activity [5-7]. In eukaryotes, sPLA$_2$s are found in the secretion of glands such as salivary, lacrimal, seminal and exocrine pancreas, as well in glands of snakes, bees and wasps, among others, where they participate in pivotal physiological and pathological functions [8]. Despite sharing primary, secondary and tertiary structures and common catalytic properties, differences in the sequence of amino acids, confer to sPLA$_2$ a wide spectrum of pharmacological effects. The venom of snakes may contain myotoxins that provoke important muscle necrosis at the snakebite site. These myotoxins include small myotoxic peptides that affect Na$^+$ channels at the sarcolemma or sarcoplasmic reticulum,

cardiotoxins or cytotoxic polypeptides present in the venom of elapid snakes and myotoxins with PLA$_2$ activity or myotoxic PLA$_2$ [9].

The PLA$_2$ myotoxins are natural components of a number of snake venoms including Bothropic venoms. They usually are small proteins and peptides that induce either local or systemic necrosis of muscle tissue (rhabdomyolysis), the latter leading to myoglobinuria and acute renal failure and death [10]. Myotoxic PLA$_2$ can be divided into two broad groups: Asp49 PLA$_2$ group, which possesses an aspartic acid residue at position 49, and Lys49 PLA$_2$ group, in which a lysine residue substitutes the aspartic acid at the same 49 position [11,12]. Both types disrupt the integrity of myofibers plasma membrane, by a catalytic-dependent or -independent mechanism, respectively [13].

The present study aimed to isolate and characterize a PLA$_2$ from the venom of the arboreal *Bothriopsis taeniata* Amazonian snake (*Viperidae*), popularly known as speckled forest pit-viper. In addition, it was sought to investigate if the isolated PLA$_2$ possesses neurotoxic activity as well to evaluate its myotoxicity on *in vitro* avian nerve-muscle preparation by using pharmacological and morphological approaches.

Herein, we showed for the first time an Asp-49 PLA$_2$ isolated from *B. taeniata* venom, called as Btae TX-I (*Botrhiopsis taeniata* Toxin-I), which looks like a post-synaptic-acting myotoxin whose myotoxic activity was significant just when 50 μg of toxin was used.

Materials and Methods

Venom, chemicals and drugs

Bothriopsis taeniata venom was a pool obtained by manual compression of the venom glands. All other chemicals and reagents used in this work were of analytical or sequencing grade, and were purchased from Sigma-Aldrich Corporation (St. Louis, MO. USA).

Animals

The Animal Services Unit of the State University of Campinas (UNICAMP) supplied male chicks (4–8 days old, HY-LINE W36 lineage). Animals were housed at 25°C on a 12 h light/dark cycle and had free access to food and water. All experiments described here were done with approved protocol number 1492-1, for the use of animals in research, conducted in accordance with guidelines established by the Ethics Committee of the Biology Institute in the Animals Use - UNICAMP (CEUA, COBEA).

Biochemical Studies

Isolation and purification of phospholipase A2: sPLA$_2$ was purified after two chromatographic steps. The first step was conducted using molecular exclusion chromatography followed by reverse phase HPLC (RP-HPLC) as described by Ponce-Soto et al. [14] and Bonfim et al. [15]. Approximately 50 mg of *Bothriopsis taeniata* venom was dissolved in 1 mL of 1 M (NH$_4$)$_2$CO$_3$ buffer, pH 8, homogenized in the sonic bath, clarified by centrifugation at 9,000 rpm for 5 min, and applied to a Kontex Flex column (78x2 cm) of Sephadex G-75, which had been pre-equilibrated with the same buffer (0.2 M). The proteins were eluted at a flow rate of 0.25 ml/min and the chromatographic profile was determined by measuring absorbance at A280 nm. The fraction corresponding to main peaks were pooled, lyophilized and stored at -20°C. Five milligrams of the fraction containing PLA$_2$ activity were dissolved in 120 μl of 0.1% TFA (buffer A) until complete dissolution. The supernatant was then applied to an analytical reverse phase HPLC column, Shim Pack CLC-ODS C18 (4.6 mmx25 cm). Protein elution was carried out using a linear gradient (0-100%) of buffer B (66.5% of acetonitrile in 0.1% TFA) at a constant flow rate of 1 ml/min. The chromatographic run was monitored at 280 nm, and the fractions obtained were then collected, lyophilized and stored at -20°C.

The degree of purity of the PLA$_2$ isoform was assessed by Tricine SDS–PAGE in a discontinuous gel and a buffer system was used to estimate the molecular mass of the proteins, under reducing and non-reducing conditions [16].

Protein determination by the Bradford method (Comassie blue): Protein content of the fractions was determined using bovine gamma globulin as a standard by the Coomassie blue method [17]. The absorbances reading were made in wavelength of 595 nm in reader ELISA Versa Max microplate reader (Molecular Devices, Sunnyvale, CA, USA). These calculated protein concentrations, performed in triplicate for each fraction sample, were the basis of other analyses.

Phospholipase A2 activity: PLA2 activity was measured using the assay described by Cho and Kézdy [18] and Holzer and Mackessy [19] modified for 96-well plates by Beghini et al. [20] using 20 μl of 4-nitro-3-octanoyloxy-benzoic acid as a substrate (Biomol, USA), 200 μl of buffer (10 mM Tris-HCl, 10 mM CaCl$_2$, 100 mM NaCl, pH 8.0), 20 μl of water and 20 μl of PLA$_2$ in a final volume of 260 μl. After the addition of PLA$_2$ (20 μg), the mixture was incubated for 40 min at 37°C, and the absorbance was checked with 10 min intervals. Enzyme activity, expressed as the initial velocity of the reaction (V$_o$), was calculated based on the absorbance increase after 20 min.

Btae TX-I obtained from RP-HPLC was determined by studying the kinetic parameters. The effect of substrate concentration (20, 10, 5, 2.5, 1.0, 0.5, 0.3, 0.2 and 0.1 mM) on enzyme activity was determined by measuring the increase of absorbance after 20 min of incubation in 10 mM Tris-HCl buffer, pH 8.0, at 37°C. The optimum pH and temperature of the PLA2 were determined by incubating the enzyme in buffers (10 mM citrate, 10 mM phosphate, 10 mM Tris and 10 mM glycine) of different pH values (4 to 10) and in Tris-HCl buffer, pH 8.0, at different temperatures (25 to 45°C), respectively.

The inhibition of PLA$_2$ activity by crotapotins from *Crotalus durissus terrificus* (CdtF5 and CdtF7) and *C. d. colillineatus* (CdcolF3 and CdcolF4) were determined by incubating both proteins (Btae TX-I : crotapotins) for 30 min at 37°C prior assaying the residual enzyme activity at 425 nm.

Determination of the molecular mass of the purified protein by mass spectrometry: Purified lyophilized protein Btae TX-I PLA$_2$ from RP-HPLC was resuspended in 8 M urea containing 10 mM DTT at pH 8.0 and the disulfide bridges were then reduced by incubation at 37°C for 2 h. Iodoacetamide (IAA) was used to alkylate the free thiols of cysteine residues, based on previous experiments, a 30% molar excess of iodoacetamide relative to the total number of thiols was eventually chosen and the mixture was incubated for 1.5 h at 37°C in the dark. The reaction was stopped by injecting the mixture onto a RP-HPLC column followed by lyophilization of the collected peak.

The molecular mass of intact native and alkylated Btae TX-I PLA$_2$ were analyzed by MALDI-TOF mass spectrometry using a Voyager-DE PRO MALDI-TOF apparatus (Applied Biosystems, Foster City, CA, USA) equipped with a pulsed nitrogen laser (337 nm, pulse with 4 ns) and 1 μL of sample in 0.1% TFA was mixed with 2 μL of the matrix sinapinic acid (3,5-dimethoxy-4-hydroxycinnamic acid). The matrix was prepared with 30% acetonitrile and 0.1% TFA and its mass analyzed under the following conditions: accelerate voltage of 25 kV, the laser fixed in 2890 μJ/com^2, delay 300 ns, and linear analysis mode [21].

Electrospray ionization mass spectrometry (ESI-CID-MS/MS) analyses were performed using a quadrupole-time of flight (Q-TOF) hybrid mass spectrometer Q-TOF Ultima from Micromass (Manchester, UK) equipped with a nano Zspray source operating in a positive ion mode. The ionization conditions of usage included a capillary voltage of 2.3 kV, a cone voltage and RF1 lens of 30 V and 100 V, respectively, and collision energy of 10 eV. The source temperature was 70°C and the cone gas was N2 at a flow of 80 l/h; nebulizing gas was not used to obtain the sprays. Argon was used for collisional cooling and for fragmentation of ions in the collision cell. External calibration with sodium iodide was made over a mass range from 50 to 3000 m/z. All spectra were acquired with the TOF analyzer in "Vmode" (TOF kV=9.1) and the MCP voltage set at 2150 V [22].

Identification of tryptic digests: The protein was reduced with 5 mM DTT and alkylated with 14 mM IAA prior to addition of trypsin (Promega-Sequence Grade Modified). After trypsin addition (20 ng/μl in 0.05 M Ambic), the sample was incubated for 16 h at 37°C. To stop the reaction, 0.4% formic acid was added and the sample centrifuged at 2,500 rpm for 10 min. The pellet was discarded and the supernatant dried in a speed vac. The resulting peptides were separated by C18

(100 µm x 100 mm) RP-UPLC (nanoAcquity UPLC, Waters) coupled with nano-electrospray tandem mass spectrometry on a Q-Tof Ultima API mass spectrometer (MicroMass/Waters) at a flow rate of 600 nl/min. Before performing a tandem mass spectrum, an ESI/MS mass spectrum (TOF MS mode) was acquired for each HPLC fraction over the mass range of 400-2000 m/z, in order to select the ion of interest. Subsequently, these ions were fragmented in the collision cell (TOF MS/MS mode).

Raw data files from LC-MS/MS runs were processed using MASSlynx 4.1 software package (Waters) and analyzed using the Mascot search engine version 2.3 (Matrix Science Ltd) against the NCBI-BLAST database, using the following parameters: peptide mass tolerance of ±0.1 Da, fragment mass tolerance of ± 0.1 Da, oxidation as variable modifications in methionine and trypsin as enzyme.

Pharmacological assay

Neurotoxic activity: Chick biventer cervicis muscle preparation (BC): Male young chicks (4–8 days old, HY-LINE W36 lineage, n=5) were anesthetized and killed by halothane inhalation and *biventer cervicis* muscles were removed and mounted [23] under a tension of 1 g in a 5 ml organ bath at 37°C (Automatic organ multiple-bath LE01 Letica Scientific Instruments, Barcelona, Spain), containing carbogen-aerated (95% O_2 and 5% CO_2) Krebs solution. Contractures to exogenously applied acetylcholine (73.3 µM ACh for 60 s) and KCl (20 mM for 180 s) were recorded in the absence of field stimulation, prior to the addition of different doses (5, 10, 20 and 50 µg/ml) of Btae TX-I PLA$_2$ and at the end of the experiment. A bipolar platinum ring electrode was placed around the tendon in which runs the nerve trunk supplying the muscle. Indirect stimulation (0.1 Hz, 0.2 ms, 5-6 V) was performed with a Grass S48 stimulator (Powerlab AD Instruments, Barcelona, Spain). Muscle contractions and contractures were isometrically recorded via a force-displacement transducer (Model MLT0201 Force transducer 5 mg-25 g Panlab s.l. AD Instruments Pty Ltd, Barcelona, Spain) connected to a Power Lab/4SP (OUAD Bridge AD Instruments, Barcelona, Spain).

Myotoxic Activity: Morphological and morphometric analyses: After 120 minutes of Btae TX-I incubation (10 and 50 µg), biventer

cervicis muscles (n=5/concentration) were immersed for 24 h in 4% paraformaldehyde, washed three times with saline solution, dehydrated in increasing ethanol concentration series (70, 80, 95 and 100%, v/v), clarified in xylene and embedded in paraffin. Sections (5 µm thick) obtained using a Leica RM2035 microtome were stained with hematoxylin-eosin (HE) and analyzed with a Olympus BX51 microscope equipped with image analysis software (Image ProPlus 6.0, Media Cybernetics, Inc.). Control preparations were prepared from muscle incubated with Krebs solution. The extent of damage in control and treated muscles was assessed by counting the total number of normal and damaged fibers per histological section and then expressing the number of damaged fibers as a percentage of the total number of fibers counted. Normal fibers were defined as those with a polygonal appearance, peripheral nucleus and evenly distributed myofibrils.

Statistics

Results were reported as mean±SEM. Statistical comparisons were done using ANOVA followed by Tukey-Kramer test. Values of $p<0.05$ indicated significance.

Results

Purification and biochemical characterization of the Btae TX-I PLA$_2$

Fractionation of crude *B. taeniata* venom on Sephadex G-75 at pH 7.8 resulted in four main peaks (I-IV; Figure 1A). The whole venom, with fractions detected by molecular exclusion, was monitored for phospholipasic activity on specific chromogenic substrate and peak III showed PLA2 activities (12.075 ± 0.138 nmoles/min/mg). Subsequently, the peak III was pooled, dialyzed, lyophilized and fractionated in an analytical shim-pack CLC-ODS (C18) column (4.6 mm x 25 cm x 0.5 µm) by RP-HPLC and resulted in the purification of three well-defined peaks (III-1 to III-3), followed by several smaller peaks (Figure 1B).

Step	Volume (ml)	Protein (mg/ml)	Activity (U/ml)	Total Activity (U.T.)	Specific Activity (U/mg)	Recovery (%)	Purification
Whole Venom	12	0.1966	109.26	1311.0	555.85	100.00	1.00
Sephadex G-75 (peak III)	3.6	0.0144	284.39	1023.8	19746.97	78.08	35.53
HPLC-FR (Btae TX-I)	1	0.0151	772.30	772.3	51303.31	58.90	92.30

Table 1: Parameters of Btae TX-I purification.

The purification procedures of PLA$_2$ Btae TX-I are summarized in Table 1 and this purified protein was selected for further biochemical and pharmacological characterization. The crude venom had catalytic activity of 2.185 ± 0.078 nmol/min/mg, which increased to 5.668 ± 0.091 mol/min/mg for peak III (Sephadex G75), resulting in a yield of 78.08%, with a purification factor of 35.53. The second chromatographic step (RP-HPLC) yielded 58.90% in relation to the whole venom with purified factor of 92.30.

After SDS-PAGE analysis, the enzyme showed a single chain with molecular mass (Mr) around 14 kDa, under reducing (1M DTT) and no reducing conditions, suggesting that it is a monomeric protein (Figure 2). The Btae TX-I homogeneity was confirmed by MALDI-TOF mass spectrometry analysis, to be determined an intact molecular weight of 13,889.98 Da, as well as, an exact molecular mass in reduced and alkylated samples of 14,701.98 Da (Figure 3A).

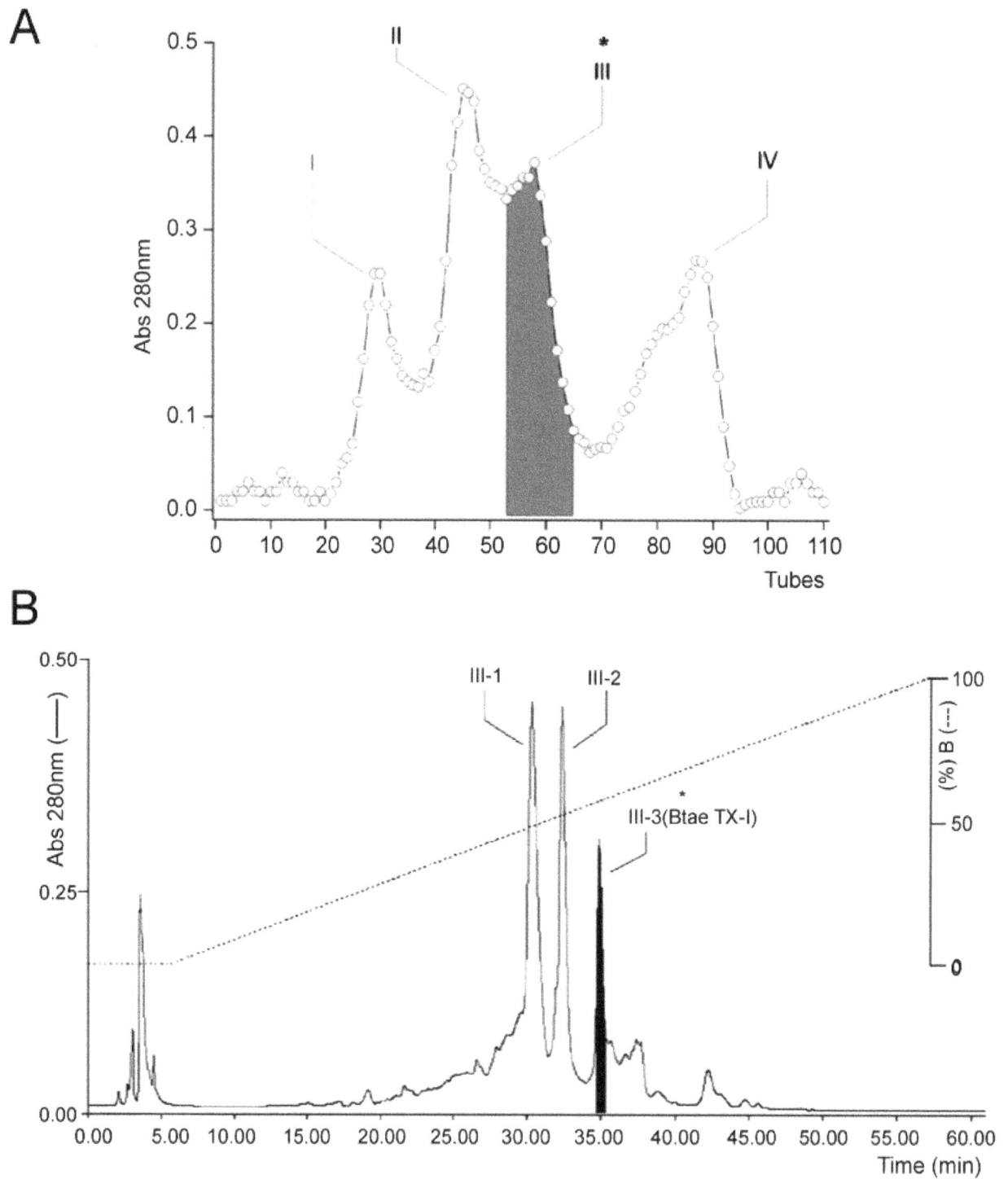

Figure 1: (A) Elution profile of *Bothriopsis taeniata* venom by molecular exclusion chromatography on a Sephadex G-75 column (Kontex Flex Column 78x2 cm). Fraction III contained PLA$_2$ activity. (B). Elution profile of peak III following RP-HPLC on a reversed-phase column, shim-pack CLC-ODS (C18), 4.6 mmx25 cmx0.5 μm. The peak corresponding to the phospholipase A$_2$ (Btae TX-I) from *Bothriopsis taeniata* venom is indicated (*).

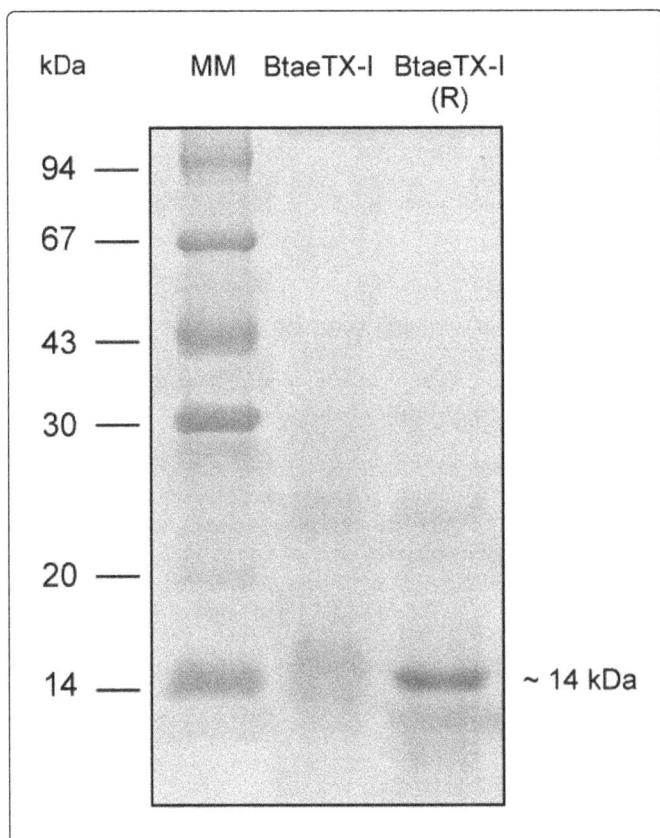

Figure 2: Electrophoretic profile of Btae TX-I protein (PLA2) by SDS-PAGE (12.5% gel). Lane 1. Molecular mass markers (MM); Lane 2. Btae TX-I not reduced (NR); Lane 3. Btae TX-I reduced with 1M DTT (R). Protein standards and their molecular weights are: phosphorylase b–94, albumin–67, ovalbumin–43, carbonic anhydrase–30, trypsin inhibitor–20.1, α-lactalbumin–14.4.

Additionally the amino acid composition determined was: N,D/11; Q,E/12; S/2; G/12; H/2; R/4; T/8; A/6; P/7; Y/10; V/4; M/2; C/14; I/5; L/6; F/4; K/13; W/not determined. This analysis revealed a high content of Lys, Tyr, Gly, Thr, and 14 half-Cys residues-typical of a basic PLA2 protein. The basic amino acids (His, Lys and Arg) represent 20.74% of the total amino acids of Btae TX-I. Also, this enzyme possesses 41.48% of hydrophobic amino acids.

Identification of tryptic peptides from Btae TX-I PLA2 by ESI-MS/MS

Alkylated Btae TX-I PLA2 was digested with trypsin and its tryptic peptides were fractionated by RP-HPLC. All tryptic digests submitted to the analysis in electrospray ionization-tandem mass spectrometry (ESI-MS/MS) were searched using the Mascot MS/MS Ion Search software (www.matrixscience.com). Table 2 shows some of these alkylated peptides with their deduced sequences and measured masses. Isoleucine and leucine residues were not discriminated in any of the sequences reported since they were indistinguishable in low energy CID spectra. Because of the external calibration applied to all spectra, it was also not possible to resolve the 0.036 Da difference between glutamine and lysine residues, except for the lysine that was deduced

based on the cleavage and missed cleavage of the enzyme. Each of the peptides identified from Btae TX-I PLA2 were submitted to NCBI database search, using the program BLAST-p with a search restricted to sequenced proteins from the basic phospholipase A_2 family.

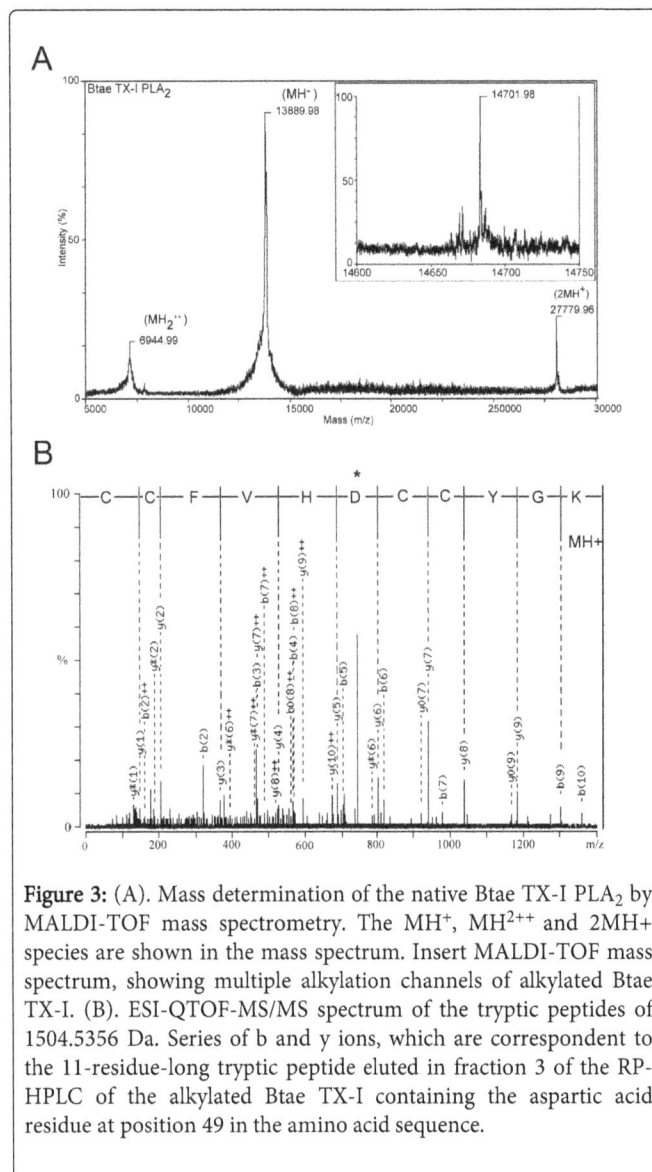

Figure 3: (A). Mass determination of the native Btae TX-I PLA2 by MALDI-TOF mass spectrometry. The MH+, MH2++ and 2MH+ species are shown in the mass spectrum. Insert MALDI-TOF mass spectrum, showing multiple alkylation channels of alkylated Btae TX-I. (B). ESI-QTOF-MS/MS spectrum of the tryptic peptides of 1504.5356 Da. Series of b and y ions, which are correspondent to the 11-residue-long tryptic peptide eluted in fraction 3 of the RP-HPLC of the alkylated Btae TX-I containing the aspartic acid residue at position 49 in the amino acid sequence.

The *tandem mass* spectra shown in Figure 3B, relative to the peptide 3 of the digest (sequence C C F V H D C C Y G K), allows classifying the protein as an Asp49 PLA2. A comparison of the sequence of Btae TX-I deduced peptides with others myotoxic PLA2s from *Bothrops* genus was shown. Sequences of the other peptides would indicate that they are part of regions highly conserved as well as also of variable regions. Such conserved residues are involved in the binding of Ca^{2+} (Tyr28, Gly30, Gly32 and Asp49) and the His48 residue, a key component of the active site, is also conserved in Btae TX-I (Figure 4). Furthermore, a majority of residues involved in the formation of a hydrophobic channel (Leu2, Phe5, and Ile9) are also conserved in Btae TX-I.

Btae TX-I (PLA₂)			
HPLC Fraction	Measured Mass (Da)	Amino acid sequence	Theorical Mass (Da)
1	1377.7115	DL/IWQ/KFGQ/KMI/LL/IK/Q	1377.6687
2	2599.1301	L/ IPFPYYTTYGCYCGWGGQ/KGQ/KPK/Q	2599.1233
3	1504.5356	CCFVHDCCYGK/Q	1504.4954
4	1661.7389	ENGVI/LI/LCGEGTPCEK/Q	1661.6716
5	951.3790	Q/KI/LCECDK/Q	951.3886
6	793.3905	AAAVCFR	793.3890
7	1414.6737	RYMAYPDVL/ICK/Q	1414.6905
8	975.4549	I/LDSYTYSK/Q	975.4623

Table 2: Measured molecular masses and deduced amino acid sequences obtained by ESI-MS/MS based on the alkylated tryptic peptides of Btae TX-I. The peptides were separated by RP-HPLC and sequenced by mass spectrometry. C = alkylated cysteine, lysine residues shown in bold were deduced on the cleavage and missed cleavage by trypsin. All molecular masses are reported as monoisotopic.

Enzymatic characterization of Btae TX-I

The activity of Btae TX-I was examined using the synthetic substrate 4-nitro-3-(octanoyloxy) benzoic acid. Btae TX-I showed to be a typical PLA_2, since it hydrolyzes synthetic substrates at position 2. Under the conditions used, this enzyme showed classic Michaelis–Menten kinetics with a discrete sigmoidal behavior, mainly at low substrate concentrations (Figure 5A).

Kinetic analysis of PLA_2 activity at different concentrations of 4N3OBA showed apparent Michaelis-Menten constant (Km) value of 0.168 mM and apparent maximum velocity ($Vmax$) value of 0.115 nmol/min (Figure 5B), and optimum pH set at 8.0 (Figure 5C). Maximum enzyme activity occurred between 35°C and 45°C, temperature. At 25°C, the enzyme showed decreased activity relative to first ones (Figure 5D). The *in vitro* phospholipase activity of Btae TX-I at equimolar ratios with each of crotalic crotapotins from *C. d. terrificus* and *C. d. collilineatus* was inhibited around 65-70% (Figure 5E). The PLA2 activity required Ca^{2+}, at 1 and 10 mM concentrations (Figure 5F). The substitution of Ca^{2+} by other cations (10 mM) alone or in presence of Ca^{2+} 1 mM reduced the enzymatic activity. However, when Mg^{2+} (10 mM) was added in presence of Ca^{2+} (1 mM) it did not reduce significantly the activity of Btae TX-I PLA_2 (Figure 5F).

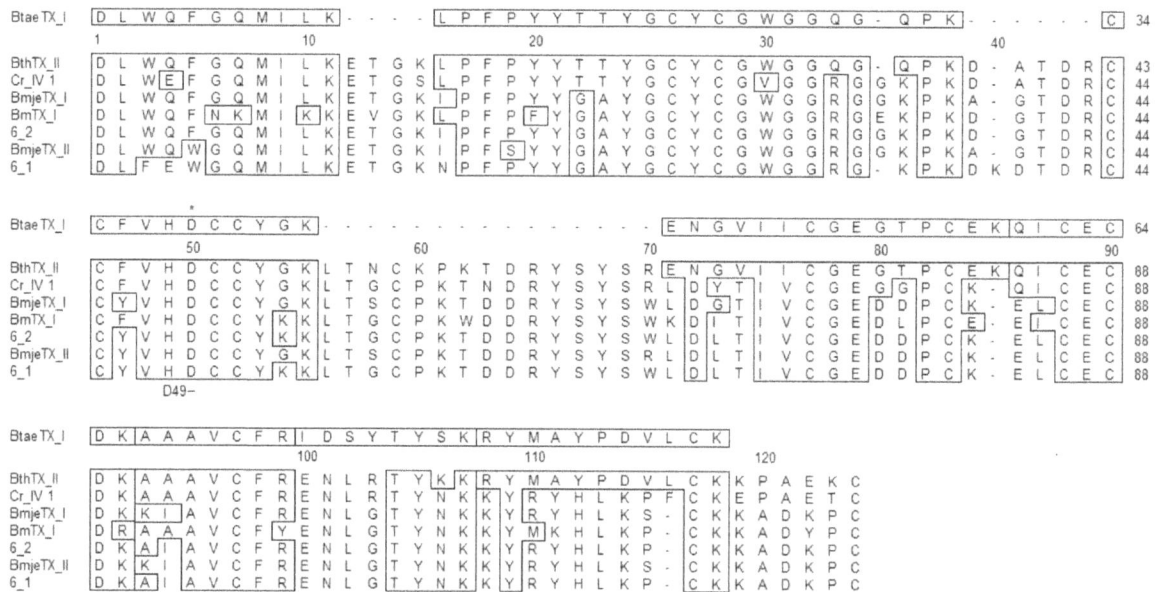

Figure 4: Comparison of the obtained amino acid sequence from tryptic peptides of the Btae TX-I with others Asp49 PLA_2. BthTX-II of bothropstoxin II from *Bothrops jararacussu* [50], Cr-IV-1 from *Calloselasma rhodostoma* [51], PLA_2 isoforms (6-1 and 6-2) of the fraction BthTX-II from *Bothrops jararacuçu* [21], PLA_2 isoforms (BmjeTX-I and BmjeTX-II) from *Bothrops marajoensis* [34] and PLA_2 (BmTX-I) from *Bothrops moojeni* [31]. The spaces are inserted in the sequences to reach the maxim homology.

Pharmacological characterization of the Btae TX-I PLA2

Neurotoxic *in vitro* activity was tested in isolated chick *biventer cervicis* preparation indirectly stimulated. Btae TX-I concentrations of 5, 10, 20 and 50 µg/mL produced a slow and discreet decrease in the twitch muscle responses (Figure 6A) and induced partial neuromuscular blockade at 120 min incubation even using the highest concentration. The time required for Btae TX-I to cause 50% blockade was 103.6 ± 2 min and 85.5 ± 2.5 min at 10-20 µg/mL and 50 µg/mL concentrations, respectively. Five µg/mL of toxin concentration was ineffective in inducing 50% blockade within 120 min incubation (data not shown).

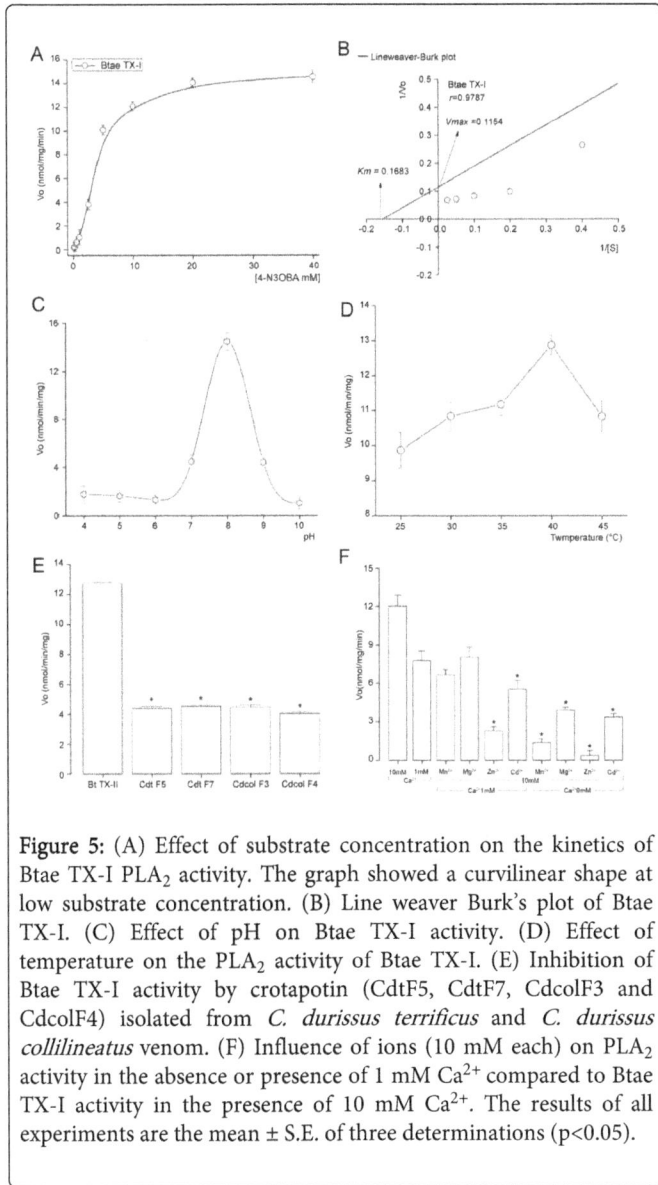

Figure 5: (A) Effect of substrate concentration on the kinetics of Btae TX-I PLA_2 activity. The graph showed a curvilinear shape at low substrate concentration. (B) Line weaver Burk's plot of Btae TX-I. (C) Effect of pH on Btae TX-I activity. (D) Effect of temperature on the PLA_2 activity of Btae TX-I. (E) Inhibition of Btae TX-I activity by crotapotin (CdtF5, CdtF7, CdcolF3 and CdcolF4) isolated from *C. durissus terrificus* and *C. durissus collilineatus* venom. (F) Influence of ions (10 mM each) on PLA_2 activity in the absence or presence of 1 mM Ca^{2+} compared to Btae TX-I activity in the presence of 10 mM Ca^{2+}. The results of all experiments are the mean ± S.E. of three determinations (p<0.05).

The toxin showed a discreet action on the nicotinic receptors since the contractures induced by ACh were reduced in just 1 ± 6.1% and 13 ± 4.7% with 10 µg/mL and 50 µg/mL concentrations, respectively after 120 min (n=5/concentration; p<0.05).

Myotoxicity: KCl and histopathological analysis

The criteria used to determine the myotoxicity was through KCl-induced contractures and by counting the number of degenerating muscle fibers against the number of normal-looking fibers. The KCl-induced contractures were reduced in 37.8 ± 3% and 59.7 ± 5.8% at 10 µg/mL and 50 µg/mL Btae TX-I concentrations, respectively. Control preparations showed contracture induced by ACh and KCl stable after the experiments (Figure 6B).

Morphologically, fibers considered normal were those presenting polygonal cross-sectional profile, peripheral nuclei, homogeneous

myofibrils distribution inside the sarcoplasm and continuous sarcolemma. Biventer cervicis muscle incubated with Krebs solution showed 1 ± 0.6% of altered fibers. BC incubated with 10 µg/mL Btae TX-I PLA2 showed 6±3.4% of altered fibers which showed to be statistically equal to the number found in controls. However, Btae TX-I at 50 µg/mL concentration caused a 27.4±0.3% of damaged fibers, which was significantly different from both Krebs solution- and 10 µg/mL toxin-incubated BC. Muscles treated with 50 µg/mL Btae TX-I presented fibers with different pathologic states, the more frequent of which being ghost fibers (when myofibrils and sarcolemma were lysed and only the basement membrane persisted) or damaged fibers (when part of the fibers were lysed) (Figures 7,8).

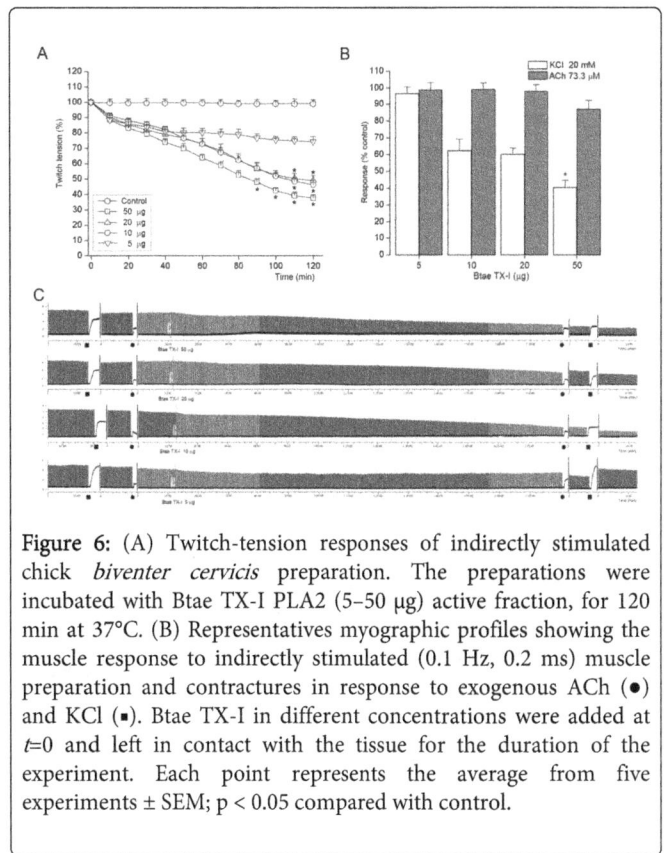

Figure 6: (A) Twitch-tension responses of indirectly stimulated chick *biventer cervicis* preparation. The preparations were incubated with Btae TX-I PLA2 (5–50 µg) active fraction, for 120 min at 37°C. (B) Representatives myographic profiles showing the muscle response to indirectly stimulated (0.1 Hz, 0.2 ms) muscle preparation and contractures in response to exogenous ACh (●) and KCl (■). Btae TX-I in different concentrations were added at t=0 and left in contact with the tissue for the duration of the experiment. Each point represents the average from five experiments ± SEM; p < 0.05 compared with control.

Discussion

The characterization of snake venom containing-$sPLA_2$ is of importance because the enzyme is the major responsible for local and systemic degeneration and inflammation of skeletal muscle tissue [24]. Apart from that, the biochemical characterization of the molecule is important not only for evolutionary purposes but also in relation to structure-function studies. Although significant progress has been made to characterize the structural basis related with the diverse PLA_2 toxic activities, further researches are required. In the present study, we report for the first time a biochemical and pharmacological characterization of a PLA_2 isolated from the venom of *B. taeniata*, named as Btae TX-I. The enzyme was isolated through two chromatographic steps: in column of molecular exclusion and hydrophobic column coupled to a system of reverse phase HPLC. This methodological combination was efficient to preserve the selectivity, resolution capacity, high degree of molecular homogeneity and biological activity [25,26].

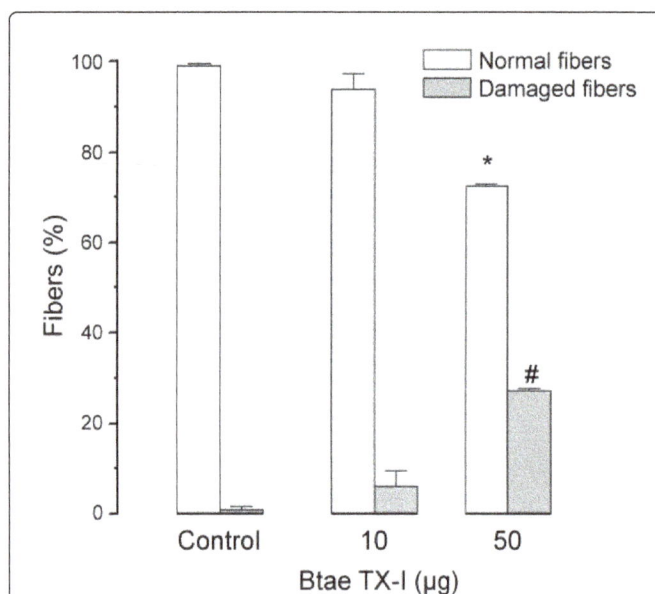

Figure 7: Percentage values of damaged and normal fibers in the whole area of the transverse section of *biventer cervicis* muscle control and treated with the concentrations of 10 µg and 50 µg Btae TX-I; *: $p < 0.05$ in relation to control; #: $p < 0.05$ in relation to 10 µg.

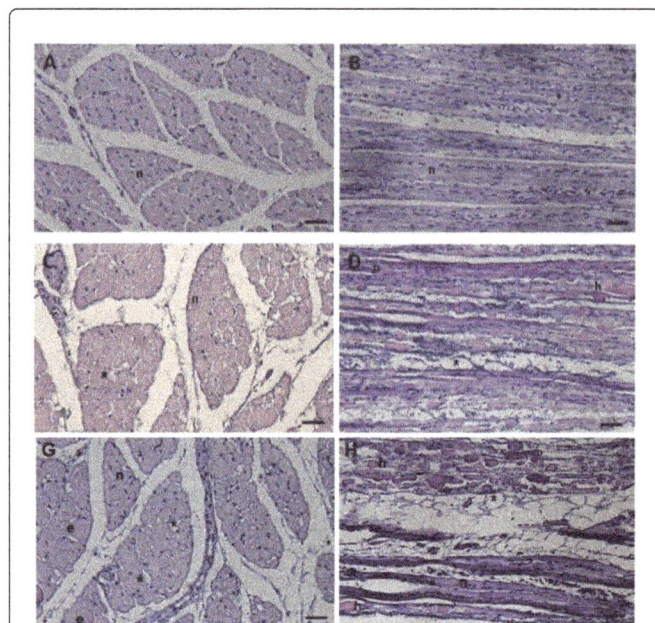

Figure 8: Transverse (A) and longitudinal section (B) of biventer cervicis muscle treated with Krebs solution (Control) showing normal (n) morphology of the muscular fibers. Transverse (C) and longitudinal section (D) of biventer cervicis muscle treated with 10 µg of Btae TX-I and 50 µg Btae TX-I (E) and (F), respectively. Observe normal fibers (n) between edematous (e), discontinuous or hipercontracted (h) and ghost fibers (*). Bar= 50 µm.

A variety of PLA2s isolated from *Bothrops sp* venoms are oligomers constituted by two or more subunits [27]. Nevertheless, SDS-PAGE under non-reducing conditions showed Btae TX-I running as a monomer and possessing a single polypeptidic chain of ~14 kDa (13,889.89 Da) after reduction, what was confirmed by MALDI-TOF mass spectrometry. Such configuration of Btae TX-I is similar to other basic Asp49 PLA_2s that also have monomeric structure like the PhTX-I from *Porthidium hyoprora* [28], blD-PLA_2 from *Bothrops leucurus* [29] and LmTX-I from *Lachesis muta muta* venoms [22]. The amino acid composition of the toxin revealed a high content of basic and hydrophobic residues, with 14 half-Cys, in agreement with the reported composition and primary structure of PLA_2 myotoxins isolated from *Bothrops* venoms [21,30,31]. In effect, the amino acid composition of Btae TX-I PLA_2 revealed the presence of 14 half-Cys residues so providing the basis for a common structural feature of PLA_2 in the formation of its seven disulfide bridges [30,32-34].

The high stability of snake venom PLA_2s, including Btae TX-I, is probably due to the relatively small molecular size of these proteins (121 amino acid residues), the presence of disulfide bridges and a high content of basic and hydrophobic residues. Such structural characteristics make this protein a compact and highly denaturation resistant molecule. PLA_2 remains active through a large temperature range as demonstrated by its highest activity at temperatures as high as 37°C and with optimum activity at pH 8.0. Temperature is another kinetic parameter utilized to characterize the Asp49 PLA_2. It has been shown that PLA_2 from *Naja naja naja* is very stable in extreme temperatures such as 100°C [35].

Together, these characteristics constitute the basis for the successful interaction between basic PLA_2 and negatively-charged phospholipids of cell membranes [36]. Such interaction is important to explain the hydrolyzing effect of these enzymes on different cell membrane types [37].

The effect of bivalent cations (Mn^{2+}, Mg^{2+}, Zn^{2+}, and Cd^{2+}) on the enzymatic activity of Btae TX-I revealed that the Ca^{2+} is an obligatory co-factor for PLA_2 catalysis role since its replacement prevents substrate binding to the enzyme. Studies have shown that is the presence of the Ca^{2+} which determines the electrophilic behavior of the catalytic site, as well as stabilizes the otherwise flexible Ca^{2+}-binding loop and appears to optimize the interaction enzyme-substrate [38-40].

Crotapotins (CA), the non-toxic subunit of *Crotalus* venom, are pharmacologically inactive and non-enzymatic acid protein; the toxin forms a non-covalent association with PLA_2 crotoxin complex (CB, toxic subunit). Crotapotins bind specifically to PLA_2 as a natural inhibitor of catalytic activity [41]. We suggest that crotapotin might interact in a less stable way, thus partially avoiding the substrate access to the catalytic site and hiding several key amino acid residues involved in the interfacial binding surface of PLA_2s. Crotapotin isoforms from *Crotalus d. collilineatus* (Cdcol F3 and Cdcol F4) and *Crotalus d. terrificus* (CdtF5 and Cdt F7) significantly inhibit the Btae TX-I activity by approximately 60%. Our results are in agreement with findings of Landucci and co-workers [42], who reported that highly purified crotapotin can inhibit pancreatic, bee, and other snake venom PLA2, and Bonfim et al. [15] and Calgarotto et al. [31], who reported that crotapotins from *C. d. terrificus* (F7), *C. d. cascavella* (F3 and F4) and *C. d. collilineatus* (F3 and F4) decreased by 50% the catalytic activity of BJ IV PLA_2 from *B. jararacussu* and BmTX-I PLA_2 from *B. moojeni* snake venoms. Together, these results suggest that crotapotin may bind to bothropic PLA$_2$ in a manner similar to that from crotalic PLA$_2$.

Although accidents caused by *Bothrops venoms* show non visible clinical signs of neurotoxicity, experimentally a number of *in vivo* or *in vitro* studies have shown that motor nerve fibers, nerve terminals or nicotinic receptor can be affected by Bothropic venoms [43]. Venom of diverse Bothrops snakes abolishes contractions caused by direct and indirect electrical stimulation of skeletal muscle in mouse [44-46]. Herein, we found that Btae TX-I PLA$_2$ causes discreet and slow concentration-dependent decrease of elicited twitch muscle responses in the chick *biventer cervicis* preparation. Btae TX-I PLA$_2$ low concentration did not interfere with the muscle contractures to exogenous ACh. Also, only a slight decrease was observed with 10 µg/mL toxin concentration, indicating that the toxin had a minor action on nicotinic receptors. In fact, the blockade of the contracture induced by ACh is compatible with the neuromuscular blocking effect produced by the toxin at the concentrations used. However, 10 µg/mL Btae TX-I inhibited the contracture responses to KCl suggesting that Btae TX-I PLA$_2$ presents specially a post-synaptic action. A similar finding was obtained in BC with BmjeTX-I and II PLA$_2$s from *B. marajoensis* venom [34] and PhTX-I PLA$_2$ from *Porthidium hyoprora* [28].

Myotoxicity induced by *Bothrops* venoms, may result from the direct action of myotoxins on the plasma membrane of muscle cells, or indirectly, as consequence of blood circulation failure and resulting ischemia caused by hemorrhagins or metalloproteases [13,30, 47-48]. Our present results suggest that Btae TX-I PLA$_2$ showed a moderate, although significant local myotoxicity in avian muscle preparation *in vitro*, as observed by histopathological analysis and morphometric data. The data are in accordance to other venoms such as from *B. atrox, B. jararaca* and *B. alternatus*, which show a low to moderate myotoxicity [49]. This study is the first experimental evidence of a PLA$_2$ myotoxin isolated from *Bothriopsis taeniata* snake venom. The toxin exhibited a moderate myotoxicity and neurotoxic activity in avian biventer cervicis preparation; the findings suggest that the sarcolemma is a target for this BTae-TX-1 Asp49 PLA$_2$.

Acknowledgements

This study was supported by Conselho Nacional de Aperfeiçoamento de Pessoal de Ensino Superior (CAPES). The authors thank Mr. Paulo A. Baldasso for general technical assistance and Professor Luis Alberto Ponce-Soto, Ph.D., for supplying crotalic crotapotin isoforms. The study is part of Doctorate thesis of Frey F. Romero-Vargas.

References

1. Chakraborti S, Chakraborti T, Alam N, Shaikh S, Roy S (2011) Role of protein kinase C-a in leukotriene D4 - mediated stimulation of cytosolic phospholipase A2 in pulmonary smooth muscle cells. IIOABJ 2: 85–90.

2. Cao J, Burke JE, Dennis EA (2013) Using hydrogen/deuterium exchange mass spectrometry to define the specific interactions of the phospholipase A2 superfamily with lipid substrates, inhibitors, and membranes. J Biol Chem 288: 1806-1813.

3. Samel M, Vija H, Kurvet I, Künnis-Beres K, Trummal K, et al. (2013) Interactions of PLA2-s from Vipera lebetina, Vipera berus berus and Naja naja oxiana venom with platelets, bacterial and cancer cells. Toxins (Basel) 5: 203-223.

4. Matoba Y, Sugiyama M (2003) Atomic resolution structure of prokaryotic phospholipase A2: Analysis of internal motion and implication for a catalytic mechanism. Proteins: Structure, Function, and Genetics 51: 453–469.

5. Cummings BS, McHowat J, Schnellmann RG (2000) Phospholipase A(2)s in cell injury and death. J Pharmacol Exp Ther 294: 793-799.

6. Cummings BS (2007) Phospholipase A2 as targets for anti-cancer drugs. Biochem Pharmacol 74: 949-959.

7. Schaloske RH, Dennis EA (2006) The phospholipase A2 superfamily and its group numbering system. Biochim Biophys Acta 1761: 1246-1259.

8. Murakami M, Taketomi Y, Miki Y, Sato H, Hirabayashi T, et al. (2011) Recent progress in phospholipase Aâ„‚ research: from cells to animals to humans. Prog Lipid Res 50: 152-192.

9. Harris JB, Cullen MJ (1990) Muscle necrosis caused by snake venoms and toxins. Electron Microsc Rev 3: 183-211.

10. Lomonte B, Angulo Y, Calderón L (2003) An overview of lysine-49 phospholipase A2 myotoxins from crotalid snake venoms and their structural determinants of myotoxic action. Toxicon 42: 885-901.

11. Rosenberg P (1990) Phospholipases: Handbook of Toxinology. Shier WT, Mebs D (ed) Marcel Dekker, New York, 67-277.

12. Pereira MF, Novello JC, Cintra AC, Giglio JR, Landucci ET, et al. (1998) The amino acid sequence of bothropstoxin-II, an Asp-49 myotoxin from Bothrops jararacussu (Jararacucu) venom with low phospholipase A2 activity. J Protein Chem 17: 381-386.

13. Gutiérrez JM, Ownby CL (2003) Skeletal muscle degeneration induced by venom phospholipases A2: insights into the mechanisms of local and systemic myotoxicity. Toxicon 42: 915-931.

14. Ponce-Soto LA, Toyama MH, Hyslop S, Novello JC, Marangoni S (2002) Isolation and preliminary enzymatic characterization of a novel PLA2 from Crotalus durissus collilineatus venom. J Protein Chem 21: 131-136.

15. Bonfim VL, Toyama MH, Novello JC, Hyslop S, Oliveira CR, et al. (2001) Isolation and enzymatic characterization of a basic phospholipase A2 from Bothrops jararacussu snake venom. J Protein Chem 20: 239-245.

16. Schägger H, von Jagow G (1987) Tricine-sodium dodecyl sulfate-polyacrylamide gel electrophoresis for the separation of proteins in the range from 1 to 100 kDa. Anal Biochem 166: 368-379.

17. Bradford MM (1976) A rapid and sensitive method for the quantitation of microgram quantities of protein utilizing the principle of protein-dye binding. Anal Biochem 72: 248-254.

18. Cho W, Kézdy FJ (1991) Chromogenic substrates and assay of phospholipases A2. Methods Enzymol 197: 75-79.

19. Holzer M, Mackessy SP (1996) An aqueous endpoint assay of snake venom phospholipase A2. Toxicon 34: 1149-1155.

20. Beghini DG, Toyama MH, Hyslop S, Sodek LC, Novello JC, et al. (2000) Enzymatic characterization of a novel phospholipase A2 from Crotalus durissus cascavella rattlesnake (maracambóia) venom. J Protein Chem 19: 679–684.

21. Ponce-Soto LA, Bonfim VL, Rodrigues-Simioni L, Novello JC, Marangoni S (2006) Determination of primary structure of two isoforms 6-1 and 6-2 PLA2 D49 from Bothrops jararacussu snake venom and neurotoxic characterization using in vitro neuromuscular preparation. Protein J 25: 147–155.

22. Damico DC, Lilla S, de Nucci G, Ponce-Soto LA, Winck FV, et al. (2005) Biochemical and enzymatic characterization of two basic Asp49 phospholipase A2 isoforms from Lachesis muta muta (Surucucu) venom. Biochim Biophys Acta 1726: 75-86.

23. Ginsborg BL, Warriner J (1960) The isolated chick biventer cervicis nerve-muscle preparation. Br J Pharmacol Chemother 15: 410-411.

24. Montecucco C, Gutiérrez JM, Lomonte B (2008) Cellular pathology induced by snake venom phospholipase A2 myotoxins and neurotoxins: common aspects of their mechanisms of action. Cell Mol Life Sci 65: 2897-2912.

25. Fuly AL, de Miranda AL, Zingali RB, Guimarães JA (2002) Purification and characterization of a phospholipase A2 isoenzyme isolated from Lachesis muta snake venom. Biochem Pharmacol 63: 1589-1597.

26. Ponce-Soto LA, Lomonte B, Gutiérrez JM, Rodrigues-Simioni L, Novello JC, et al. (2007) Structural and functional properties of BaTX, a new Lys49 phospholipase A2 homologue isolated from the venom of the snake Bothrops alternatus. Biochim Biophys Acta 1770: 585-593.

27. Magro AJ, Fernandes CA, dos Santos JI, Fontes MR (2009) Influence of quaternary conformation on the biological activities of the Asp49-phospholipases A2s from snake venoms. Protein Pept Lett 16: 852-859.

28. Huancahuire-Vega S, Ponce-Soto LA, Martins-de-Souza D, Marangoni S (2011) Biochemical and pharmacological characterization of PhTX-I a new myotoxic phospholipase A2 isolated from Porthidium hyoprora snake venom. Comp Biochem Physiol C Toxicol Pharmacol 154: 108-119.

29. Higuchi DA, Barbosa CM, Bincoletto C, Chagas JR, Magalhaes A, et al. (2007) Purification and partial characterization of two phospholipases A2 from Bothrops leucurus (white-tailed-jararaca) snake venom. Biochimie 89: 319-328.

30. Gutiérrez JM, Lomonte B (1995) Phospholipase A2 myotoxins from Bothrops snake venoms. Toxicon 33: 1405-1424.

31. Calgarotto AK, Damico DC, Ponce-Soto LA, Baldasso PA, Da Silva SL, et al. (2008) Biological and biochemical characterization of new basic phospholipase A(2) BmTX-I isolated from Bothrops moojeni snake venom. Toxicon 51: 1509-1519.

32. Gutiérrez JM, Lomonte B (1997) Phospholipase A2 myotoxins from Bothrops snake venoms. In Venom Phospholipase A2 Enzymes, Structure, Function and Mechanism (Ed. Kini RM), pp. 321-352. Wiley, Chichester.

33. Soares AM, Fontes MRM, Giglio JR (2004) Phospholipase A2 myotoxins from Bothrops snake venoms: structure–function relationship. Curr Org Chem 8: 1677–1690.

34. Ponce-Soto LA, Martins-de-Souza D, Marangoni S (2010) Neurotoxic, myotoxic and cytolytic activities of the new basic PLA(2) isoforms BmjeTX-I and BmjeTX-II isolated from the Bothrops marajoensis (Marajó Lancehead) snake venom. Protein J 29: 103-113.

35. Kini RM (1997) Phospholipase A2 a complex multifunctional protein puzzles. In: Kini RM (Eds), Enzymes: Structure, Function and Mechanism. Wiley, Chichester, England, pp. 1–28.

36. Murakami MT, Arni RK (2003) A structure based model for liposome disruption and the role of catalytic activity in myotoxic phospholipase A2s. Toxicon 42: 903-913.

37. Kini RM (2003) Excitement ahead: structure, function and mechanism of snake venom phospholipase A2 enzymes. Toxicon 42: 827-840.

38. Scott DL, Otwinowski Z, Gelb MH, Sigler PB (1990) Crystal structure of bee-venom phospholipase A2 in a complex with a transition-state analogue. Science 250: 1563–1566.

39. Janssen MJ, Burghout PJ, Verheij HM, Slotboom AJ, Egmond MR (1999) Introduction of a C-terminal aromatic sequence from snake venom phospholipases A2 into the porcine pancreatic isozyme dramatically changes the interfacial kinetics. Eur J Biochem 263: 782–788.

40. Pan YH, Epstein TM, Jain MK, Bahnson BJ (2001) Five coplanar anion binding sites on one face of phospholipase A2: relationship to interface binding. Biochemistry 40: 609-617.

41. Faure G, Xu H, Saul FA (2011) Crystal structure of crotoxin reveals key residues involved in the stability and toxicity of this potent heterodimeric Î²-neurotoxin. J Mol Biol 412: 176-191.

42. Landucci EC, Toyama M, Marangoni S, Oliveira B, Cirino G, et al. (2000) Effect of crotapotin and heparin on the rat paw oedema induced by different secretory phospholipases A2. Toxicon 38: 199-208.

43. de Souza Queiróz L, Marques MJ, Santo Neto H (2002) Acute local nerve lesions induced by Bothrops jararacussu snake venom. Toxicon 40: 1483-1486.

44. Brazil OV (1966) Pharmacology of crystalline crotoxin. II. Neuromuscular blocking action. Mem Inst Butantan 33: 981-992.

45. Oshima-Franco Y, Hyslop S, Cintra AC, Giglio JR, da Cruz-Höfling MA, et al. (2000) Neutralizing capacity of commercial bothropic antivenom against Bothrops jararacussu venom and bothropstoxin-I. Muscle Nerve 23: 1832-1839.

46. Zamunér SR, da Cruz-Höfling MA, Corrado AP, Hyslop S, Rodrigues-Simioni L (2004) Comparison of the neurotoxic and myotoxic effects of Brazilian Bothrops venoms and their neutralization by commercial antivenom. Toxicon 44: 259-271.

47. Prianti AC Jr, Ribeiro W, Lopes-Martins RA, Lira-Da-Silva RM, Prado-Franceschi J, et al. (2003) Effect of Bothrops leucurus venom in chick biventer cervicis preparations. Toxicon 41: 595-603.

48. Abreu VA, Dal Belo CA, Hernandes-Oliveira SS, Borja-Oliveira CR, Hyslop S, et al. (2007) Neuromuscular and phospholipase activities of venoms from three subspecies of Bothrops neuwiedi (B. n. goyazensis, B. n. paranaensis and B. n. diporus). Comp Biochem Physiol A Mol Integr Physiol 148: 142-149.

49. Andrião-Escarso SH, Soares AM, Rodrigues VM, Angulo Y, Díaz C, et al. (2000) Myotoxic phospholipases A2 in Bothrops snake venoms: Effect of chemical modifications on the enzymatic and pharmacological properties of bothropstoxins from Bothrops jararacussu. Biochimie 82: 755-763.

50. Moura-da-Silva AM, Paine MJ, Diniz MR, Theakston RD, Crampton JM (1995) The molecular cloning of a phospholipase A2 from Bothrops jararacussu snake venom: evolution of venom group II phospholipase A2's may imply gene duplications. J Mol Evol 41: 174-179.

51. Bonfim VL, Ponce-Soto LA, Martins de Souza D, Souza GH, Baldasso PA, et al. (2008) Structural and functional characterization of myotoxin, Cr-IV 1, a phospholipase A2 D49 from the venom of the snake Calloselasma rhodostoma. Biologicals 36: 168-176.

25

The Intensive Care Management of Children with Scorpion Envenomation

Yuval Cavari[1], Shaul Sofer[1*], Natalya Bilenko[2], Guy Beck[3] and Isaac Lazar[1]

[1]Pediatric intensive care unit, Soroka Medical Center, the Faculty of Health Sciences Ben-Gurion University of the Negev, Beer Sheva, Israel

[2]Department of public health, the Faculty of Health Sciences Ben-Gurion University of the Negev, Beer Sheva, Israel

[3]Division of Pediatrics, Soroka Medical Center, the Faculty of Health Sciences Ben-Gurion University of the Negev, Beer Sheva, Israel

*Corresponding author: Shaul Sofer, Pediatric Intensive care unit, Soroka Univerity Medical Center, Israel, E-mail: shsofer@bgu.ac.il

Abstract

Objective: Scorpion envenomation is a serious health problem worldwide, and a common health hazard in the southern region of Israel. Cardiac dysfunction is the leading cause of morbidity and death. Early bedside echocardiography showed to identify all victims with cardiac involvement. We looked for our management of stung children using clinical evaluation, serum troponin, and early echocardiography in cases of moderate and severe envenomation.

Materials and methods: Retrospective cohort study of children admitted to the Pediatric Intensive Care Unit after scorpion sting during 5 years, 2008-2013. Review of electronic medical records for demography, clinical and laboratory data, especially echocardiography and serum troponin T level, treatment and outcome.

Results: Total number of envenomated children was 185. Age ranged between 1 month and 18 years, 53 were below 3 years of age. Main clinical presentation included decrease level of consciousness (22%) and respiratory failure (15%). Echocardiography on arrival was performed on 117 (63%) children and was abnormal in 29, of whom 25 received inotropic support and 10 required mechanical ventilation. Serum troponin T was measured on arrival in 170 (92%) children and was elevated in 29, of whom 15 (52%) had abnormal echocardiogram; Comparing troponin results to echocardiography; it had a low sensitivity (52%) in identifying cardiac dysfunction. 17 infants below 3 years of age required ventilation for (central) hypopnea and apneic episodes. All children below age 3 had normal echocardiogram. All 185 children survived the envenomation and discharged without sequel.

Conclusion: Early echocardiography should be preferably performed in all scorpion envenomated children. Early serum troponin misses sensitivity for cardiac dysfunction. In our patient population cardiac involvements was not present in children under age 3. Respiratory failure is mainly secondary to central CNS effect in young infants and cardiac dysfunction in older children.

Keywords: Sting; Cardiac dysfunction; Echocardiography; Pediatric; Troponin; Respiratory failure

Introduction

Scorpion sting is a common medical hazard in certain parts of the world. It is estimated that the annual number of scorpion stings worldwide exceeds 1.2 million patients, leading to morbidity and mortality [1]. Most victims of scorpion sting suffer only from localized pain. Systemic intoxication when occur may include stimulation or depression of the central nervous system (CNS), stimulation of the autonomic nervous system (sympathetic and/or parasympathetic), and activation of the inflammatory cascade [1-3]. Thus, irritability and restlessness, hypothermia or hyperthermia, tachycardia or bradycardia, hypertension, excessive sweating, salivation and vomiting are common symptoms. CNS, cardiac and respiratory failures are less common but may lead to death [1,2,4-9]. Children experience more severe envenomation and their mortality rate is higher [1,2,10]. The most dreadful harm of intoxication are heart failure, tachyarrhythmia, cardiogenic pulmonary edema and shock. Clinical signs of heart failure may start within minutes after the sting or may develop hours later [4,7,11-13].

Previous prospective study from our institution showed that left ventricular hypokinesia, decrease fractional shortening and left ventricle ejection fraction (LVEF) detected on echocardiography (echo) of victims shortly after the sting, provided early hemodynamic support. Normal echo study upon hospital arrival excluded the possibility of subsequent heart failure [14].

In comparison to the previous study where echo was part of the protocol and had to be done within three hours of admission, echo examination in our current study was done at the discretion of the attending pediatric intensive care unit (PICU) physician who decided to call upon a senior cardiologist. In this retrospective study we sought to evaluate our everyday practice, and to assess again the need of echo examination in all cases of scorpion envenomation. In addition, we wanted to evaluate again the relevance of early blood troponin measurement upon arrival.

We also sought to confirm our previous observation that hemodynamic changes are uncommon in young children and that respiratory failure at this age is mainly related to bradypnea and apneic episodes that are apparently secondary to CNS effect of the venom [4,6,14]

In view of our excellent clinical results in the management of scorpion envenomation in children, we briefly report our main approach to management and therapy.

The most common and dangerous scorpion in the southern Negev desert of Israel is the "yellow scorpion" *Leiurus quinquestriatus hebraeus*. About 30-50 scorpion envenomated children, are admitted to the PICU annually.

Materials and Methods

This retrospective study involved all children admitted to the PICU of the Soroka University Medical Center with signs and symptoms of general intoxication after scorpion sting. Children arrived to the emergency department (ED) with local manifestation alone (class 1) [15] were not admitted to the PICU and excluded from the study. Data was collected from the medical records of all envenomated children during 5 year period between July 2008 and June 2013.

Our medical center is the only hospital in the Negev southern region of Israel, serving population of about 600,000; among them 180,000 are Bedouin Arabs, native inhabitants of the Negev desert. The study was approved by the hospital's Ethics Committee.

The electronic medical records (Metavision, iMDSoft, Needham Heights, MA) of children stung by scorpion were reviewed for their demographic and clinical data. Laboratory results were reviewed for serum troponin T level taken within 15 minutes of ED admission, during the first intravenous access placement-as a marker of cardiac injury. When repeated, second troponin sample was taken on the second admission day. Echo was performed within two hours of arrival and evaluated by a senior pediatric cardiologist. It was repeated on the next day of admission according to clinical judgment.

Bedside echocardiography evaluation was done as previously described [14]. Left chamber dimensions measurements at end systole and end diastole. Left ventricular systolic function was assessed by means of ejection fraction (EF) and factional shortening (FS) and calculated in the standard manner. Abnormal systolic function was defined as FS below 28% and/or EF below 54% and/or borderline-normal FS and EF with poorly contracting wall motion (Hypokinesia).

In this study we concentrated mainly on the more seriously envenomated children. Therefore, we focused our data collection to the level of consciousness, the present or absent of respiratory distress, cardiac failure and the need for inotropic support, mechanical ventilation, length of stay in the PICU and hospital. Mechanical ventilation was initiated in cases of respiratory failure due to bradypnea/apneic episodes and or tachypnea and dyspnea in cases of cardiac failure. Continuous intravenous dobutamine was initiated in children with abnormal echo. Dopamine, milrinone and adrenaline were used if cardiac dysfunction aggravated despite dobutamine therapy. Antivenom serotherapy was administered according to the decision of the attending physician.

We described qualitative variables by mean and standard deviations (SD) and qualitative variables by absolute numbers and percent. We compared between continuous and categorical variables echo groups using one-way Anova and chi-square, respectively. Differences with P value under 0.05 were accepted as statistically significant.

Results

185 children with signs and symptoms of general envenomation after scorpion sting were admitted to the PICU and included in our study. Demographic and major clinical characteristics upon PICU admission are presented in Table 1. Age distribution ranged between 1 month and 18 years. 53 (29%) of the children were three years old or younger. Bedouin origin and male gender were more prone to be stung. Three major life threatening indications for PICU admission were recognized: Decrease level of consciousness in 40 (22%) patients. Respiratory failure secondary to hypopnea or apneic episodes in 17 (9%) children and respiratory instability with cardiac dysfunction in 10 (5.4%) children. All these 27 children required mechanical ventilation. 25 (14%) children were given inotropic support for hypokinesia and decrease fractional shortening documented on early echocardiography.

Patients age 3 years' old and younger showed different characteristics than older envenomated children. Decrease level of consciousness was more common in younger children (36%) in comparison to older children (16%) (p<0.008). 25% of younger children were mechanically ventilated in comparison to 11% in the older children group (p<0.02). All ventilated children in the younger group had respiratory failure due to apnea or hypopnea and none had any signs of cardiac failure.

117 out of 185 (63%) patients had an echo study shortly after arrival. All 68 patients that did not have an echo examination were mildly symptomatic and their PICU and hospital length of stay was significantly shorter than patients who had an echo examination (p<0.001) (Table 2). Therefore we assumed that their echo examination would have been normal. 29/185 (16%) patients had notable pathological findings in their echo examination. In most of the children with an echo examination, troponin was measured (107/117). Compering to echo results, troponin level upon arrival had low sensitivity in identifying cardiac involvement (sensitivity 52%, specificity 88%, PPV 63% and NPV 83%). Moreover, among the 14 children with abnormal echo and normal troponin level, 10 children were in need for inotropic support and 5 of them required mechanical ventilation. Ultimately, all patients' echo returned to normal on follow up examination.

Repeated troponin taken 24 hours post envenomation, had higher sensitivity than troponin on admission for cardiac injury. In 46 patients which a second troponin sample was taken (in correlation with clinical signs and the echo results), the second troponin level was raised in all patients with abnormal echo. Compared to their matched admission troponin level, these repeated troponin levels had higher sensitivity and lower specificity (first troponin sensitivity 57% and specificity 83% in comparison to second troponin sensitivity 96% and specificity 65%).

Regarding mechanical ventilation, comparison between the 17 patients with normal echo (group 1) to the 10 patients with abnormal echo (group 2), showed that these groups vary significantly. Group 2 patients were older, had higher troponin level, longer ventilation time and longer PICU and hospital length of stay (Table 3).

Antivenom was given to 11 patients, 3 with normal echo and 8 with abnormal echo. Inotrope support was started in all cases with dobutamine. It was given at a dose of 5-10 mcg/kg/min to 26 patients, all but one, with abnormal echo. In addition, dopamine drip 5-25 mcg/kg/min was given to 5 patients, and adrenaline drip 0.1-1.3 mcg/kg/min to 3 patients. Milrinon drip was added to 6 patients.

Mean hospital length of stay for all children was 42.6 ± 50.6 hours. All survived and discharged home with no sequel. PICU and hospital length of stay were significantly longer in patients with abnormal echo in comparison to children with normal echo or those in whom echo was not performed. The group of patients that had no echo examination had the shortest length of stay (Table 3).

Discussion

Scorpion envenomation is a common medical hazard in many areas of the world and an important cause of morbidity and mortality, especially among children [1,2,9,10].

Heart failure and cardiogenic shock are known to be the most hazardous complications, [1,2,4,7-13,16] and as such need to be recognized and treated as soon as possible. Symptoms of hemodynamic compromise may occur shortly after the sting or delayed for several hours, with the appearance or worsening of tachycardia, tachypnea, dyspnea, hypotension, and signs of reduced peripheral perfusion [4,7,8,11-13] Therefore admission in a PICU is of paramount importance as well as finding ways to early recognize those patients with cardiac dysfunction. Bahloul et al. [9], reported analysis of 685 cases of scorpion envenomation from Tunisie, and found that children are in high risk of life threatening cardiac depression, which initially may be missed and remained unnoticed until patient deterioration. Delay in diagnosis of high risk children, may adversely affect their outcome. Previous studies showed that early bedside echo has 100% sensitivity and specificity in identifying myocardial dysfunction in cases of scorpion envenomation [14,17,18]. This allow early initiation of targeted hemodynamic monitoring and support. As suggested by Sagarad et al. [17,18] apparently not all patients with decrease left ventricular ejection fraction (LVEF) on early echo required inotropic support. Those with only mild LVEF decrease might be closely clinically and echographicly observed. This should be done however in a PICU environment as showed in Sagarad study where 10% of the patients with initial, mild LVEF decrease who were sent to the ward, required later on, inotropic support for hemodynamic deterioration. In our current study only 4 of the 29 patients who had left ventricular dysfunction on echo were treated without inotropic support. All were closely observed in the PICU and did well. In all other 25 children dobutamine drip was started. It was changed to dopamine in 5 and to adrenaline drip in 3 due to severe hemodynamic deterioration. 6 children received in addition milrinon drip. Dobutamine has been shown to have a quick therapeutic effect in these cases, enhancing LVEF, cardiac output and oxygen delivery to the tissues [7,19]. Our practice of treatment initiation with dobutamine is based both on published literature and our past 15 years experience in treating these children, while our unpublished experience with initial adrenaline treatment seemed to cause ventricular arrhythmias. In agreement with our previous study, serum troponin was not helpful in detecting early injury as 10 of the 14 patients that had normal troponin despite pathological echo required inotropic support and 5 of them were ventilated as well. These findings are also in agreement with Cupo and Hering [20] who found low correlation between troponin and echo findings upon arrival. Meki et al. [21] and Sagarad et al. [17,18] however found 100% sensitivity and specificity between troponin level and echo results. This differences can be explained by the different time gap between the sting and troponin measurement in the different studies. In Sagarad studies all patients were initially admitted to a local hospital and then referred to the hospital where the study was held. In Meki's study mean arrival

time after the sting was 15.9 h, whereas in our center most patients arrive within 3 h of sting [14].

Children that present to the ED within few hours after the sting with no clear clinical symptoms of cardiac dysfunction might show troponin level that does not correlate well with the degree of the cardiac depression seen on echo. Whereas echo is a mirror image of the envenomation affect, troponin is a biochemical marker that its build up is time sensitive. Second day troponin, in more severe envenomated children, had higher sensitivity than admission troponin, and when in doubt a repeat troponin test may be helpful [14,17,18,21].

Our current and previous studies strongly suggest that in any case of severe envenomation an early echo should be performed. This can be easily done in institutions providing 24/7 in-house cardiology services. Fulfilling this task in other institutions, would enclose educational approach and training of non-cardiologist physician in ED and PICU to identify hypokinesia and decrease contractility on echo. Children with mild symptoms of intoxication and normal echo, might be sent from the ED to the pediatric ward [20-22].

The natural history of envenomation varies by age: hemodynamic changes are uncommon in babies and infants younger than 2 years old [4,7,8,12,14,23,24]. In our current study none of the 53 children below age 3 years had cardiac dysfunction. This explain also the differences among the 2 groups of ventilated children: group 1 consisted of young infants with normal heart function, who presented in respiratory failure with hypopnea and apneic episodes presumably related to the toxic effect of the venom on the CNS, causing severe encephalopathy [4,6]; group 2-older children with cardiac dysfunction, where respiratory failure was characterized by tachypnea and dyspnea as part of the failing heart. Patients from group 1 had no pulmonary pathology, had a much shorter course of ventilation; they recovered earlier and had shorter PICU and hospital length of stay.

Only 11 patients in our study received anti-venom sero-therapy. This modality of therapy in scorpion envenomation is controversial [1,2,13,25-27] and therefore we allow the attending physician to decide whether to use it or not.

This retrospective observational study suffers from all limitations of retrospective studies. It is however a recording of our everyday practice based on implementation of conclusions drowns from a previous structured prospective study [14] and therefore we believe it may be valuable for clinicians dealing with scorpion envenomation.

Using the parameters above, such as age, type of failure (cardiac vs. respiratory), clinical presentation and echocardiography allow the clinician to anticipate who is prone to complications and who isn't and to treat accordingly.

Mortality rate among scorpion envenomated children in our institution decreased with time from 11% in the 60's (20th century) [16], to 2% in the 90's [13] and 0% in last decade (323 children). We reflect this achievement to the practice described above.

Conclusion

Early echocardiography should be preferably performed in all scorpion envenomated children. Early serum troponin misses sensitivity for cardiac dysfunction. Cardiac involvements are not common in children under age 3.

References

1.   Chippaux JP, Goyffon M (2008) Epidemiology of scorpionism: a global appraisal. Acta Trop 107: 71-79.

2.   Isbister GK1, Bawaskar HS (2014) Scorpion envenomation. N Engl J Med 371: 457-463.

3.   Petricevich VL1 (2010) Scorpion venom and the inflammatory response. Mediators Inflamm 2010: 903295.

4.   Sofer S, Gueron M (1988) Respiratory failure in children following envenomation by the scorpion leiurus quinquestriatus: Hemodynamic and neurological aspects. Toxicon 26: 931-939.

5.   Gueron M, Ilia R, Sofer S (1992) The cardiovascular system after scorpion envenomation. A review. J Toxicol Clin Toxicol 30: 245-258.

6.   Sofer S, Gueron M (1990) Vasodilators and hypertensive encephalopathy following scorpion envenomation in children. Chest 97: 118-120.

7.   Abroug F, Ayari M, Nouira S, Gamra H, Boujdaria R, et al. (1995) Assessment of left ventricular function in severe scorpion envenomation: combined hemodynamic and echo-Doppler study. Intensive Care Med 21: 629-635.

8.   Abroug F, Boujdaria R, Belghith M, Nouira S, Bouchoucha S (1991) Cardiac dysfunction and pulmonary edema following scorpion envenomation. Chest 100: 1057-1059.

9.   Bahloul M, Chabchoub I, Chaari A, Chtara K, Kallel H, et al. (2010) Scorpion envenomation among children: clinical manifestations and outcome (analysis of 685 cases). Am J Trop Med Hyg 83: 1084-1092.

10. Chippaux JP (2012) Emerging options for the management of scorpion stings. Drug Des Devel Ther 6: 165-173.

11. Hering SE, Jurca M, Vichi FL, Azevedo-Marques MM, Cupo P (1993) Reversible cardiomyopathy' in patients with severe scorpion envenoming by tityus serrulatus: Evolution of enzymatic, electrocardiographic and echocardiographic alterations. Ann Trop Paediatr 13: 173-182.

12. Bahloul M, Ben Hamida C, Chtourou K, Ksibi H, Dammak H, et al. (2004) Evidence of myocardial ischaemia in severe scorpion envenomation. Myocardial perfusion scintigraphy study. Intensive Care Med 30: 461-467.

13. Sofer S, Shahak E, Gueron M (1994) Scorpion envenomation and antivenom therapy. J Pediatr 124: 973-978.

14. Sofer S, Zucker N, Bilenko N, Levitas A, Zalzstein E, et al. (2013) The importance of early bedside echocardiography in children with scorpion envenomation. Toxicon 68: 1-8.

15. Khattabi A, Soulaymani-Bencheikh R, Achour S, Salmi LR (2011) Scorpion Consensus Expert Group. Classification of clinical consequences of scorpion stings: Consensus development. Trans R Soc Trop Med Hyg 105: 364-369.

16. Gueron M, Yaron R (1970) Cardiovascular manifestations of severe scorpion sting. Clinicopathologic correlations. Chest 57: 156-162.

17. Sagarad SV, Kerure SB, Thakur B, Reddy SS, K B, et al. (2013) Echocardiography guided therapy for myocarditis after scorpion sting envenomation. J Clin Diagn Res 7: 2836-2838.

18. Sagarad SV, Thakur BS, Reddy SS, Balasubramanya K, Joshi RM, et al. (2012) Elevated cardiac troponin (cTnI) levels correlate with the clinical and echocardiographic evidences of severe myocarditis in scorpion sting envenomation. J Clin Diagn Res 6: 1369-1371.

19. Elatrous S, Nouira S, Besbes-Ouanes L, Boussarsar M, Boukef R, et al. (1999) Dobutamine in severe scorpion envenomation: effects on standard hemodynamics, right ventricular performance, and tissue oxygenation. Chest 116: 748-753.

20. Cupo P, Hering SE (2002) Cardiac troponin I release after severe scorpion envenoming by Tityus serrulatus. Toxicon 40: 823-830.

21. Meki AR, Mohamed ZM, Mohey El-deen HM (2003) Significance of assessment of serum cardiac troponin I and interleukin-8 in scorpion envenomed children. Toxicon 41: 129-137.

22. Mohamad IL, Elsayh KI, Mohammad HA, Saad K, Zahran AM, et al. (2014) Clinical characteristics and outcome of children stung by scorpion. Eur J Pediatr 173: 815-818.

23. Cupo P, Figueiredo AB, Filho AP, Pintya AO, Tavares Júnior GA, et al. (2007) Acute left ventricular dysfunction of severe scorpion envenomation is related to myocardial perfusion disturbance. Int J Cardiol 116: 98-106.

24. Amaral CF, Lopes JA, Magalhães RA, de Rezende NA (1991) Electrocardiographic, enzymatic and echocardiographic evidence of myocardial damage after Tityus serrulatus scorpion poisoning. Am J Cardiol 67: 655-657.

25. Abroug F, Ouanes-Besbes L, Ouanes I, Dachraoui F, Hassen MF, et al. (2011) Meta-analysis of controlled studies on immunotherapy in severe scorpion envenomation. Emerg Med J 28: 963-969.

26. Foëx BA (2011) Meta-analysis of controlled studies on immunotherapy in severe scorpion envenomation: a commentary. Emerg Med J 28: 915-916.

27. Skolnik AB, Ewald MB (2013) Pediatric scorpion envenomation in the United States: morbidity, mortality, and therapeutic innovations. Pediatr Emerg Care 29: 98-103.

26

The Reproductive Health and Liver Functions of Occupationally Exposed Female Pesticide Sprayers of Mango Plantations

Farrukh Jamal*and Quazi S. Haque*

Department of Biochemistry, Dr. Ram Manohar Lohia Avadh University, Faizabad-224001, India

*Corresponding authors: Dr. Farrukh Jamal, Assistant Professor, Department of Biochemistry, Dr. Ram Manohar Lohia Avadh University, Faizabad-224001, India, E-mail: farrukhrmlau@gmail.com

Quazi S. Haque, Dr. Ram Manohar Lohia Avadh University, Faizabad-224001, U.P, India, Fax: E-mail: haq.biochem06@gmail.com

Abstract

The present study explores the effect of pesticide exposure on the reproductive health and liver function of females participating in agricultural related work. Blood samples were obtained from thirty-five (35) females (out of one hundred females of reproductive age) who were willing donors. Fifty (50) females matched for age and socio economic status was recruited as a control group to compare levels of hormones (estradiol, progesterone and follicle stimulating hormone), liver enzymes-alanine aminotransferase (ALT), and aspartate aminotransferase (AST). Results showed that 56% of the females were illiterate with 48% representing agricultural work. Females who helped in farming operations showed a higher incidence of adverse pregnancy outcome such as abortions and stillbirths compared to non-participants. There was a significant elevation in estradiol and progesterone levels among female agricultural workers. While there was an elevation in serum liver enzymes (AST and ALT) there was a significant decrease in FSH level in females engaged in agricultural activities. The study suggests that participation of females in agricultural activities with potential exposure to pesticides endangers their reproductive health and liver functions.

Keywords: Liver enzymes; Reproductive health; Female workers; Agriculture; Occupational exposure

Introduction

Indian economy is largely based on agricultural products and consequently the output primarily depends on extensive use of pesticides. Agricultural practices involve the use of a diverse group of agro-chemicals that is indiscriminately sprayed by the farmers for pest control. Pesticides are a threat to the environment and capable of eliminating a variety of organism without discrimination. Organophosphorus pesticides (OPs) alone or in combination with organochlorines (OCs) are frequently used and sprayed in mango plantation of Malihabad (Lucknow, U.P.) which is a mango belt in north India and therefore remains an important source of poisoning. These agro-chemicals are popularly termed as pesticides and have been broadly classified in to organophosphorus, organochlorines, carbamates and pyrethroids [1]. While India ranks 12th globally, it is the largest manufacturer of basic pesticides in Asia. Of the total pesticide consumption insecticides account for ~75% followed by fungicides (~12%) and herbicides (~ 10%) [2]. In mango field the common pesticide sprayed includes Dichlorovas 76% EC, Monocrotophos 36% EC, Dimethoate 30% EC, Phosphamidon 85% SL Endosulfan 35% EC, Carbaryl, 25% EC, Monocrotophos 36% SL, Methomyl [1].

In rural Malihabad Lucknow, one of the main activities of women, besides their household duties, is extending assistance in agricultural work. This is due to change in the economic conditions of families. A large family in which the chances of increasing cultivated land is remote; a high prevalence of labor migration predisposes the involvement of women in agricultural work. In many parts of the world women constitute a large proportion of farmers and therefore represents a considerable force in agricultural work [3]. They are exposed to a wide variety of health hazards including toxic chemicals used to boost crop yield. This exposure to pesticides can occur directly from occupational and environmental sources and indirectly through diet. Although there is a growing public concern about the impact of exposure to pesticides on human health, lack of knowledge, careless attitude and appalling safety practices in handling pesticides pose a serious health risk to the farmers. Some pesticides were classified as reproductive and developmental toxins in the Pan American Pesticide Database [4]. Exposure to pesticides has been associated with several disease conditions including hypertension, hepatomegaly, dermatitis, neurological and immunological effects, chromosomal aberrations and elevated cancer risks [5,6]. The actual exposures to insecticides can be assessed by biological monitoring of human tissues and body fluids [7].

The pesticide exposure causes cellular leakage of enzymes from hepatocytes and other affected body organs [8]. A high degree of abnormal liver function in agricultural workers may indicate toxic effects of pesticides as well as its presence in blood. Altered liver enzyme activities have been reported among occupational workers exposed to organophosphorus pesticides alone or in combination with organochlorines [9]. In women, exposure to pesticides have been associated with reproductive malfunctioning which includes decrease in fertility, spontaneous abortions, stillbirth premature birth, low birth weight, developmental abnormalities, ovarian disorders, and disruption of the hormonal function [10,11]. Women's health is gaining attention with the realization that men's and women's bodies react differently to environmental agents. As the number of women participants is increasing worldwide and a considerable proportion of them are of reproductive age; attention is required to note any reproductive dysfunction due to occupational exposure. This study exposes the relevance and influence of pesticides on females engaged in agricultural practices.

Material and Methods

We conducted a cross-sectional study in female pesticide sprayers of mango plantation in rural Malihabad, Lucknow. This is a cross-sectional comparative study that was conducted at the end of spraying day among the female sprayers. Rural Malihabad village consists of 100 families living in two small satellites (one composed of 60 families and the other of 40 families). The purpose of the study was explained to all the participants and their consent was obtained. The requisite clearance of institutional human ethics committee was obtained for the study.

Sample collection

All families in the village were surveyed and from each family one female in reproductive age was randomly selected to participate.

Data collection

Detailed information regarding socio-economic status, family history, type of physical activity, personal habits were recorded for each subject on a pre-tested questionnaire. The questionnaire was in local language and data entered was done by investigators. Questionnaire covers the following points: socio-demographic data, agricultural activities, exposure to pesticides, menarche history, and outcome of pregnancy (abortion, stillbirth, preterm labour, low birth weight or congenital anomalies), dysfunctional uterine bleeding, and tumor of the uterus or ovaries.

Exposed females named a lot of pesticides like monocrotophos, phosphomidon, dichlorvos, malathion, endosulfan, thiodon, methyl parathion, dimethoate and carbaryl etc. used frequently in the form of mixtures by applicators. Exposure was considered chronic because the females included in the study are always engaged in pesticide application (mixing and spraying). The females were considered exposed if they shared in preparing, mixing or spraying pesticides on a regular basis.

The exposed females did not report any co-existing exposure. They did not use any protective measures during spraying or mixing. Fifty females matched for age and socio economic status were recruited as a control group to compare levels of hormones (estradiol, progesterone and follicle stimulating hormone), liver enzymes alanine aminotransferase and aspartate aminotransferase. The control group was chosen from a neighbouring village whose main occupation was not related to any agricultural activities. All the studied populations were non-smokers and non-alcohol drinkers receiving no medications on a regular basis.

Approval consent was obtained from all participants. Under complete aseptic conditions, a blood sample of 5 mL was taken from each subject. Samples were centrifuged for separation of serum to be used for analysis. The estimation of serum liver enzymes (ALT and AST) following the methods of Reitman and Frankel [12]. The hormones (estradiol, progesterone and follicle stimulating hormone) was determined by immunologic methods (Elisa technique) using commercial kits (Panbio, Australia) [13,14]. To overcome variation in hormone levels in different phases of the menstrual cycle, samples were taken from both groups during the follicular phase of the menstrual cycle (starting from the first day of menstruation to mid cycle). Also, pregnant females were not included in the study to exclude high progesterone level during pregnancy.

Statistical analysis

The statistical significance of mean values of different parameters in exposed and control were performed using the SPSS package system version 16.

Results

Table 1 show that more than half of the females in the village were illiterate. Only 4% of the females were graduates from the university. In the study, agricultural work represented 48% of the occupations. Females who helped in preparing pesticides represented 67.16%. Females who shared in spraying pesticides represented 13.43%. Duration of work exceeded 10 years in 58.21% of the studied females as shown in table 2.

Socio-demographic status	No.	Percentage
Education		
Can write and read	6	6
Illiterate	56	56
Primary	9	9
Preparatory	2	2
Secondary or diploma	21	21
Two years after secondary school	2	2
Graduation	4	4
Total	100	100
Occupation		
Agricultural workers	48	48
Others	52	52
Total	100	100

Table 1: Detailed information regarding socioeconomic status of the female workers in Rural Malihabad, Lucknow.

All studied populations were non-smokers, non-alcohol drinkers, apparently in good health and taking no medication on a regular basis. Agricultural workers showed higher levels of progesterone and estradiol compared to the controls and the difference was statistically significant with p values of <0.001 and <0.001, respectively. However, FSH level was significantly lower in female agricultural workers with p value <0.001. Liver functions were affected as evidenced by high enzyme levels with significant difference at p values <0.001 and <0.05 for AST and ALT, respectively, as shown in table 3. There was no correlation between the duration of work and the tested parameters. It is clear from table 4 that females sharing in agricultural work gave birth to a lower percentage of well-born babies (62.69%) compared to working females (78.79%). Females exposed to pesticides reported higher incidences of uterine bleeding but the difference was not statistically significant compared with those not sharing in the agricultural work.

Discussion

In the pesticide sprayers of rural Malihabad Lucknow, the health protection has been overlooked for many years despite the health risks associated with occupational exposure to agrochemicals. Of main concern are the most frequently used OP and CB pesticides, such as methamidophos, chlorpyrifos, diazinon, ethyl parathion, dimethoate, mancozeb, zineb, carbendazim, carbofuran, propineb and propamocarb. Most of these pesticides belong to extremely hazardous and highly hazardous category, which have been either banned or strictly controlled in developed countries. With regard to the most common pesticide-related symptoms, pesticide sprayers of mango plantation in Malihabad, Lucknow reported dizziness, headache, nausea, blurring of vision and skin and throat irritation, which were similar to other reports associated with exposure to OP and CB pesticides.

	Yes/No	No.	%
Helping in farming operations	No	33	33
	Yes	67	67
	Total	100	100
Preparation of Pesticides for spraying	Help or do it by herself	45	67.16
	No	22	32.84
	Total	67	100
Helping in spraying pesticides	No	9	13.43
	Yes	58	66.57
	Total	67	100
Duration of exposure	Less than 10 years	28	41.79
	10 years and more	39	58.21

Table 2: Agricultural activities conducted by the female workers (studied group) in rural Malihabad, Lucknow.

Parameter	Group	No.	Mean	Std. deviation	P value
FSH (mIU/ml)	Agricultural worker	35	4.229	1.584	<0.001
	Control	50	6.024	2.218	
Progesterone (ng/ml)	Agricultural worker	35	3.283	4.238	<0.001
	Control	50	0.716	0.757	
Estradiol (pg/ml)	Agricultural worker	35	55.369	13.815	<0.001
	Control	50	47.284	10.001	
Aspartate aminotransferase (AST)	Agricultural worker	35	28.343	5.434	<0.001
	Control	50	24.52	3.079	
Alanine aminotransferase (ALT)	Agricultural worker	35	24.429	3.363	<0.05
	Control	50	21.68	5.56	

Table 3: Comparison between female agricultural workers and controls concerning hormone levels namely (progesterone, FSH and estradiol) and liver enzymes namely (AST and ALT).

	Helping in farming operations						
Pregnancy Outcome	No		Yes		Total		P value
	No.	%	No.	%	No.	%	
Well born fetus (no preterm labour, low birth weight or congenital anomalies)	26	78.79	42	62.69	68	68	<0.05
Adverse outcome (abortion, Stillbirth, preterm labour, low birth weight or congenital anomalies)	7	21.21	25	37.31	32	32	
Total	33	100	67	100	100	100	

Table 4: Pregnancy outcome in females involved in agricultural activities in rural Malihabad, Lucknow.

In undertaking this kind of study, we must first consider the difficulty of quantification and assessment of the effects of the exposure that may lead to chronic intoxication. Multiple exposures of different pesticides which might interact in an additive or multiplicative way and so could affect the pattern of health effects expected in the case of mono-exposures. The other important points that have also affected this study include the large number of spraying done and the usage of various pesticides during the period of study, often in combinations, some commercially available but the majority made by the sprayers themselves. Despite all these limitations, it is possible to draw conclusions about the overall health risks of these complex exposures.

Our study revealed a high percentage of illiterate females in the studied village. Illiteracy, especially among females, still constitutes a major problem in and around rural Malihabad. The study pointed to the large number of females engaged in agricultural activities (67%). The questionnaire showed their unawareness of the health hazards of pesticide exposure on their reproductive health. Only a few of them knew the guidelines for the safe usage and storage of pesticides. None of them gave information about the mixtures of pesticides they use. They only reported that they use different types of pesticides and usually apply them in combinations. Measuring hormone levels in females helping in agricultural activities and exposed to pesticides during their work demonstrated higher progesterone, estradiol and lower FSH levels as compared to controls. Moreover the progesterone level (3.283 ng/ml) is higher than the normal range during the follicular phase, which is 0.2-1.4 ng/ml. This high progesterone level could be attributed to a possible disturbance in hormone level associated with exposure. Those females might be exposed to organophosphorus pesticides in the pesticide mixtures they apply. OPs are suspected to alter reproductive function by reducing brain acetylcholinesterase (AChE) activity and secondarily influencing the gonads. Experiments on animals have shown that repeated doses of OP significantly decreased brain AChE activity and significantly increased acetylcholine, gamma-aminobutyric acid, epinephrine, nor-epinephrine, dopamine, and 5-hydroxyttyptamine concentrations, altering reproductive function by reducing brain acetylcholinesterase activity and monoamine levels, thus impairing hypothalamic and/or pituitary endocrine functions and gonadal processes [15].

The present study, suggest more detailed study of reproductive hormones must be done to clarify the cause for this marked rise of progesterone. The low FSH level is explained by a negative feedback mechanism of the pituitary gland resulting from high estradiol. These findings were in accordance with previous studies that proposed about pesticides induce hormone disruption [16,17]. This alteration of hormone levels may interfere with the menstrual cycle and lead to adverse reproductive health effects [18-20].

It also explains the increased number of females complaining of dysfunctional uterine bleeding in those exposed to pesticides [15] showed negative associations between OP exposure and serum levels of FSH and LH in Mexican agricultural workers, but they did not observe significant associations between testosterone or estradiol serum levels and urinary OP metabolites [21] reported that in adult men, an inverse association exists between urinary levels of OP and CB metabolites and serum LH and testosterone levels.

This study supported the possible association between pesticide exposure and adverse pregnancy outcome. Females involved in agricultural work reported a higher percentage of adverse outcomes of pregnancy (abortion, stillbirth and congenital anomalies) compared to females not engaged in agriculture, which agrees with other studies [22-26]. The intricate processes of the menstrual cycle, ovum production, fertilization, implantation, growth and development of the foetus may be particularly susceptible to low-dose exposures to endocrine disruptors. The study suggests that the reproductive health and liver functions of female pesticide sprayers in agricultural activities is adversely affected and adequate information and safety measures must be imposed to reduce it.

Acknowledgment

This research received no specific grant from any funding agency in the public, commercial, or not-for-profit sectors. The infrastructure support to the Department of Biochemistry, Dr. RML Avadh University, Faizabad, under the DST-FIST programme from the Ministry of Science & Technology, Govt. of India is thankfully acknowledged.

References

1. Haque QS, Jamal F, Rastogi SK (2012) Effect of organo-phosphorus on biochemical parameters on agricultural workers. Asian Journal of Biochemistry 7: 37-45.

2. Indira DP, Bellamy R, Shyamsunder P (2007) Facing hazards at work-agricultural workers and pesticide exposure in Kuttanad, Kerala. South Asian Network for Development and Environmental Economics p.1-4.

3. Rice HR, Baker BA (2007) Workplace hazards to women's reproductive health. Minn Med 90: 44-47.

4. Kegley SE, Hill BR, Orme S, Choi AH (2010) PAN pesticide database, Pesticide Action Network, North America (Oakland, CA, 2014).

5. Horrigan L, Lawrence RS, Walker P (2002) How sustainable agriculture can address the environmental and human health harms of industrial agriculture. Environ Health Perspect 110: 445-456.

6. Raschke AM, and Burger AE (1997) Risk assessment as a management tool used to assess the effect of pesticide use in an irrigation system situated in a semi-desert region. Arch Environ Contam Toxicol 32: 42–49.

7. Abu Mourad T (2005) Adverse impact of insecticides on the health of Palestinian farm workers in the Gaza Strip: a hematologic biomarker study. Int J Occup Environ Health 11: 144-149.

8. Dewan A, Bhatnagar VK, Mathur ML, Chakma T, Kashyap R, et al. (2004) Repeated episodes of endosulfan poisoning. J Toxicol Clin Toxicol 42: 363-369.

9. Amr MM (1999) Pesticide monitoring and its health problems in Egypt, a Third World country. Toxicol Lett 107: 1-13.

10. Nurminen T (1995) Maternal pesticide exposure and pregnancy outcome. J Occup Environ Med 37: 935-940.

11. Clementi M, Causin R, Marzocchi C, Mantovani A, Tenconi R (2007) A study of the impact of agricultural pesticide use on the prevalence of birth defects in northeast Italy. Reprod Toxicol 24: 1-8.

12. Reitman S, Frankel S (1957) A colorimetric method for the determination of serum glutamic oxalacetic and glutamic pyruvic transaminases. Am J Clin Pathol 28: 56–63.

13. Ratcliffe WA, Carter GD, Dowsett M, Hillier SG, Middle JG, et al. (1988) Oestradiol assays: applications and guidelines for the provision of a clinical biochemistry service. Ann Clin Biochem 25: 466-483.

14. Uotila M, Ruoslahti E, Engvall E (1981) Two-site sandwich enzyme immunoassay with monoclonal antibodies to human alpha-fetoprotein. J Immunol Methods 42: 11-15.

15. Recio R, Gomez GO, Martinez J M, Aburto VB, Cervante ML et al. (2005) Pesticide exposure alters follicle-stimulating hormone levels in Mexican agricultural workers. Environmental Health Perspectives 113: 1160-1163.

16. Cooper GS, Klebanoff MA, Promislow J, Brock JW, Longnecker MP (2005) Polychlorinated biphenyls and menstrual cycle characteristics. Epidemiology 16: 191-200.

17. Bretveld RW, Thomas CM, Scheepers PT, Zielhuis GA, Roeleveld N (2006) Pesticide exposure: the hormonal function of the female reproductive system disrupted? Reprod Biol Endocrinol 4: 30.

18. Farr SL, Cooper GS, Cai J, Savitz DA, Sandler DP (2004) Pesticide use and menstrual cycle characteristics among premenopausal women in the agricultural health study. Am J Epidemiol 160: 1194-1204.

19. Figà-Talamanca I (2006) Occupational risk factors and reproductive health of women. Occup Med (Lond) 56: 521-531.

20. Mendola P, Messer LC, Rappazzo K (2008) Science linking environmental contaminant exposures with fertility and reproductive health impacts in the adult female. Fertil Steril 89: e81-94.

21. Meeker JD, Singh NP, Ryan L, Duty SM, Barr DB, et al. (2004) Urinary levels of insecticide metabolites and DNA damage in human sperm. Hum Reprod 19: 2573-2580.

22. Arbuckle TE, Lin Z, and Mery LS (2001) An exploratory analysis of the effect of pesticide exposure on the risk of spontaneous abortion in an Ontario farm population. Environ Health Perspect 109: 851-857.

23. García AM (2003) Pesticide exposure and women's health. Am J Ind Med 44: 584-594.

24. Windham GC, Lee D, Mitchell P, Anderson M, Petreas M, et al. (2005) Exposure to organochlorine compounds and effects on ovarian function. Epidemiology 16: 182-190.

25. Andersen HR, Schmidt IM, Grandjean P, Jensen TK, Jørgensen EB et al. (2008) Impaired reproductive development in sons of women occupationally exposed to pesticides during pregnancy. Environ Health Perspect 116: 566–572.

26. Shirangi A, Fritschi L, Holman CD, Bower C (2009) Birth defects in offspring of female veterinarians. J Occup Environ Med 51: 525-533.

27

Toxic Metal Contamination of Banked Blood Designated for Neonatal Transfusion

Sripriya Sundararajan[1], Allison M Blatz[2], Dorr G Dearborn[2,3,4], Arthur W Varnes[3], Cynthia F Bearer[1], and Dina El Metwally[1*]

[1]Department of Pediatrics, University of Maryland, Baltimore, MD 21201, USA

[2]Departments of Pediatrics, Case Western Reserve University, Cleveland, OH 44106, USA

[3]Environmental Health Sciences, Case Western Reserve University, Cleveland, OH 44106, USA

[4]Mary Ann Swetland Center for Environmental Health, Case Western Reserve University, Cleveland, OH 44106, USA

*Corresponding author: Dina El Metwally, Division of Neonatology, Department of Pediatrics, University of Maryland School of Medicine, 110 S Paca St. 8th floor, Baltimore, MD 21201, E-mail: dmetwally@peds.umaryland.edu

Abstract

Objective: Very low birth weight (VLBW) infants frequently receive blood transfusions. We hypothesize that toxic metals in donor blood may pose a health risk with potential adverse neurologic effects on the developing brain of a vulnerable VLBW infant.

Study design: Samples from 100 donor blood units were collected from a large urban hospital. Blood was analyzed for aluminum, arsenic, beryllium, cadmium, manganese, mercury, nickel, lead and polonium. The estimated upper limit of acceptable metal concentration in donor blood was calculated assuming a transfusion volume of 20 ml/kg and using either previously published acceptable intravenous doses or oral reference doses with a conservative estimate of 10% gastrointestinal absorption. Ingested mercury was assumed to be 95% absorbed.

Results: Eight of the nine metals were detectable. Concentrations of arsenic, beryllium, cadmium, mercury and polonium were not of concern for any single blood transfusion. Concentrations of aluminum, manganese, nickel and lead exceeded the estimated upper limit of acceptable concentration in 5, 11, 4 and 26 units respectively. Of the 100 units, 31 had at least one toxic metal concentration high enough to pose a potential health risk.

Conclusions: VLBW infants are exposed to heavy metals that are toxic from blood transfusion. The number of units with concerning levels of toxic metals was higher than expected. Neonatologists should be aware of this potential exposure to toxic metals from donor blood when decision is made to administer blood transfusion. Neurodevelopmental studies of toxic metal exposed infants from blood transfusion are warranted.

Keywords Blood bank; Blood transfusion; VLBW; Heavy metal contamination

Abbreviations

VLBWs: Very Low Birth Weight Infants; ELBW: Extremely Low Birth Weight Infants; CDC: Centers for Disease Control and Prevention; ETC: Estimated Tolerable Concentration; PRBCs: Packed Red Blood Cells

Introduction

Blood transfusion is a critical part of neonatal intensive care and is life saving for neonates with severe anemia or hemorrhage [1]. During the first 2 weeks of life, approximately 50% of infants weighing less than 1000g at birth will receive their first transfusion [2] and without the use of erythropoiesis-stimulating agents, 85% to 90% of VLBW infants receive blood transfusions [3,4]. All blood products administered to VLBWs is subject to universal screening for infectious agents as directed by the Food and Drug Administration [5]. Additional procedures of blood processing may be required by the individual institutions, such as irradiation [6] and leukoreduction [7]

before transfusing blood to neonates. VLBW infants are transfused with blood that has been donated by adults 17 years of age or older. These donors may have had a variety of exposures to substances including toxic heavy metals from environmental and occupational sources [8]. VLBWs are especially vulnerable to these toxic metal exposures [9-14]. The federal government has codified exposure levels acceptable to adult workers and to children exposed to environmental contaminants. These exposures occur mainly via ingestion or inhalation.

In contrast, toxic heavy metals present in transfused blood are administered intravenously. Safe levels for intravenous administration of most of these toxic metals are unknown. Lead in donor blood has previously been shown to be present at concentrations that pose a health risk for VLBW infants [12,15]. Aluminum (Al), arsenic (As), beryllium (Be), cadmium (Cd), mercury (Hg), Lead (Pb), Manganese (Mn) and Nickel (Ni) have been studied extensively due to the known serious adverse health effects associated with human exposure to these metals. According to the Agency for Toxic Substance and Disease Registry's (ATSDR) priority list of hazardous substances, the latent effects from these heavy metals include carcinogenesis, neurotoxicology and developmental deficits in humans and animals ([16 10]. Toxic metals tend to stay in the body for long periods of time and may cause detrimental adverse effects on human growth and development [19,20]. Therefore, it is an urgent and high priority to explore and determine the burden of exposure of toxic metals from human blood to the developing VLBW infants. We hypothesized that `metals, known to have especially detrimental neurotoxic health effects, could be present in donor blood used for VLBW infants at potentially toxic concentrations. The above metals were prioritized based on carcinogenicity, neurotoxicity, teratogenicity, and prevalence in the greater Cleveland area as this was the source of the donor blood samples, and published literature suggest increased susceptibility of adverse neurological effects in children [9,12,15,21-51]. Toxic metals meeting one or more of these criteria were selected to be the focus of this study. They were Al, As, Be, Cd, Pb, Mn, Hg, Ni, and polonium (Po).

Methods

Blood collection

Donor blood units were selected from a convenience sample obtained from University Hospitals of Cleveland blood bank over a period of 2 weeks. Upon review by the Institutional Review Board (IRB), the study was deemed not human subjects research and thus was exempt from IRB review. Donor blood was collected by the blood bank, mixed with citrate phosphate dextrose (standard anti-coagulant) solution, and stored in standard blood bank bags which included a section of tubing divided into segments that could be reserved for any future tests. For this study, one segment was collected by cutting through the plastic connecting two of the segments. 2 mL of blood within the segment was transferred into blue-top, trace-mineral-free vacutainers (Vacutainer Brand, #369737) using Fenwal Hematype Segment Devices (Baxter, 4R5128). Blood was subsequently stored at -20°C until further analysis.

Metal analysis

An inductively coupled plasma – mass spectroscopy method (Using Perkin-Elmer 9000 (ELAN DRC II, SCIEX, INC SHELTON, CT) was used to determine blood metal concentrations that had an ability to measure all 9 metals simultaneously. Donor blood samples that were to be analyzed were removed from the freezer and allowed to thaw at room temperature. After vigorous mixing, 500 uL of whole blood was withdrawn with an Eppendorf pipette and discarded to clean the tip. A second 500 uL aliquot was transferred to a clean, dry 23-mL Parr acid digestion bomb. The cleanliness of each Parr bomb was established before each set of sample analysis by adding 1000 uL of nitric acid (vide infra) to each bomb. If any analyte was found to be above its detection limit, the bomb was re-cleaned prior to being used to digest a blood sample.

Following addition of whole blood to the Parr bomb, 1000 uL of concentrated nitric acid (GFS Chemical double-distilled from Vycor) was then added. The bomb was then sealed and placed in an oven at 120oC for two hours. After digestion was complete, the bombs were cooled to room temperature and opened. The contents were quantitatively transferred to clean, dry 1-oz. polyethylene bottles. The sample was then diluted to 10 mL volume with deionized water and subsequently analyzed by inductively coupled plasma – mass spectroscopy (Perkin-Elmer 9000). All reagents including water and acids were high-purity grade.

To ensure quality and control of the heavy metal analysis, each batch of 10 blood samples from donors also contained 1 standard sample (NBS Standard Reference Material 1557a). For accuracy and precision, the standard sample was analyzed 10 times. The mean values and standard deviations for each metal (ug/L) in the standard sample are: Al, 2300 ±700; As, 57 ± 5; Be, 1.0 ± 0.5; Cd, 350 ± 30; Pb, 230 ± 70; Mn, 8300 ± 500; and Hg, 10 ± 7.

Statistical analysis

Statistical analyses were performed using Excel Statistical software. Descriptive statistics was used to determine the median, range and mean of the detectable values of the various heavy metal concentrations (Al, As, Be, Cd, Pb, Mn, Hg, Ni and Po) from banked donor blood.

Calculations of estimated tolerable acute intravenous dose

To estimate the safety of the concentrations of metals in the blood units, an estimated tolerable acute intravenous dose was calculated from available literature. If no specific literature was available pertaining to intravenous doses considered tolerable, the acute oral reference dose given by the ATSDR was used. If the acute oral reference dose was not given, the chronic oral reference dose was used. Oral reference doses were converted to intravenous doses based on a conservative assumption that only 10% of a gastrointestinal dose of heavy metal would be absorbed with the exception of Hg [52-54]. Thus, an "intravenous reference dose" would be 1/10th of the oral reference dose. Using 20 mL/kg as the blood volume of a transfusion used in many neonatal intensive care units, the concentration of each metal in the donor blood that would yield a tolerable dose was calculated (estimated tolerable concentration (ETC), ng/mL (or µg/L)=(tolerable dose (µg/kg)/20 mL/kg).

Hg absorption was treated differently as it is known that Hg is highly absorbed and results from dietary intake of forms of organic Hg, particularly methylmercury (Centers for Disease Control and Prevention). For calculation of the ETC of Hg, the assumption was made that most Hg in blood is methylmercury, and the EPA's oral reference dose of 0.1 µg/kg/day (100 ng/kg/day) was used as the tolerable oral dose [55,56].

Results

All units had detectable concentrations of at least one heavy metal. The descriptive statistics are given in Table 1. Po was the only metal not detected in any unit. Arsenic (As) was the only toxic metal to be detected in all 100 donor blood units. Pb was detected in 26 of the 100 units. The distributions of the concentrations of the individual metals are shown in the Figure. For 7 of the 9 metals, the majority of the units had metal concentrations below the limit of detection. In contrast, the majority of values for both As and Be were above the limit of detection.

Units with metal concentrations above the ETC are shown in Table 2. Al, Mn, Ni and Pb concentrations were high enough that in multiple units they were above their ETCs. Several units were greater than twice the ETC for Al, Ni and Pb. Thirty-one units had at least one metal above its ETC (Table 3), and 10 units had more than one metal above the ETC. Pb was present in 84% (26 units) of the 31 units with at least one metal above the ETC.

Discussion

In this descriptive study, we show that whole blood concentration for toxic metals may exceed ETC. For one particular unit, the concentration of Al was 10 times the ETC. Our results fell within the ranges of blood metal concentrations reported by the NHANES for Pb and Cd in the 2009-2010 survey under laboratory data (1.8 to 435.2 µg/L and 0.14 to 8.67 µg/L for Pb and Cd respectively) [57]. The limit of detection (LOD) was different for each metal because multiple factors, such as the analytical sensitivity of a mass spectral line and inter-element and physical interferences are different for each metal [58]. For example, Be was detected at any concentration above 0.08 ng/ml, whereas Mn was detected at a concentration above 30 ng/ml. Thus, 97% of the samples had Be over the limit of detection, yet only 11% had Mn concentrations above the limit of detection. This difference in distribution does not necessarily represent a higher level of exposure to Be, but rather a limitation of the analytical method. Despite Po being established as a human carcinogen, environmental levels of Po are extremely low. It was reassuring to not detect Po in any of the donor blood samples, despite the fact that very low levels of Po are found naturally in the body particularly in first-hand smokers[42].

The results of this study may underestimate the dose of toxic heavy metal exposure to a VLBW infant because these infants 1) often receive multiple transfusions of packed red blood cells (pRBC) rather than whole blood as was used in this study, and 2) often receive multiple transfusions from the same donor. Because Pb binds exclusively to hemoglobin molecule in erythrocytes [59], a VLBW infant who might have been transfused with pRBC would receive nearly double the concentration of heavy metals initially present in the donor blood [15]. Several studies suggest that other metals also bind to hemoglobin [60-65]. The difference in metal concentrations between whole blood versus pRBCs may not be a trivial issue. In a recent study [66], 40 of 49 (82%) pRBC units had detectable Hg, compared to 16% of whole blood units reported here. In addition, 6.8% of the pRBC units exceeded the EPA reference dose on the day of transfusion [66]. If the concentration of Hg were doubled in pRBCs prepared from whole blood reported here, 4 units (4%) would have exceeded the reference dose for Hg on the day of transfusion. Similarly, 11 (11%) of transfusions would exceed the Mn ETC.

Another factor to consider when estimating exposure is the practice of assigning a donor unit to an infant. VLBW infants are generally assigned a dedicated unit of blood from a single donor and several transfusions can be administered from the same donor unit. This practice limits exposure of VLBW infants to multiple donor units and thereafter the risk of infection and allo-immunization to foreign antigens from various blood donors is mitigated. On the contrary, VLBW infants receiving multiple transfusions from one donor unit may be chronically exposed to the cumulative effect of toxic metals from that donor blood unit.

Any concentration higher than the calculated ETC could potentially be harmful to VLBW infants. In this study, at least 31% of the blood bank blood had metal concentrations greater than the ETC. Several strategies exist to identify such donor blood units. The first strategy will be to adopt a universal screening program of blood collected by blood banks for heavy metal concentrations. Sensitive, inexpensive assays for blood lead are readily available due to the American Academy of Pediatrics and CDC recommended blood lead screening program [53]. Screening for this one metal would identify 81% of those units with one or more metal concentrations higher than the

acceptable level. The addition of screening for Al would identify 94% of unacceptable units.

The second strategy would be a targeted screening of blood units donated by members of communities known to be at high risk for elevated metal concentrations in the blood. In this study, all 100 units of banked blood had As detected above the LOD. According to the 2013 ATSDR priority list of hazardous substances, arsenic ranks at number one as the hazardous substance determined to pose the most significant potential threat to human health due to its known toxicity. For most people, diet is the predominant source of As exposure, which includes, fish, shellfish and drinking water. Other sources of inorganic As exposure include use of arsine gas in the microelectronics industry, semiconductor manufacturing units, and workers in metal smelters exposed to above-average inorganic As levels from arsine released into the air. Elevated levels of inorganic As may also be present in soil, either from natural mineral deposits or contamination from human activities, which may lead to dermal or ingestion exposure [67]. All the above listed sources and exposures could potentially lead to elevated levels of inorganic As in the human body and therefore in donor blood. As CDC continues to gather data in the Biomonitoring program, geographically relevant data will be available (Centers for Disease Control and Prevention). Such data might be used to determine which potential toxic metals, especially As, should be tested in blood donors from a given community.

A third strategy would be the development of a questionnaire to identify donors at high risk for elevated metal concentrations in their blood. An example of such a questionnaire is that developed by the CDC to identify children at risk for elevated blood Pb concentrations [23]. The results of the questionnaire would be used to target donor units for analysis of blood metals.

In conclusion, at least 31% of the donor blood in the blood bank had metal concentrations above an estimated tolerable concentration. This exposure could potentially pose a grave health risk to a vulnerable VLBW infant, especially of the developing nervous system. The number of donor blood units with concerning levels of metal(s) was higher than expected. It is suggested that neonatologists consider the potential threat of toxic metal exposure to neonates when deciding whether their patients should receive blood transfusions. Future research to determine the actual impact and burden of these toxic heavy metal exposures from blood products is imperative.

Acknowledgments

We thank Michelle Walsh for editorial comments, John Holcomb, Ph.D. (Cleveland State University), Lori Pollak, M.A.T., and Richard Woodman, M.S. for assistance with the statistical analysis. We thank Elizabeth Bamford for editorial assistance.

References

1. Kirpalani H, Whyte R (2011) Truths, associations, and hypotheses. J Pediatr 159: 359-361.

2. Bifano EM, Curran TR (1995) Minimizing donor blood exposure in the neonatal intensive care unit. Current trends and future prospects. Clin Perinatol 22: 657-669.

3. Ohlsson A, Aher SM (2012) Early erythropoietin for preventing red blood cell transfusion in preterm and/or low birth weight infants. Cochrane Database Syst Rev 9: CD004863.

4. Widness JA, Seward VJ, Kromer IJ, Burmeister LF, Bell EF, et al. (1996) Changing patterns of red blood cell transfusion in very low birth weight infants. J Pediatr 129: 680-687.

5. Requirements for testing human blood donors for evidence of infection due to communicable disease agents (2001). Final rule. Federal register 66: p31146-31165.

6. Strauss RG1 (1997) Practical issues in neonatal transfusion practice. Am J Clin Pathol 107: S57-63.

7. Fergusson D, Hébert PC, Lee SK, Walker CR, Barrington KJ, et al. (2003) Clinical outcomes following institution of universal leukoreduction of blood transfusions for premature infants. JAMA 289: 1950-1956.

8. Crinnion WJ (2010) The CDC fourth national report on human exposure to environmental chemicals: what it tells us about our toxic burden and how it assist environmental medicine physicians. Altern Med Rev 15: 101-109.

9. Steuerwald U, Weihe P, Jørgensen PJ, Bjerve K, Brock J, et al. (2000) Maternal seafood diet, methylmercury exposure, and neonatal neurologic function. J Pediatr 136: 599-605.

10. Al-Saleh I, Shinwari N, Mashhour A, Rabah A (2014) Birth outcome measures and maternal exposure to heavy metals (lead, cadmium and mercury) in Saudi Arabian population. Int J Hyg Environ Health 217: 205-218.

11. Menai M, Heude B, Slama R, Forhan A, Sahuquillo J, et al. (2012) Association between maternal blood cadmium during pregnancy and birth weight and the risk of fetal growth restriction: the EDEN mother-child cohort study. Reprod Toxicol 34: 622-627.

12. Bearer CF, Linsalata N, Yomtovian R, Walsh M, Singer L (2003) Blood transfusions: a hidden source of lead exposure. Lancet 362: 332.

13. Elabiad MT, Hook RE (2013) Lead content of blood transfusions for extremely low-birth-weight infants. Am J Perinatol 30: 765-770.

14. Klein GL, Alfrey AC, Shike M, Sherrard DJ (1991) Parenteral drug products containing aluminum as an ingredient or a contaminant: response to FDA notice of intent. ASCN/ASPEN Working Group on Standards for Aluminum Content of Parenteral Nutrition Solutions. The American journal of clinical nutrition 53: 399-402.

15. Bearer CF, O'Riordan MA, Powers R (2000) Lead exposure from blood transfusion to premature infants. J Pediatr 137: 549-554.

16. ATSDR C, CERCLA (2007) Priority List of Hazardous Substances. Agency for Toxic Substances and Disease Registry.

17. Ostrowski SR, Wilbur S, Chou CH, Pohl HR, Stevens YW, Allred PM, et al. (1999) Agency for Toxic Substances and Disease Registry's 1997 priority list of hazardous substances. Latent effects-carcinogenesis, neurotoxicology, and developmental deficits in humans and animals. Toxicol Ind Health 15: 602-644.

18. Pugh KH, Zarus GM (2012) The Burden of Environmental Disease in the United States J Environ Health 74: 30-34.

19. Horton LM, Mortensen ME, Iossifova Y, Wald MM, Burgess P (2013) What do we know of childhood exposures to metals (arsenic, cadmium, lead, and mercury) in emerging market countries? Int J Pediatr 2013: 872596.

20. Rahbar MH, Samms-Vaughan M, Dickerson AS, Hessabi M, Bressler J (2015) Concentration of lead, mercury, cadmium, aluminum, arsenic and manganese in umbilical cord blood of Jamaican newborns. Int J Environ Res Public Health 12: 4481-4501.

21. Rice D, Barone S Jr (2000) Critical periods of vulnerability for the developing nervous system: evidence from humans and animal models. Environ Health Perspect 3: 511-533.

22. Ostrowski SR, Wilbur S, Chou CH, Pohl HR, Stevens YW, et al. (1999) Agency for Toxic Substances and Disease Registry's 1997 priority list of hazardous substances. Latent effects--carcinogenesis, neurotoxicology, and developmental deficits in humans and animals. Toxicol Ind Health 15: 602-44.

23. Buratti M, Valla C, Pellegrino O, Rubino FM, Colombi A (2006) Aluminum determination in biological fluids and dialysis concentrates

via chelation with 8-hydroxyquinoline and solvent extraction/ fluorimetry. Anal Biochem 353: 63-68.

24. Gura KM, Puder M (2006) Recent developments in aluminium contamination of products used in parenteral nutrition. Current opinion in clinical nutrition and metabolic care 9: 239-246.

25. Vahter M (2009) Effects of arsenic on maternal and fetal health. Annu Rev Nutr 29: 381-399.

26. Mamtani R, Stern P, Dawood I, Cheema S (2011) Metals and disease: a global primary health care perspective. J Toxicol 2011: 319136.

27. Sutton M, Burastero SR (2003) Beryllium chemical speciation in elemental human biological fluids. Chem Res Toxicol 16: 1145-1154.

28. Verma DK, Ritchie AC, Shaw ML (2003) Measurement of beryllium in lung tissue of a chronic beryllium disease case and cases with sarcoidosis. Occup Med (Lond) 53: 223-227.

29. Al-Saleh I, Shinwari N, Mashhour A, Mohamed Gel-D, Ghosh MA, et al. (2006) Cadmium and mercury levels in Saudi women and its possible relationship with hypertension. Biol Trace Elem Res 112: 13-29.

30. Cerulli N, Campanella L, Grossi R, Politi L, Scandurra R, et al. (2006) Determination of Cd, Cu, Pb and Zn in neoplastic kidneys and in renal tissue of fetuses, newborns and corpses. J Trace Elem Med Biol 20: 171-179.

31. Risher JF, De Rosa CT, Jones DE, Murray HE (1999) Summary report for the expert panel review of the toxicological profile for mercury. Toxicol Ind Health 15: 483-516.

32. Risher JF, De Rosa CT, Jones DE, Murray HE (1999) Updated toxicological profile for mercury. Toxicol Ind Health 15: 480-482.

33. Debes F, Budtz-Jørgensen E, Weihe P, White RF, Grandjean P (2006) Impact of prenatal methylmercury exposure on neurobehavioral function at age 14 years. Neurotoxicol Teratol 28: 536-547.

34. Faroon O, Ashizawa A, Wright S, Tucker P, Jenkins K, et al. (2012) Toxicological Profile for Cadmium. Atlanta (GA).

35. Williams M, Todd D, Roney N, Crawford J, Coles C (2012)Toxicological Profile for Manganese. Atlanta (GA).

36. Erikson KM, Thompson K, Aschner J, Aschner M (2007) Manganese neurotoxicity: a focus on the neonate. Pharmacol Ther 113: 369-377.

37. Wasserman GA, Liu X, Parvez F, Factor-Litvak P, Ahsan H, et al. (2011) Arsenic and manganese exposure and children's intellectual function. Neurotoxicology 32: 450-457.

38. Ozmen H, Erulas FA, Karatas F, Cukurovali A, Yalcin O (2006) Comparison of the concentration of trace metals (Ni, Zn, Co, Cu and Se), Fe, vitamins A, C and E, and lipid peroxidation in patients with prostate cancer. Clin Chem Lab Med 44: 175-179.

39. Abadin H, Ashizawa A, Stevens WY, Llados F, Diamond G, et al. (2007) Toxicological Profile for Lead. Atlanta (GA).

40. Jusko TA, Henderson CR, Lanphear BP, Cory-Slechta DA, Parsons PJ, et al. (2008) Blood lead concentrations < 10 microg/dL and child intelligence at 6 years of age. Environ Health Perspect 116: 243-248.

41. Henshaw DL, Keitch PA, James PR (1995) Lead-210, polonium-210, and vehicle exhaust pollution. Lancet 345: 324-325.

42. Khater AE (2004) Polonium-210 budget in cigarettes. J Environ Radioact 71: 33-41.

43. Skwarzec B, Ulatowski J, Struminska DI, Borylo A (2001) Inhalation of 210Po and 210Pb from cigarette smoking in Poland. J Environ Radioact 57: 221-230.

44. Substances AFT, Registry D (2008) Toxicological Profile for Aluminum. US Department of Health and Human Services, Public Health Service Atlanta, GA.

45. Taylor JR, Woskin De, Ennever FK (1999) Toxicological profile for cadmium. US Agency for Toxic Substances and Disease Registry, Atlanta, GA.

46. ATSDR U (2007) Toxicological Profile for lead. US Department of Health and Human Services 1: 582.

47. Risher J, Woskin R De (1999) Toxicological profile for mercury. Agency for Toxic Substances and Disease Registry.

48. Health UDo, Services H (2000) Toxicological profile for arsenic.

49. Williams M, Daniel G, Roney N, Crawford J, Coles C, et al. (2012) Toxicological Profile for Manganese, 201, US Department of Health and Human Services, Public Service Atlanta GA.

50. ATSDR I (2002) Toxicological profile for beryllium. Atlanta, Agency for Toxic Substances and Disease Registry.

51. Fay M (2005) Toxicological profile for nickel: Agency for Toxic Substances and Disease Registry.

52. Aschner JL, Aschner M (2005) Nutritional aspects of manganese homeostasis. Mol Aspects Med 26: 353-362.

53. Etzel RA (2003) Pediatric environmental health competencies for specialists. Ambulatory pediatrics: the official journal of the Ambulatory Pediatric Association 3: 60-63.

54. Gulson BL, Mahaffey KR, Vidal M, Jameson CW, Law AJ, et al. (1997) Dietary lead intakes for mother/child pairs and relevance to pharmacokinetic models. Environ Health Perspect 105: 1334-1342.

55. Rice DC, Schoeny R, Mahaffey K (2003) Methods and rationale for derivation of a reference dose for methylmercury by the U.S. EPA. Risk Anal 23: 107-115.

56. Rice DC (2004) The US EPA reference dose for methylmercury: sources of uncertainty. Environ Res 95: 406-413.

57. CDC (2015) NHANES 2009-2010.

58. Jenner G, Longerich HP, Jackson SE, Fryer BJ (1999) ICP-MS a powerful tool for high-precision trace-element analysis in earth sciences: evidence from analysis of selected USGS reference samples. Chemical Geology 83: 133-148.

59. Simons TJ (1986) Passive transport and binding of lead by human red blood cells. J Physiol 378: 267-286.

60. Bramanti E, D'Ulivo A, Lampugnani L, Zamboni R, Raspi G (1999) Application of mercury cold vapor atomic fluorescence spectrometry to the characterization of mercury-accessible -SH groups in native proteins. Anal Biochem 274: 163-173.

61. Levine J, Weickert M, Pagratis M, Etter J, Mathews A, et al. (1998) Identification of a nickel (II) binding site on hemoglobin which confers susceptibility to oxidative deamination and intramolecular cross-linking. The Journal of biological chemistry, 273: 13037-13046.

62. Lu M, Wang H, Li XF, Arnold LL, Cohen SM, et al. (2007) Binding of dimethylarsinous acid to cys-13alpha of rat hemoglobin is responsible for the retention of arsenic in rat blood. Chem Res Toxicol 20: 27-37.

63. Missy P, Lanhers MC, Grignon Y, Joyeux M, Burnel D (2000) In vitro and in vivo studies on chelation of manganese. Hum Exp Toxicol 19: 448-456.

64. THOMAS RG (1964) THE BINDING OF POLONIUM BY RED CELLS AND PLASMA PROTEINS. Radiat Res Suppl 5: SUPPL 5:29-39.

65. Vittori D, Nesse A, Pérez G, Garbossa G (1999) Morphologic and functional alterations of erythroid cells induced by long-term ingestion of aluminium. J Inorg Biochem 76: 113-120.

66. Elabiad MT, Hook RE (2011) Mercury content of blood transfusions for infants with extremely low birth weight. Pediatrics 128: 331-334.

67. Freire C, Koifman RJ, Fujimoto D, de Oliveira Souza VC, Barbosa F Jr, et al. (2015) Reference values of cadmium, arsenic and manganese in blood and factors associated with exposure levels among adult population of Rio Branco, Acre, Brazil. Chemosphere 128: 70-78.

28

Wound Healing Effects of a Lipocalin-Derived Peptide

Luana Wlian[1], **Linda Christian Carrijo-Carvalho**[1], **Sonia Aparecida Andrade**[1], **Silvia Vanessa Lourenço**[2], **Consuelo Junqueira Rodrigues**[3], **Durvanei Augusto Maria**[1] **and Ana Marisa Chudzinski Tavassi**[1*]

[1]*Butantan Institute, São Paulo, Brazil*

[2]*Dental School, University of São Paulo, São Paulo, Brazil*

[3]*University of São Paulo, São Paulo, Brazil*

*Corresponding author: Ana Marisa Chudzinski Tavassi, Instituto Butantan, Laboratório de Bioquímica e Biofísica , Av. Vital Brazil, 1500, 05503-900, São Paulo, SP, Brazil, E-mail: ana.chudzinski@butantan.gov.br

Abstract

The role of lipocalins in wound healing is currently unknown, although the involvement of these proteins in injury response has been reported. This study aimed to investigate the effects of a peptide comprising the sequence of a previously described lipocalin conserved motif (pM2b), in an experimental model of skin lesion. Circular full-thickness wounds in the skin of rat dorsum were treated with pM2b or saline as control, and allowed to heal, keeping the wound occluded and moist. During wound healing, the following parameters were evaluated in the regenerating tissue: wound closure, collagen content, glycosaminoglycans (GAGs) and metalloproteinase (MMP) activity. In addition, tissue sections were subjected to histological analysis. Treatment with pM2b promoted an overall improvement in wound healing and tissue repair, with distinctly marked signals in the early stages of wound healing, such as the presence of histiocytes, fibroblasts and thick collagen bundles, as well as early reepithelization in the recovering tissue. In the latter stages, pM2b-treated wounds showed a better resolution of wound healing, with evidence of regeneration and reduced scars. The regenerating tissue showed collagen increase, no significant changes in the total amount of GAGs, and increased MMP-2 activity, in comparison with control lesions. The results suggest that lipocalins which share the sequence motif related to pM2b can play a role in wound healing. The lipocalin-derived peptide can serve as a tool to develop new pharmaceuticals and formulations to aid wound healing.

Keywords Lipocalin; Lopap; Amino acid motif; Signature sequence; Peptide; Wound healing

Introduction

A diversity of biological molecules is involved in triggering and regulation of wound healing and tissue repair processes. Interaction between extracellular matrix (ECM) and cells, as well as modulation of cell responses play important roles in the dynamic regulation of wound healing and establishment of normal tissue morphology and function [1-3]. Among the decisive events distinguished in wound healing are the primary hemostasis, wound contraction, cell recruitment, orchestrating of cell responses by growth factors and cytokines, and the synthesis of ECM components [4].

Collagen is the main ECM component, important to maintaining tissue integrity. During tissue repair, fibroblasts and myofibroblasts are recruited to the new forming tissue and synthesize collagen. Rapid collagen synthesis and arrangement in a well-organized pattern, equilibrated with tissue remodeling that involves the activation of matrix metalloproteinase are critical factors, which determine the success of tissue repair, and scar prevention [5,6].

Recently, lipocalins have arisen in literature as players in injury response and morphogenic processes [7-12]. Lipocalins are multifunctional proteins that can modulate cell survival, differentiation and immune responses [13-15]. We have previously demonstrated that a signature sequence is involved in the modulation of cell responses by lipocalins and have described a peptide (pM2b), which comprises the conserved sequence motif related to the lipocalin signature sequence [16,17]. In vitro assays showed this lipocalin-derived peptide triggers anti-apoptotic activity in endothelial cells and neutrophils, and is able to modulate fibroblast responses, inducing the synthesis of ECM proteins, and expression of inflammatory and cell survival mediators [16,18]. In vivo assays, pM2b also induced increased collagen synthesis in normal dermis [18]. In the present study, we evaluated the healing effects of pM2b in skin full-thickness wound.

Materials and Methods

Peptide and reagents

The synthetic peptide (pM2b) with the amino acid sequence YAIGYSCKDYK-OH was obtained from Orpegen Pharma (Heidelberg, Germany). All other reagents were of analytical grade.

Full-thickness skin lesion model

Male Wistar rats aged 6-8 weeks and weighing 120-150 g were obtained from the Central Animal Breeding House, Butantan Institute. The animals were fed with standard pellet diet and water ad libitum. All procedures were approved by the institutional animal care and use committee. Rats were anesthetized with a mixture of ketamine (75 mg.kg^{-1} im) and xylazine (10 mg.kg^{-1} im). The dorsum was shaved and disinfected with ethanol. Six full-thickness round sections (three wounds on each side) of 6 mm diameter were aseptically made on the skin using a metallic punch. The wounds on the right side were topically treated with a single dose of the peptide (50 µl, 230 nM pM2b) while the wounds on the left side were treated with the vehicle (saline) as control. Each wound was dressed with Bioclusive transparent dressing (Johnson & Johnson, Arlington, TX, USA). Full-thickness excisions were taken as a reference of normal intact skin, considered as control of intact dermis. At intervals of 3, 7, 14, and 21 days after wounding rats (n=8) were euthanized, and full-thickness skin samples from the healing wounds were excised for posterior analyses. Before excision, the size of each lesion was measured and the wounds were examined to evaluate wound contraction and the healing tissue. The wound area was measured using the formula: wound area (mm^2) = (a x b) x π/4, were a and b are the major and minor axes (mm diameter) of the wounds, respectively [19]. Data are presented as percentage of the initial wound area.

Histological analysis

Skin samples collected at the time of wounding and at all-time intervals after wounding were immediately fixed in a solution of 10% neutral buffered formalin, embedded in paraffin, sectioned at a thickness of 3 µm, and stained with hematoxilin-eosin (HE) to analyze tissue morphology, and picrosirius red for collagen analysis. Slides were examined under light microscopy. Images were acquired at 250x magnification. Peptide-treated lesions were compared with saline-treated lesions at each time intervals.

Collagen analysis

Collagen analysis was done as previously described [20]. Skin samples collected at the intervals of 7, 14, and 21 days after wounding were incubated for 4 h at room temperature with pepsin in 0.5 M acetic acid, pH 2.5, and then maintained at 4°C during 20 h. Then, the samples were centrifuged at 8 000 g for 30 min. The supernatants were lyophilized and dissolved with 0.5 M acetic acid. The total amount of protein was measured by the method of Bradford, using a standard curve of bovine serum albumin [21].

Analysis of glycosaminoglycans

Glycosaminoglycans (GAGs) were extracted as previously described [22]. Skin samples collected at the intervals of 7, 14, and 21 days after wounding were incubated for 24 h in acetone and delipidated in methanol: chloroform (1:2). Dry tissues were rehydrated in 100 mM sodium acetate, pH 5.0, with 5 mM cysteine and 5 mM EDTA and incubated with 20 mg/mL papain for 24 h at 60°C. After 20 min centrifugation at 3000 g, supernatants were collected and GAGs were precipitated by addition of 0.5% cetylpyridinium chloride (CPC). The CPC-GAG complex was dissociated with 2 M sodium chloride with ethanol (100:15). GAGs were washed in ethanol and quantified by the carbazole method, using a galacturonic acid standard curve [23].

Matrix metalloproteinase activity assay

Matrix metalloproteinases (MMPs) were extracted from the recovering tissue collected at all-time intervals and analyzed by gelatin zymography, as previously described [24]. The samples were homogenized (1/10, w/v) in 100 mMTris-HCl, pH 7.6, containing 200 Mm NaCl, 100 mM CaCl$_2$ and 1 % Triton X-100, at 4°C for 24 h. After centrifugation at 12000 g for 15 min, the supernatants were collected and the protein concentration was measured by the method of Bradford, using a standard curve of bovine serum albumin [21]. The samples were subjected to electrophoresis at 100 V, 4°C, using 7.5% polyacrylamide gels containing 1 mg/mL co-polymerized gelatin. The

MMP activity was visualized as clear bands against a dark-blue background.

Statistical analysis

Statistical analysis was performed using Student's t-test. P values less than 0.05 were regarded as statistically significant.

Results

Wound closure and macroscopic changes

A slight improvement in wound closure was observed in the peptide-treated lesions, with significant differences at the third and fourteenth day after treatment (Figure 1).

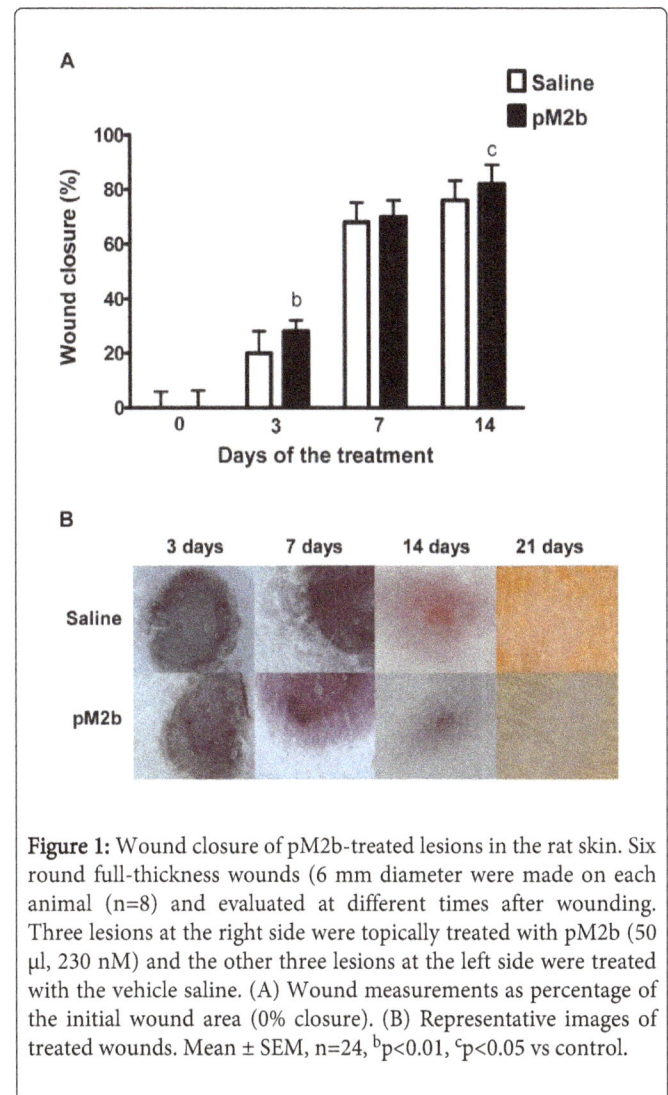

Figure 1: Wound closure of pM2b-treated lesions in the rat skin. Six round full-thickness wounds (6 mm diameter were made on each animal (n=8) and evaluated at different times after wounding. Three lesions at the right side were topically treated with pM2b (50 µl, 230 nM) and the other three lesions at the left side were treated with the vehicle saline. (A) Wound measurements as percentage of the initial wound area (0% closure). (B) Representative images of treated wounds. Mean ± SEM, n=24, [b]p<0.01, [c]p<0.05 vs control.

Dermoscopy is a non-invasive diagnostic tool that allows the recognition of morphologic structures not visible skin. Were analyzed and highlighted the following structures in the skin include hair shafts, hair follicle openings, the peri-follicular epidermis and cutaneous microvasculature. After three days, the control group lesions presented bleeding, discrete epithelial disarrangement and edematous areas in the wound edges. On the other hand, pM2b treated lesions showed only discrete bleeding points and markedly retracted edges (Figure 1). At the seventh day, control lesions showed few retracted edges, intense bleeding points, vascular congestion and discrete necrosis segments, while peptide-treated lesions showed reepithelization and markedly retracted edges. Fourteen days after wounding, control lesions had accentuated vascularization with partial contraction and pM2b-treated lesions showed wound contraction and poor vascularization when compared with control. After twenty one days, peptide-treated lesions showed repaired tissue of normal appearance and absence of scars. Hypertrophic scars were accounted in approximately 30% of the wounds treated with saline.

Histological aspects of HE stained sections

The dermis control rats were composed by dense connective tissue, intermingled by skin appendages. Deep aspects of the specimens show striated muscle bundles and adipose tissue (Figure 2).

(Group saline – initial) ulcerated fragment of skin covered with a leuco-fibrinouspseudo membrane. Acute and chronic inflammatory infiltrate and edema, extending to the deep aspects of the dermis are also observed; (Group treated pM2b – 0 Day) ulcerated fragment of skin covered with a leuco-fibrinouspseudo membrane, present inflammatory infiltrate, with presence of histiocytes and edema.

(Group saline – 7Days) ulcerated fragment of skin covered with a leuco-fibrinouspseudo membrane over well-organized granulation tissue. Note the perpendicular distribution of blood vessels; (Group pM2b - 7Days) Well-organized granulation tissue under area of early reepitelization. Note the presence of fibroblasts and the perpendicular distribution of blood vessels.

(Group saline - 14Days) Fragment of skin with evidence of early reepithelization. In the dermis, remnants of granulation tissue, mild inflammatory infiltrate and hemorrhagic exsudate are observed. Collagen fibres are organized in parallel bundles; (Group pM2b - 14Days) Fragment of skin with evidence of intenseregeneration. In the dermis, mild, mild inflammatory infiltrate and small hemorrhagic foci are observed. Collagen fibers are organized in parallel bundles.

(Group saline - 21Days) Fragment of re-epithelized skin with areas ortho keratinized epidermis. Dermis is composed by dense connective tissue with parallel thick collagen bindles intermingled with small blood vessels, mild inflammatory infiltrate and edema. (Group pM2b - 21Days: Fragment of re-epithelized skin with extensive ortho keratinized epidermis. Dermis is composed by dense connective tissue with parallel thick collagen bindles intermingled with small blood vessels, absence inflammatory infiltrate and edema.

The HE-stained slides of samples from saline-treated lesions, obtained three days after wounding, showed ulcerated fragment of skin covered with a leuco-fibrinouspseudo membrane. Acute and chronic inflammatory infiltrate and edema, extending to the deep aspects of the dermis were also observed. Samples from pM2b-treated wounds showed intense ulcerated fragment of skin covered with a leuco-fibrinouspseudo membrane. Acute and chronic inflammatory infiltrate, with presence of histiocytes and edema, extending to the deep aspects of the dermis were also observed (Figure 2).

After seven days, ulcerated fragment of skin covered with a leuco-fibrinouspseudo membrane over well-organized granulation tissue was observed in control samples. Note the perpendicular distribution of blood vessels. The pM2b peptide-treated lesions showed well-organized granulation tissue under area of early reepithelization. Note

the presence of proliferation fibroblasts and the perpendicular distribution of blood vessels (Figure 2).

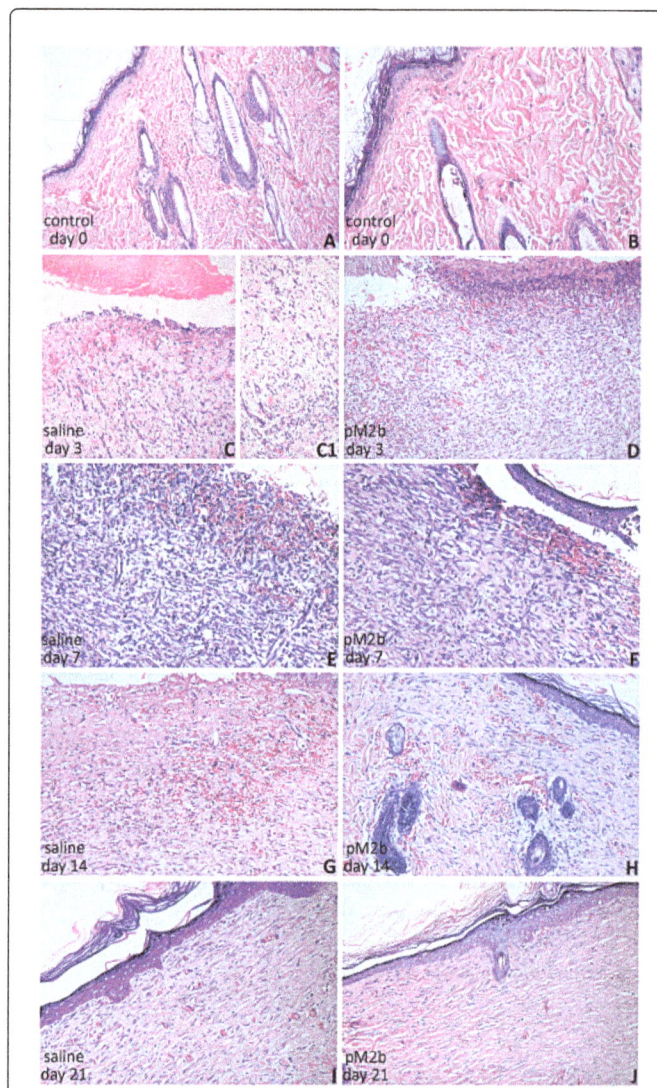

Figure 2: HE stained sections of post-wounding recovering tissue. Photomicrographs of mice skin and scar tissue with or without treatment, stained with HE technique. Full-thickness excisions from the wounding site topically treated with pM2b (50 μl, 230 nM) or saline were subjected to histological analysis. Fragment of control skin with ortho keratinized epidermis. Dermis is composed by dense connective tissue, intermingled by skin appendages. Deep aspects of the specimens show striated muscle bundles and adipose tissue.

At the fourteenth day, control samples showed fragment of skin with evidence of discrete reepithelization cutaneous process. In the dermis, remnants of granulation tissue, mild inflammatory infiltrate and hemorrhagic exudate were observed. Collagen fibers were organized in parallel bundles. Samples from pM2b-treated lesions showed fragment of skin with evidence of active regeneration. In the dermis, mild inflammatory infiltrate and rare hemorrhagic foci were observed. Collagen fibers were organized in parallel bundles (Figure 2).

Twenty one days after wounding, both control and peptide-treated samples presented fragment of reepithelized skin with ortho keratinized epidermis. In groups peptide treated, dermis was composed by dense connective tissue with parallel thick collagen bundles intermingled with small blood vessels, absence inflammatory infiltrate and edema (Figure 2).

Histological aspects of picrosirius-stained sections

Picrosirius-stained slides of recovering tissue from group control lesions three days after wounding had thin collagen bundles (stained red), separated by edema extending to the entire dermis. Lesions treated with pM2b showed thin collagen bundles, separated by edema extending to the superficial portion of the dermis (Figure 3).

(Group saline - initial): thin collagen bundles (stained red), separated by edema extending to the entire dermis; (Group saline - 3Days) thin collagen bundles (stained red), separated by edema extending to the superficial portion of the dermis.

(Group pM2b - 3Days) thin collagen bundles (stained red), organized in a parallel architecture. Compare with the normal thick collagen bundles (stained bright red) in the adjacent area.

(Group pM2b - 7Days) thin collagen bundles (stained red), organized in a parallel architecture. In some areas of the surgical defect, nodules of more mature collagen (bright red) can be observed. Compare with the normal thick collagen bundles (stained bright red) in the adjacent area.

(Group pM2b - 14Days) thin collagen bundles (stained red), organized in a parallel architecture, intermingled by mild edema. Compare with the normal thick collagen bundles (stained bright red) in the adjacent area.

(Group saline - 21Days) dermis showing thick bundles of collagen, stained in red, intermingled by mild edema; (Group pM2b 21Days) dermis showing thick bundles mature of collagen, intermingled by mild edema.

At the seventh day, thin collagen bundles, organized in a parallel architecture were observed in control. Compare with the normal thick collagen bundles in the adjacent area. Samples from peptide-treated lesions presented thin collagen bundles, organized in a parallel architecture. In some areas of the surgical process, nodules of more mature collagen (bright red) were observed. Compare with the normal thick collagen bundles in the adjacent area (Figure 3).

At the fourteenth day, control samples presented thin collagen bundles, organized in a parallel architecture, intermingled by mild edema. Compare with the normal thick collagen bundles in the adjacent area. On the other hand, pM2b-treated samples showed thick collagen bundles, organized in a parallel architecture, intermingled by mild edema (Figure 3).

Twenty one days after wounding, the recovering tissue from control and pM2b-treated wounds presented dermis showing thick bundles of collagen, stained in red, intermingled by mild edema (Figure 3). Compare with normal dermis prior to wounding showing thick bundles of collagen (Figure 3).

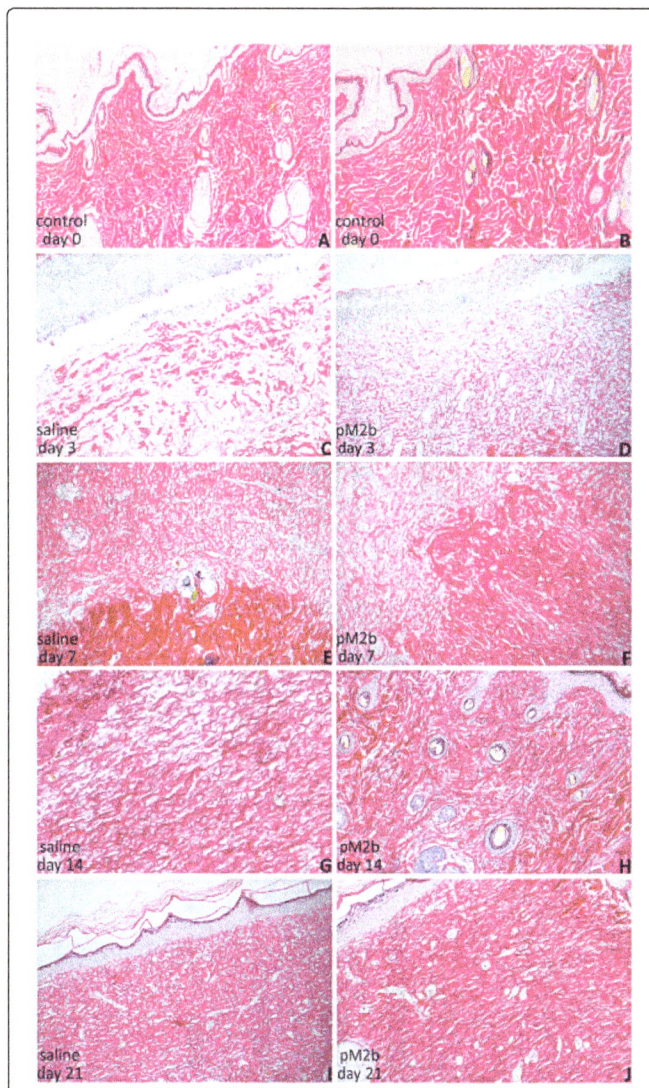

Figure 3: Picrosirius stained sections of post-wounding recovering tissue. Full-thickness excisions from the wounding site topically treated with pM2b (50 µl, 230 nM) or saline were subjected to histological analysis. Slides containing mice skin were stained with picrosirius red, and examined by bright field. The samples dermis group controls showing thick bundles of collagen, stained in red.

Extracellular matrix components

Analysis of protein extracts showed a significant increase of collagen content in pM2b-treated wounds, seven and fourteen days after wounding (Figure 4).

The total amount of GAGs measured were 5.33 ± 2.8 µg/mL and 5.99 ± 2.5 µg/mL seven days after wounding, in control and pM2b-treated samples, respectively. After fourteen days, samples from saline-treated wounds showed 5.86 ± 1.81 µg/mL and samples from pM2b-treated wounds 6.25 ± 2.0 µg/mL. After twenty one days, measures of 1.79 ± 0.59 µg/mL and 1.84 ± 0.55 µg/mL were observed in control and pM2b samples, respectively. Despite a slight increase in the total amount of GAGs were observed in the samples from peptide-treated wounds, there were no significant differences.

A significant increase of protein concentration was observed in the MMP extracts from pM2b-treated lesions, three days after wounding (Figure 5).

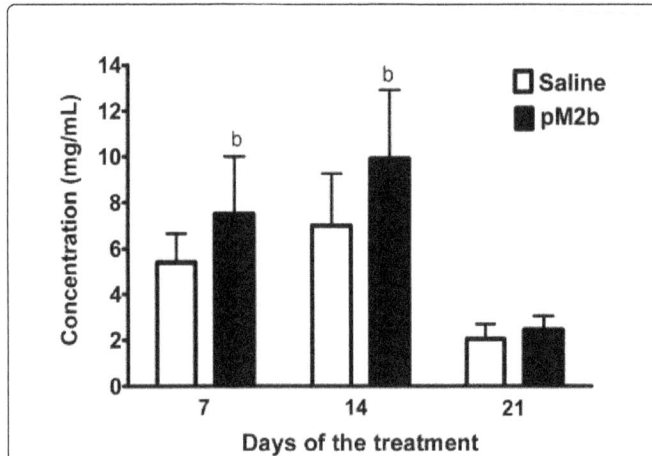

Figure 4: Effect of pM2b on collagen content in the healing tissue. Protein measurements in collagen extracts of tissue samples from the wounds topically treated with pM2b (50 µl, 230 nM) or saline, measured by Bradford assay. Mean ± SEM, n=8, [b]p<0.01 vs control.

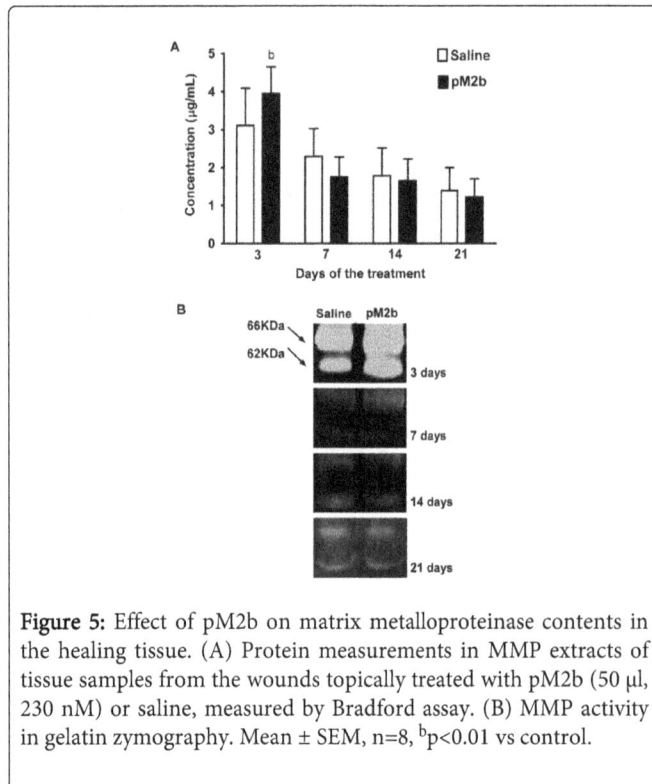

Figure 5: Effect of pM2b on matrix metalloproteinase contents in the healing tissue. (A) Protein measurements in MMP extracts of tissue samples from the wounds topically treated with pM2b (50 µl, 230 nM) or saline, measured by Bradford assay. (B) MMP activity in gelatin zymography. Mean ± SEM, n=8, [b]p<0.01 vs control.

In addition, the zymography analysis showed an increase in proteolytic activity of extracts from the peptide-treated wounds (Figure 5B), with higher intense bands, in the samples collected at the third day after wounding. Two clear bands of approximately 66 and 62

kDa were observed, which corresponds to the molecular mass of the intermediate and active forms of MMP-2, respectively.

Discussion

Healing is the interaction of a complex cascade of cellular events that generates resurfacing, reconstitution, and restoration of the tensile strength of injured skin. Wound healing occurs in overlapping steps recognized as hemostasis, inflammation, proliferation and remodeling, which involves interactions between cells and biochemical mediators around the injury site [2,4]. Growth factors and cytokines are the main described endogenous factors mediating such events [25]. However, the lipocalin roles in these processes are not known so far. The present study was carried out to investigate the possible beneficial effects of a lipocalin-derived peptide (pM2b) in wound healing following a lesion-induced model in rats. The peptide was designed based on the amino acid sequence of Lopap (Lonomiaobliqua prothrombin activator protease), a lepidop teranlipocalin [26] previously reported that displays anti-apoptotic activity, also inducing a set of cell responses, which involves increased expression of cell adhesion molecules, nitric oxide, PGI2 and IL-8, in addition to leukocyte recruitment [27-29].

This peptide reproduced the anti-apoptotic activity of Lopap and other lipocalins, such as purpurin and prostaglandin D synthase [16]. In addition, pM2b was able to induce the synthesis of extracellular matrix proteins in fibroblast culture and modulate pro-inflammatory cytokine signaling [18]. pM2b is related to a conserved lipocalin sequence motif, which has been proposed as a signature sequence with roles in cell modulation [16,17].

This study corroborates with the previous findings, indicating that pM2b displays modulation effects in wound healing in vivo. Macroscopic observations of the recovering wounds are in accordance with the results of histological analysis. The cell modulation activity displayed by pM2b might be involved in the chronic inflammatory infiltrate observed and the migration of histiocytes and fibroblasts to the site of injury.

The modulation effect of pM2b in fibroblasts inducing cytokine signaling, such as IL1-β, IL-6R, CXCR-1 and CXCR-2 [16], could contribute to the beneficial effect of peptide treatment in wound healing herein observed. Indeed, a decrease of these mediators has been associated with delayed wound healing [30,31].

Activated fibroblasts present in the recovering wounds that were treated with the peptide can be responsible for the increase in collagen production and organization fibrilar. Collagen is the most abundant component of extracellular matrix synthesized by fibroblasts. During wound healing, collagen deposits provide a matrix for anchorage and migration of cells and generate tension forces [2].

Other effect observed in pM2b-treated wounds was the increased levels of MMPs, especially active MMP2. The increase of MMP2 activity observed in pM2b-treated wounds, in the early stage of wound healing, may be associated with cell migration and reepithelization. MMPs play important roles in wound healing, regulating tissue remodeling, ECM composition, cell migration, and the function of non-ECM molecules, such as growth factors and their receptors, cytokines and chemokines, and adhesion receptors [32]. MMP2 is expressed by keratinocytes and fibroblasts and its level is increased by the interaction between these cells during wound healing [33].

Despite the involvement of lipocalins in tissue regeneration and developmental process has been widely suggested, this is the first description of a lipocalin-derived molecule being evaluated for its potential effects in wound healing. Further studies should focus on the investigation of signaling pathways involved in tissue responses to pM2b treatment, the optimized dosage, absorption and half-life. Results altogether suggest that lipocalins, through a conserved motif, can play a role in healing and tissue repair, through fibroblast modulation and extracellular matrix remodeling. The data presented here indicate the lipocalin-derived peptide is an active molecule, which can be useful to develop new the therapeutic medications for healing and regeneration.

Acknowledgements

This work was supported by grants from CAT/CEPID-FAPESP and INCTTOX - CNPq/FAPESP program. Luana WLIAN held a scholarship from FAPESP (grant no. 07/52155-7). Linda CARRIJO-CARVALHO has a Postdoctoral fellowship from CAT/CEPID – FAPESP (grant no. 2010/00600-0).

References

1. Widgerow AD (2011) Cellular/extracellular matrix cross-talk in scar evolution and control. Wound Repair Regen 19: 117-133.

2. Schultz GS, Davidson JM, Kirsner RS, Bornstein P, Herman IM (2011) Dynamic reciprocity in the wound microenvironment. Wound Repair Regen 19: 134-148.

3. Adams PD (2009) Healing and hurting: molecular mechanisms, functions, and pathologies of cellular senescence. Mol Cell 36: 2-14.

4. Baum CL, Arpey CJ (2005) Normal cutaneous wound healing: clinical correlation with cellular and molecular events. Dermatol Surg 31: 674-686.

5. Namazi MR, Fallahzadeh MK, Schwartz RA (2011) Strategies for prevention of scars: what can we learn from fetal skin? Int J Dermatol 50: 85-93.

6. Ferguson MW, O'Kane S (2004) Scar-free healing: from embryonic mechanisms to adult therapeutic intervention. Philos Trans R SocLond B Biol Sci 359: 839-850.

7. Petta S, Tripodo C, Grimaudo S, Cabibi D, Cammà C, et al. (2011) High liver RBP4 protein content is associated with histological features in patients with genotype 1 chronic hepatitis C and with nonalcoholic steatohepatitis. Dig Liver Dis 43: 404-410.

8. Ganfornina MD, Do Carmo S, Martínez E, Tolivia J, Navarro A, et al. (2010) ApoD, a glia-derived apolipoprotein, is required for peripheral nerve functional integrity and a timely response to injury. Glia 58: 1320-1334.

9. Li Z, Korzh V, Gong Z (2007) Localized rbp4 expression in the yolk syncytial layer plays a role in yolk cell extension and early liver development. BMC Dev Biol 7: 117.

10. Kim HJ, Je HJ, Cheon HM, Kong SY, Han J, et al. (2005) Accumulation of 23 kDalipocalin during brain development and injury in Hyphantriacunea. Insect BiochemMol Biol 35: 1133-1141.

11. Pagano A, Giannoni P, Zambotti A, Randazzo N, Zerega B, et al. (2002) CALbeta, a novel lipocalin associated with chondrogenesis and inflammation. Eur J Cell Biol 81: 264-272.

12. DescalziCancedda F, Dozin B, Zerega B, Cermelli S, Cancedda R (2000) Ex-FABP: a fatty acid binding lipocalin developmentally regulated in chicken endochondral bone formation and myogenesis. BiochimBiophysActa 1482: 127-135.

13. Grzyb J, Latowski D, StrzaÅ‚ka K (2006) Lipocalins - a family portrait. J Plant Physiol 163: 895-915.

14. Lögdberg L, Wester L (2000) Immunocalins: a lipocalin subfamily that modulates immune and inflammatory responses. BiochimBiophysActa 1482: 284-297.

15. Flower DR (1996) The lipocalin protein family: structure and function. Biochem J 318 : 1-14.

16. Chudzinski-Tavassi AM, Carrijo-Carvalho LC, Waismam K, Farsky SH, Ramos OH, et al. (2010) A lipocalin sequence signature modulates cell survival. FEBS Lett 584: 2896-2900.

17. Mesquita Pasqualoto KF, Carrijo-Carvalho LC, Chudzinski-Tavassi AM (2013) Rational development of novel leads from animal secretion based on coagulation and cell targets: In silico analysis to explore a peptide derivative as lipocalins' signature. Toxicon 69: 200-10.

18. Carrijo-Carvalho LC, Maria DA, Ventura JS, Morais KL, Melo RL, et al. (2012) A lipocalin-derived Peptide modulating fibroblasts and extracellular matrix proteins. J Toxicol 2012: 325250.

19. Komi-Kuramochi A, Kawano M, Oda Y, Asada M, Suzuki M, et al. (2005) Expression of fibroblast growth factors and their receptors during full-thickness skin wound healing in young and aged mice. J Endocrinol 186: 273-289.

20. Rhodes RK, Miller EJ (1978) Physicochemical characterization and molecular organization of the collagen A and B chains. Biochemistry 17: 3442-3448.

21. Bradford MM (1976) A rapid and sensitive method for the quantitation of microgram quantities of protein utilizing the principle of protein-dye binding. Anal Biochem 72: 248-254.

22. Cardoso LE, Erlich RB, Rudge MC, Peraçoli JC, Mourão PA (1992) A comparative analysis of glycosaminoglycans from human umbilical arteries in normal subjects and in pathological conditions affecting pregnancy. Lab Invest 67: 588-595.

23. Taylor KA, Buchanan-Smith JG (1992) A colorimetric method for the quantitation of uronic acids and a specific assay for galacturonic acid. Anal Biochem 201: 190-196.

24. Heussen C, Dowdle EB (1980) Electrophoretic analysis of plasminogen activators in polyacrylamide gels containing sodium dodecyl sulfate and copolymerized substrates. Anal Biochem 102: 196-202.

25. Barrientos S, Stojadinovic O, Golinko MS, Brem H, Tomic-Canic M (2008) Growth factors and cytokines in wound healing. Wound Repair Regen 16: 585-601.

26. Reis CV, Andrade SA, Ramos OH, Ramos CR, Ho PL, et al. (2006) Lopap, a prothrombin activator from Lonomiaobliqua belonging to the lipocalin family: recombinant production, biochemical characterization and structure-function insights. Biochem J 398: 295-302.

27. Waismam K, Chudzinski-Tavassi AM, Carrijo-Carvalho LC, Pacheco MT, Farsky SH (2009) Lopap: a non-inflammatory and cytoprotective molecule in neutrophils and endothelial cells. Toxicon 53: 652-659.

28. Carrijo-Carvalho LC, Chudzinski-Tavassi AM (2007) The venom of the Lonomia caterpillar: an overview. Toxicon 49: 741-757.

29. Reis CV, Farsky SH, Fernandes BL, Santoro ML, Oliva ML, et al. (2001) In vivo characterization of Lopap, a prothrombin activator serine protease from the Lonomiaobliqua caterpillar venom. Thromb Res 102: 437-443.

30. Pradhan L, Cai X, Wu S, Andersen ND, Martin M, et al. (2011) Gene expression of pro-inflammatory cytokines and neuropeptides in diabetic wound healing. J Surg Res 167: 336-342.

31. Devalaraja RM, Nanney LB, Du J, Qian Q, Yu Y, et al. (2000) Delayed wound healing in CXCR2 knockout mice. J Invest Dermatol 115: 234-244.

32. Stamenkovic I (2003) Extracellular matrix remodelling: the role of matrix metalloproteinases. J Pathol 200: 448-464.

33. Gill SE, Parks WC (2008) Metalloproteinases and their inhibitors: regulators of wound healing. Int J Biochem Cell Biol 40: 1334-1347.

29

Benefic Interactive Effects between Garlic Consumption and Serum Iron Excess

Hela Ghorbel[1*], Ines FKI[1], Choumous Kalel[2], Jamoussi Kamel[3] and Sami Sayadi[1]

[1]Laboratory of Bioprocess Environnemtaux, Pole regional excellence AUF (PER-LBP), Sfax Biotechnology Centre (CBS), PO Box 11773038 Sfax, Tunisia

[2]Laboratory of Hematology, CHU, Habib Bourguiba, 3029 Sfax, Tunisia

[3]Laboratory of Biochemistry, University Hospital, Habib Bourguiba, 3029 Sfax, Tunisia

*Corresponding author: Hela Ghorbel, Bioprocess Laboratory, Division of Regional Excellence AUF (PER-LBP), Centre of Biotechnology of Sfax (CBS), University of Sfax, BP: 11773038 Sfax, Tunisia, E-mail: ghorbelh1@yahoo.fr

Abstract

Hemochromatosis is the most common form of iron overload disease. In case of pathological serum iron increase, kidney is the first organ directly affected. Moreover, anemia is the major symptom of most cases of kidney failure and oxidative stress is thought to be a significant factor in the pathogenesis of iron-overload disease. Garlic, was recently demonstrated as inhibitor of intestinal iron absorption. The purpose of this study was to show that crude garlic consumption in case of serum iron increase could prevents biochemical and histological kidney perturbations and ameliorates hematological parameters. For this, four groups of young rats were treated for forty five days: control group C, iron overload group I, garlic overload group G and both garlic and iron overload group IG. In iron treated rats (group I) all haematological parameters showed a decrease. Moreover, kidneys showed a significant increase in protein and malondialdehyde (MDA) concentrations associated to total antioxidant capacity important decrease and deep histological changes. For group G rats, we had found a significant decrease in red blood cells and hemoglobin concentrations and in the kidney an important increase in total antioxidant capacity and in creatinine levels. After association between iron and garlic consumption (group IG) we had found positive interactive effects and important regulation of all modified parameters. In conclusion, for a great part of its effects, garlic protects from iron increase problems and could have important clinical relevance in case of hemochromatosis disease.

Keywords: Kidney; Iron excess; Anemia; Garlic; Total antioxidant capacity; MDA

Introduction

Iron, the most abundant transition metal in the body, is required by all mammalian cells for growth and survival. Iron overload has been shown to result in several structural and functional changes in various tissues of patients with primary or secondary increased iron load [1-3]. The toxic effect of iron is mediated mainly by reactive oxygen species (ROS) which formation is catalyzed by iron in the Haber–Weiss reaction and which cause inflammatory response reflected in the kidney among other organs. In fact, Zager [4] studied the potential nephrotoxic effect of iron compounds given intravenously in vitro experiments on isolated mouse proximal segments or cultured proximal tubular cells and he found variable cytotoxicity of these substances. Oxidative stress is thought to be a significant factor in the pathogenesis of iron-overload disease. Iron catalyzed lipid peroxidation which promotes the formation of highly reactive aldehydes, such as malondialdehyde (MDA) in several organs and particularly in the kidney [5]. Reactive oxygen species (ROS) form covalent links to proteins, phospholipids, and DNA which cause considerable kidney tissue damage [6].

Recent trends in controlling and treating oxidative stress tend to favor natural antioxidant compounds rather than synthetic ones [7]. The human diet, which contains large number of natural compounds, is essential in protecting the body against the development of diseases, and garlic (Allium sativum) is one of the well known plant with remarkable hypolipidemic [8], hypoglycemic [9], anti-atherosclerotic [10], antioxidant [11] and anti-carcinogenic [12] properties. Garlic is a commonly worldwide used food. In mediterranean cooking, is regularly consumed at various doses both crude and cooked, and its potential medical properties have been recognized for thousands of years [13]. Garlic in different forms has antioxidant properties. These properties are shown to be due to the existence of compounds such as water soluble organosulfure compounds, S-allylcysteine, and lipid soluble compounds like diallyl sulfide [7, 12].

Many studies had demonstrated that iron intoxication induced severe kidney damage which progress to failure [14-15]. Moreover, it has been approved that secondary hemochromatosis causes sever aplastic anemia and the complete hematopoietic recovery is possible after continuous iron chelation therapy [16]. Other studies have improved that the consumption of garlic gives renal protection and accelerates red blood cell turnover and splenic erythropoietic gene expression [17,18]. However, there are no previous investigations dealing with the curative garlic effects in case of iron overload, kidney failure and hematological disorders.In this study we state the hypothesis that crude garlic consumption has positive interactive effects with iron excess which could protects kidney and hematological parameters from iron increase.

Materials and methods

Animals

According to the European convention for the protection of vertebrate animals used for experimental and other scientific purposes (Council of Europe No. 12, Strasbourg, 1985) and according to the review committee of our institution, rats rearing and experiments of this work were approved. In the present study, Suisse strain male rats, aged 2 months were purchased from the Central Pharmacy (SIPHAT, Tunisia). They were housed at 22 ± 3°C with light/dark periods of 12 h

and a minimum relative humidity of 40%. They had free access to water and commercial diet (SICO, Sfax, Tunisia). The standard diet contained 73.44 mg of iron by gram of diet.

Parameters and Treatments	C	I	G	IG
Initial body weight	181 ± 6	183 ± 4	181 ± 9	185 ± 8
Final body weight (g)	230 ± 10	263 ± 16***	233 ± 18	254 ± 6 * +++xx
Food consumption (g/day/rat)	8.3 ± 0.6	3.7 ± 0.3 ***	7.8 ± 0.4	4.4 ± 0.5 *** +++xxx
Water consumption (ml/day/rat)	2.8 ± 0.4	1.7 ± 0.5***	3.1 ± 0,8	2.1 ± 0.6 *** ++xxx
Ingested iron (g/day/rat)	0.59 ± 0.08	3.18 ± 0.78***	0.62 ± 0.12	3.27 ± 0.46 ***
Ingested garlic (g/day/rat)	-	-	0.39 ± 0.09	0.22 ± 0.02
Treated I, G and IG vs controls C: *: $p \leq 0.05$, ***: $p \leq 0.001$; Treated IG vs treated I: ++: $p \leq 0.01$, +++: $p \leq 0.001$; Treated IG vs treated G: XX: $p \leq 0.01$, XXX: $p \leq 0.001$				

Table 1: Body weight (n=10), Daily food (n=30), water (n=30), iron and garlic intake (n=30) by 2 months aged rats: controls (group C), treated by $FeCl_2$ (group I), by garlic (group G) or by both $FeCl_2$ and garlic (group IG) for 45 days.

Experimental protocol

The initial number of young rats (weighing~180g) was 40, equally divided into four groups of ten individuals each one: controls (group C; n=10), overload with $FeCl_2$ at a dose of 150 mg/100ml of drinking water (group I; n=10), overload by garlic at a dose of 5g/100g of dampen standard diet (group G; n=10) and overload with $FeCl_2$ and garlic respectively at doses of 150mg/100ml of drinking water and 5g/

100g of dampen standard diet (group IG; n=10). Sacrifice of all groups' rats was done 45 days after beginning treatments. The daily consumed food, water and supplemented iron and garlic quantities' were precisely measured during all the treatment period (Table 1). In this study, the used doses of iron and garlic were precisely determined after a serious of experiments in which we have obtained the most important effects.

Parameters and Treatments	C	I	G	IG
RBC	7.77±0.46	7.25±0.20*	6.91±0.07**	7.36±0.59
Hb	1.51±0.28	1.51±0.15*	1.61±0.54*	1.07±0.51
HCT	40.63±0.47	3.01±0.07**	40.08±.16	4.71±.03+x
T Bil	0.55±0.03	0.78±0.18*	0.64±0.03*	0.44±0.15+
Iron	1.71 ± 0.08	1.93 ± 0.17*	.66±0.08	1.58 ± 0.05+
Number of determinations (n=10); Treated I, G and IG groups versus controls C:*: $P \leq 0.05$, **: $P \leq 0.01$; Treated IG versus treated I: +: $P \leq 0.05$; Treated IG versus treated G: x: $P \leq 0.05$				

Table 2: Red blood cells (RBC) (1012/L), hemoglobin (Hb) (g/L), hematocrite (HCT) (L/L), total bilirubin (T Bil) (µmol/l) and iron serum levels (µmol/L) of young rats: controls (group C), treated by $FeCl_2$ (group I), treated by garlic (group G) and by both $FeCl_2$ and garlic (group IG) for a period of 45 days.

Samples extraction

After anaesthesia with chloral hydrate by intraabdominal way, kidneys (twenty/group) were carefully dissected out for weight, biochemical, oxidative stress and histological analysis. All blood samples were withdrawn from the brachial artery of young rats. Some parts of them were collected on EDTA treated tube for haematological parameters determination using a Coulter Maxem machine and the rest others were centrifuged at 2200 g for 15 min. All kidneys and serum samples were kept at -80°C until analysis.

Biochemical and histological studies

Serum biochemical analysis: Serum samples were collected for iron and total bilirubin analysis using Hitachi 912 kits analyser. Commercial kits from Roche laboratories were respectively used for iron (ref: 11970747 216) and total bilirubin (ref: 11877976 190) analysis. Serum creatinin, urea and acid uric determination was realized using photometric method.

Kidney cytosol extraction: Kidneys (ten/group) were utilized for cytosol extraction. Cells fraction was realized after adding 10 ml of KCl (1.15%) to 1g of kidney by using ultra-turrax at 4°C temperature.

ABTS assay in kidney cytosol samples: The Trolox equivalent antioxidant capacity (TEAC) assay is measuring the reduction of the ABTS radical cation by antioxidants. ABTS radical cation (ABTS+) was produced by reacting 7mM ABTS stock solution with 140 mM potassium persulfate and allowing the mixture to stand in the dark at room temperature for 12-16 h before use. For the study, ABTS+ solution was diluted with ethanol to an absorbance of 0.70 (±0.02) at 734 nm. After addition of 1ml of diluted ABTS+ solution to 50µl of kidney cytosol, or Trolox standard, the reaction mixture was incubated for 2 min in a glass cuvette at 30°C. The decrease in absorbance was recorded at 734 nm. All measurements were performed in triplicate. The free radical scavenging capacity of the biological sample, calculated as inhibition percentage of ABTS+, was equated against a Trolox standard curve prepared with different concentrations (40-200 µmol/l). The results are expressed as mM of Trolox equivalents.

Kidney TBARS determination: As a marker of lipid peroxidation, the TBARS (thiobarbituric acid-reactive substances) concentrations were measured in kidney homogenates using the method of Park and his collaborators [19]. For this, 200 ml of a 10% (w/v) tissue homogenate solution was mixed with 600 ml of distilled H_2O and 200 ml of 8.1% (w/v) SDS, vortexed, and incubated for 5 min at room temperature. The reaction mixture was heated at 95°C for 1 h after the addition of 1.5ml of 20% acetic acid (pH 3.5) and 1.5ml of 0.8% (w/v) TBA. After cooling the reaction, 1ml of distilled water and 5ml of butanol:pyridine (15:1) solution were added and vortexed. The mixture was centrifuged at 1935×g for 15min and the resulting colored layer was measured at 532 nm using malondialdehyde (MDA) made by the hydrolysis of 3-tetramethoxypropane as standard.

Bradford kidney cytosol analysis: For protein determination samples were brought to a volume of 800 µl with water. Next, 200 µl of Bradford reagent (Bio-Rad laboratories catalog number 500-0006) was added to each sample to bring it to a volume of 1 ml. The samples were then analyzed in a Beckman spectrophotometer to determine their absorbance at 595 nm. Kidney protein concentrations were calculated using a standard serum albumin bovine (BSA) curve prepared with different concentrations (0-20 µg/ml).

Kidney histopathological analysis: Three kidneys were randomly selected from each group for light microscopy. They were taken and immediately fixed in a Bouin solution, embedded in paraffin and serially sectioned at 5 µm. Then, the sections were stained with hematoxylin eosin (HE) for routine histological examination, with PAS for glycoprotein revelation and with Perls' Prussian blue for iron sedimentation.

Statistical analysis: Comparisons of mean values between rats treated groups (I and IG) and control group (C) or between treated rats (group IG) and (group I). Statistical differences were calculated using a one-way analysis of variance (ANOVA) using SPSS13 logiciel, followed by Student's t-test. Statistical significance was defined as a P value of less than 0.05. Values were expressed as the means followed by ecartype.

Results

Growth and feeding

Body growth rate variation: Animals used for all groups have, at the beginning of the experience; no body weights significant differences (Table 1). During the studied period a regular increase in body growth rate was noted. However, the body growth rates of groups I and IG were more important than that of controls (Table 1). Indeed, at the sacrifice day, we have obtained respectively a significant increase by 12.5 ± 0.06 % and 6 ± 0.6 % in group I and IG rats' body weights comparatively to controls (Table 1). For group G, no difference was obtained comparatively to control rats.

Food and water consumption: Food and water consumptions were decreased in group I and IG rats. In fact, we have obtained a decrease in food consumption respectively by 55 ± 0.2 % and 48 ± 0.12 % and in water by 39 ± 0.22 % and 23 ± 0.14 % (Table 1). For group G, food and water consumptions were at the same order of magnitude comparatively to controls (Table 1).

Haematological parameters: For group I, all haematological parameters showed a decrease comparatively to control group C. Indeed, red blood cells, haemoglobin and hematocrite significantly decreased by 5 ± 0.02; 6 ± 0.08 and 19 ± 1.02% respectively. In rats of group G, we had found a decrease by 11 ± 0.12 and 7 ± 0.08% in red blood cells number and in haemoglobin levels in comparison to control rats and a partial recovery of hematocrite (Table 2). After both iron and garlic treatment (group IG), a partial recovery, without reaching control levels, in red blood cells and haemoglobin was noted and an increase by 6 ± 0.06 and 23 ± 0.12 % in hematocrite comparatively to group I and group G (Table 2).

Serum biochemical parameters: After iron treatment, group I rats showed a significant increase by 11 ± 0.09%; 33 ± 0.13% 10 ± 0.12% and 19± 0.20% in serum iron, total bilirubin, creatinine and urea levels, respectively (Table , Figure 1). After garlic treatment and comparatively to control group, serum iron total bilirubin and urea levels showed no changes but creatinine increased by 11 ± 0.13%. However, for group IG these parameters reached those of control rats (Table, Figure 1). Acid uric, in group I increased by 13± 0.13 and in G and IG groups, decreased by 23; 42 ± 0.68 and 68 ± 0.15%, respectively, comparatively to control group C (Figure 1).

Kidney weights: We have obtained an increase in kidney weights by 14 ± 0.12 and 11.5 ± 0.08% of treated rats of groups I and IG respectively comparatively to control group C. For rats treated by iron and garlic (group IG), kidney weights were 26.5 ± 0.05% less than those of group I rats and 13 ± 0,16% superior than those of group G. Group G kidney weights, show no difference comparatively to control ones' (Figure 2).

Kidney biochemical analysis: In kidneys of rats of group I, a significant increase by 10 ± 0.10 and 55 ± 0.07% of protein and MDA concentrations was obtained but total antioxidant capacity showed an important decrease by 56 ± 0.11% comparatively to control group C (Figure 2). After garlic treatment (group G) we had obtained a decrease (19 ± 1.67 and 54 ± 0.85%) in protein and MDA concentrations and an increase (24 ± 0.29%) in total antioxidant capacity comparatively to controls. For rats of group IG, protein and MDA kidney concentrations decreased by 4 ± 0.05; 19 ± 0.08% and by 14 ± 0.03 and 64 ± 0.05% comparatively to controls and group I, respectively and increased by 15 ± 0.09 and 44 ± 0.45% comparatively to group G rats. However, kidneys total antioxidant capacity significantly increased by 51 ± 0.09% comparatively to group I without reaching that of control group C and decreased comparatively to group G by 33 ± 0.75% (Figure 2).

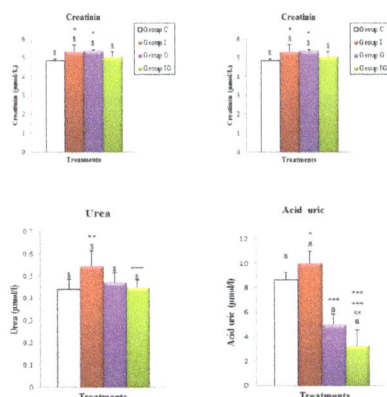

Figure 1: Creatinin (μmol/l), urea (μmol/l), and acid uric (μmol/l) serum contents of young rats: controls (group C) and treated for a period of 45 days by FeCl$_2$ (group I), by garlic (group G) or by both FeCl$_2$ and garlic (group IG). Treated I, G and IG vs controls C:*: P ≤ 0.05; **: P ≤ 0.01; ***: P ≤ 0.001, Treated IG vs treated I: +++: P ≤ 0.01, Treated IG vs treated G: xx:P ≤ 0.01

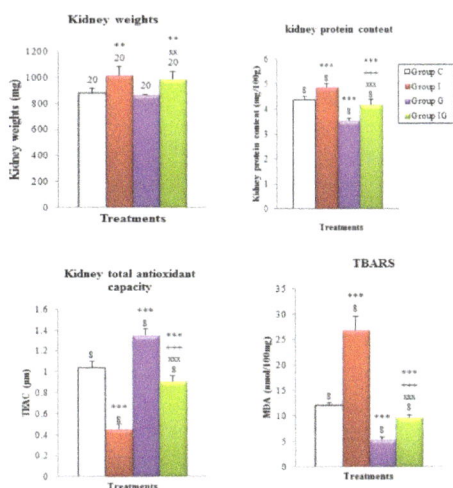

Figure 2: Kidney weights (mg), protein content (mg/100g), TEAC (μmol) and TBARS (nmol/l) kidney contents of young rats: controls (group C) and treated for a period of 45 days by FeCl$_2$ (group I), by garlic (group G) or by both FeCl$_2$ and garlic (group IG). Treated I, G and IG vs controls C: **: P≤0.01; ***: P ≤ 0.001, Treated IG vs treated I: +++: P ≤ 0.01, Treated IG vs treated G:xx:P ≤ 0.01; xxx: P≤0.001

Kidney histology: After hematoxylin-eosine and PAS staining, kidney glomeruli tissue group C rats showed normal cellularity, cell nuclei are not clustered or overlapping. The tubules are almost back to back and the tubular basement membranes are almost touching with a very little interstitium in the cortex (Figures 3C and 4C). Whereas, in iron treated group, we had observed some shrunken proximal tubules and hydropic epithelial cell damages (Figure 3I). Some tubules and glomeruli are collapsed (Figure 3I); others are surrounded by thickened tubular and glomeruli basement membranes (Figure 4I).

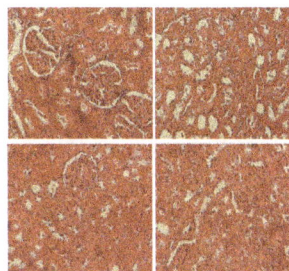

Figure 3: Haematoxyline eosin kidney-stained sections of young rats: controls (C) and treated for a period of 45 days by FeCl$_2$ (group I), by garlic (group G) or by both FeCl$_2$ and garlic (group IG). G: glomeruli, T: tubules, SPT: shrunken proximal tubules, CT: collapsed tubules, CG: collapsed glomeruli, LC: Large cavities, CBS: closed bowman space, (Gx400)

Note the laminated appearance of some tubular basement membrane segments as well as the abrupt attenuation of others in the same tubule (Figure 4I). Distal tubules delimited large clear cavities (Figure 3I, 4I). Glomeruli sizes, were little than those observed in control group with closed bowman space (Figures 3I and 4I). For rats of group G and IG, hematoxilin-eosine and PAS staining kidney sections showed the same histological aspect of controls ones' (Figures 3G; 3IG and 4G; 4IG).

The Perls' Prussian blue kidney stained sections of iron treated rats (group I) showed iron deposition in tubules comparatively to control and garlic treated groups (Figures 5C and 5I). For groups G and IG no iron deposition was observed (Figures 5G and 5IG).

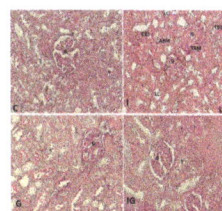

Figure 4: PAS kidney-stained sections of young rats: controls (C) and treated for a period of 45 days by FeCl$_2$ (group I), by garlic (group G) or by both FeCl$_2$ and garlic (group IG). TBM: thickened basement membranes, ABM: attenuation basement membranes, LC: Large cavities, CBS: closed bowman space, (Gx400).

Discussion

Iron is an integral part of a diverse array of biologically active molecules, which form key components of homeostatic processes that are central to life [20]. Iron homeostasis must be maintained so that cells have sufficient iron for cell growth, but not excess due to its toxicity [21].

In this study, group I treated rats showed increased serum iron concentration. This result could be explained by a total iron passage across the enterocytes apical membrane transporters divalent metal transporter 1 (DMT1) to the blood [22]. This important passage of iron via intestine provoked iron accumulation in many organs especially kidney. Indeed, acute kidney injuries after iron excess has been confirmed by several studies [23,24] but little is known about iron kidney functional impairment and garlic protective effects.

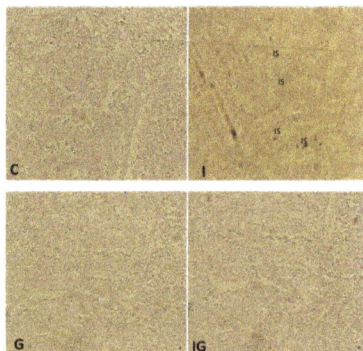

Figure 5: Perls' Prussian blue kidney-stained sections of young rats: controls (C) and treated for a period of 45 days by $FeCl_2$ (group I), by garlic (group G) or by both $FeCl_2$ and garlic (group IG). IS: Iron sedimentation, (Gx400).

The human diet, which contains large number of natural compounds, is essential in protecting the body against the development of diseases, and garlic is one of the well-known plants with remarkable antioxidant properties [7,12] and inhibitory effects on iron availability [25]. For group IG treated rats, the consumption of garlic decreased serum iron levels. This result was confirmed by the study of Ma and collaborators [26] suggesting that the Bioactive garlic polyphenols inhibit iron absorption in a dose-dependent manner in human intestinal Caco-2 cells. Moreover, Tuntipopipat and his collaborators [25] confirmed that garlic polyphenolic compounds are able, in a dose-dependent manner, to inhibit iron absorption by forming iron complexes in the intestine, making dietary iron less available for absorption.

At the beginning of our experiments, no significant body weight differences between control and treated group I rats were observed. But after forty-five days (sacrifice day) of iron treatment we had obtained a significant increase in body weights comparatively to controls. This result could not be explained by food consumption because we had found a significant decrease in daily food and water intakes. But, it may be explained, as demonstrated by previous studies, by the disturbance of endogenous insulin glucose and lipid metabolism [27,28] or by a general stimulation of collagen production [29]. However, at the sacrifice day of garlic treated rats (group G), we had found no changed body growth rate, food and water consumptions comparatively to those of controls'. In comparison, to group IG rats, for which we have obtained a decrease in body weights despite the relative increase in daily food and water consumptions. The decrease in body weights of rats of group IG comparatively to rats' of group I could be explained by a decrease in collagen production or by endogenous insulin glucose and lipid metabolism equilibration [30].

For kidney function, we had found in group I treated rats important increase in serum creatinine and urea comparatively to control group C. These results are similar to those found by Kadkhodaee and collaborators [31] who had demonstrated that rats iron dextran treatment produced kidney injuries and elevation of plasma creatinine

and urea levels. As well, Petrak and collaborators [15] identified increased levels of three enzymes of urea cycle (carbamomyl-phosphate synthase, ornithine carbamoyl transferase and arginase) in mice iron overload. These perturbations of biochemical renal function biomarkers may be explained by the important increase of oxidative stress resulted from excess iron filtration and transport via nephron. Indeed, our results showed that in iron treated group I, lipid peroxidation was importantly increased and total antioxidant capacity was significantly decreased suggesting a negative pool of antioxidant factors in kidney tissue. This result could be explained by the direct implication of iron in kidney injuries and nephrotoxicity via the formation of hydroxyl radicals [32], which play a critical role in acute as well as chronic renal diseases [33]. In fact, oxidative stress and intracellular iron metabolism share the same metabolic pathways and gene products regulated by iron and stress play a crucial role in the maintenance of cellular homeostasis [34]. Moreover, in group I, kidneys were deeply affected by iron transport which induced weights and protein content increase associated to deep histological changes. Indeed, we had observed tubular iron sedimentation, hydropic epithelial cell degeneration, modified tubule aspects and atrophic glomeruli sizes with closed bowman spaces. All these disorders could not only due the oxidative stress induced by iron transport but they also may be a result of intralysosomal storage of iron in the kidney [33].

In group G kidneys', we had found, comparatively to controls, a little increase in creatinine and urea levels and a decrease in protein content and in acid uric levels. Theses biochemical perturbations were obtained in absence of any histological changes. In fact, the histological aspect of group G kidneys' hadn't changed comparatively to control ones'. This result could be explained by improvement of the antioxidant status. Indeed, MDA concentration was significantly decreased and total antioxidant capacity was importantly increased. According, to this experimental design, the daily ingested quantities of garlic seem to have some negative effects on kidney histological aspect.

After garlic adjunction to iron treated rats (group IG), the daily ingested quantities of garlic were sufficient to protect kidney from iron increase damages. Indeed, we had obtained decreased creatinin, urea and MDA levels associated with increased renal total antioxidant capacity suggesting improvement of total renal antioxidant status and normal histological aspect. These results confirmed previous data of Pedraza-Chaverri and collaborators [35] who have demonstrated that garlic, by its antioxidant power, has nephroprotective properties, which have been attributed to the active compound S-allyl cysteine (SAC) [36]. According to Hassan and collaborators [37], garlic oil treatment induced a clear improvement of kidney function, due to its antioxidant properties in scavenging free radicals and reducing levels of lipid peroxidation. SAC is reported to suppress the formation of superoxides, while diallyldisulfide (DADS) and diallylsulfide (DAS) scavenge hydroxyl radicals, thus enhance in vivo endogenous antioxidant system and prevent oxidative stress [38].

For the haematological parameters, we had found, in group I treated rats, an increase in serum acid uric and total bilirubin associated to haematological parameters impairment. Indeed, the reduction in red blood cell (RBC), haemoglobin (Hb) and hematocrite (Ht) obtained in group I treated rats, is a situation of haematological system failure which could be a result of kidney failure. Recently, Weiss and his collaborators [39] showed that chronic renal failure anemia is due to insufficient production of renal erythropoietin. In fact, erythropoietin has been shown to increase transferrin receptor synthesis and cell surface expression in erythroid cells by activating the iron regulatory protein 1. Without sufficient erythropoietin stimulation of the erythroid cell, the number of erythroid cell surface transferrin receptor is probably down-regulated, increasing the likehood of iron uptake by nonerythroid tissues [40]. The increase of total bilirubin obtained in group I rats may be explained by hemolysis of red blood cells induced directly by serum iron increase. In fact, De Gobbi and his collaborators [41] demonstrated that juvenile hemochromatosis is associated to anemia and β thalassemia. As well, Park and Han [16] have obtained a complete hematopoietic recovery after continuous iron chelation therapy in a patient with severe aplastic anemia with secondary hemochromatosis induced by multiple packed red blood cell transfusions. So, kidney failure status obtained in group I could be explained by the association of free heme release after hemolysis and iron excess. Indeed, increased levels of free red blood cell constituents together with an exhaustion of their scavengers induced renal tubular damage [42].

In group G, the daily consumed doses of garlic induced a decrease in red blood cells and in hemoglobin concentrations and an increase in total bilirubin. These results showed that the consumption of crude garlic alone induced anemia. This disease was obtained by different mechanisms to those previously demonstrated by serum iron increase. In fact, according to Munday and his collaborators [43] and Oboh [44] crude garlic could either induces hemolytic anemia or shortens the half-live of red blood cells than the controls.

For garlic and iron treated rats (group IG), the daily consumed doses of garlic were able to induce an amelioration in all erythrocyte parameters associated to decreased total bilirubin serum levels. These results could be explained by the fact that garlic consumed quantities were appropriate to prevent hematological parameter disorders and to protect from kidney failure as it was previously demonstrated.

In conclusion, the results obtained in this study confirmed our hypothesis and showed the positive interactive effects between crude garlic consumption and iron increase in protecting rats from hematological disorders and chronic kidney failure.

Acknowledgments

This research was supported by the Laboratory of Physiology in Superior Institute of Biotechnology of Sfax Tunisia and the Laboratory of Environnemental Bioproceeds in Center of Biotechnology by EEC contract ICA3-CT2002-1003, and the 'Contracts Programmes SERST', Tunisia.

References

1. Zaino EC (1980) Pathophysiology of thalassemia. Ann N Y Acad Sci 344: 284-304.

2. Weinberg ED (1990) Cellular iron metabolism in health and disease. Drug Metab Rev 22: 531-579.

3. Bonkovsky HL (1991) Iron and the liver. Am J Med Sci 301: 32-43.

4. Zager RA (2005) Parenteral iron treatment induces MCP-1 accumulation in plasma, normal kidneys, and in experimental nephropathy. Kidney Int 68: 1533-1542.

5. Zager RA, Johnson AC, Hanson SY (2004) Parenteral iron nephrotoxicity: potential mechanisms and consequences. Kidney Int 66: 144-156.

6. Breborowicz A, Polubinska A, Górna K, Breborowicz M, Oreopoulos DG (2006) Iron sucrose induced morphological and functional changes in the rat kidney. Transl Res 148: 257-262.

7. Craig W, Beck L (1999) Phytochemicals: Health Protective Effects. Can J Diet Pract Res 60: 78-84.

8. Bordia A, Bansal HC, Arora SK, Singh SV (1975) Effect of the essential oils of garlic and onion on alimentary hyperlipemia. Atherosclerosis 21: 15-19.

9. Jain RC, Vyas CR (1975) Garlic in alloxan-induced diabetic rabbits. Am J Clin Nutr 28: 684-685.

10. Bordia A, Verma SK (1980) Effect of garlic feeding on regression of experimental atherosclerosis in rabbits. Artery 7: 428-437.

11. Banerjee SK, Mukherjee PK, Maulik SK (2003) Garlic as an antioxidant: the good, the bad and the ugly. Phytother Res 17: 97-106.

12. Agarwal MK, Iqbal M, Athar M (2007) Garlic oil ameliorates ferric nitrilotriacetate (Fe-NTA)-induced damage and tumor promotion: implications for cancer prevention. Food Chem Toxicol 45: 1634-1640.

13. Tattelman E1 (2005) Health effects of garlic. Am Fam Physician 72: 103-106.

14. Agarwal R, Vasavada N, Sachs NG, Chase S (2004) Oxidative stress and renal injury with intravenous iron in patients with chronic kidney disease. Kidney Int 65: 2279-2289.

15. Petrak J, Myslivcova D, Man P, Cmejla R, Cmejlova J, et al. (2007) Proteomic analysis of hepatic iron overload in mice suggests dysregulation of urea cycle, impairment of fatty acid oxidation, and changes in the methylation cycle. Am J Physiol Gastrointest. Liver Physiol. 292: G1490-G1498.

16. Park SJ, Han CW (2008) Complete hematopoietic recovery after continuous iron chelation therapy in a patient with severe aplastic anemia with secondary hemochromatosis. J Korean Med Sci 23: 320-323.

17. Akgül B, Lin KW, Ou Yang HM, Chen YH, Lu TH, et al. (2010) Garlic accelerates red blood cell turnover and splenic erythropoietic gene expression in mice: evidence for erythropoietin-independent erythropoiesis. PLoS One 5: e15358.

18. Bagheri F, Gol A, Dabiri S, Javadi A (2011) Preventive effect of garlic juice on renal reperfusion injury. Iran J Kidney Dis 5: 194-200.

19. Park SY, Bok SH, Jeon SM, Park YB, Lee SJ, et al, (2002) Effect of rutin and tannic acid supplements on cholesterol metabolism in rats. Nutr Res. 22: 283-295.

20. Wareing M, Ferguson CJ, Green R, Riccardi D, Smith CP (2000) In vivo characterization of renal iron transport in the anaesthetized rat. J Physiol 524 Pt 2: 581-586.

21. De Domenico I, Ward DM, Kaplan J (2007) Hepcidin regulation: ironing out the details. J Clin Invest 117: 1755-1758.

22. Bleackley MR, Wong AY, Hudson DM, Wu CH, Macgillivray RT (2009) Blood iron homeostasis: newly discovered proteins and iron imbalance. Transfus Med Rev 23: 103-123.

23. Kudo H, Suzuki S, Watanabe A, Kikuchi H, Sassa S, et al. (2008) Effects of colloidal iron overload on renal and hepatic siderosis and the femur in male rats. Toxicology 246: 143-147.

24. Haase M, Bellomo R, Haase-Fielitz A (2010) Novel biomarkers, oxidative stress, and the role of labile iron toxicity in cardiopulmonary bypass-associated acute kidney injury. J Am Coll Cardiol 55: 2024-2033.

25. Tuntipopipat S, Zeder C, Siriprapa P, Charoenkiatkul S (2009) Inhibitory effects of spices and herbs on iron availability. Int J Food Sci Nutr 60 Suppl 1: 43-55.

26. Ma Q, Kim EY, Lindsay EA, Han O (2011) Bioactive dietary polyphenols inhibit heme iron absorption in a dose-dependent manner in human intestinal Caco-2 cells. J Food Sci 76: H143-150.

27. Lonardo A (1999) Fatty liver and nonalcoholic steatohepatitis. Where do we stand and where are we going? Dig Dis 17: 80-89.

28. Sanyal AJ, Campbell-Sargent C, Mirshahi F, Rizzo WB, Contos MJ, et al, (2001) Nonalcoholic steatohepatitis: association of insulin resitance and mitochondria abnormalities. Gastroenterology 120: 1281-1285.

29. Gardi C, Arezzini B, Fortino V, Comporti M (2002) Effect of free iron on collagen synthesis, cell proliferation and MMP-2 expression in rat hepatic stellate cells. Biochem Pharmacol 64: 1139-1145.

30. Baluchnejadmojarad T, Roghani M, Homayounfar H, Hosseini M (2003) Beneficial effect of aqueous garlic extract on the vascular reactivity of streptozotocin-diabetic rats. J Ethnopharmacol 85: 139-144.

31. Kadkhodaee M, Gol A (2004) The role of nitric oxide in iron-induced rat renal injury. Hum Exp Toxicol 23: 533-536.

32. Baliga R, Zhang Z, Baliga M, Ueda N, Shah SV (1998) In vitro and in vivo evidence suggesting a role for iron in cisplatin-induced nephrotoxicity. Kidney Int 53: 394-401.

33. Dimitriou E, Kairis M, Sarafidou J, Michelakakis H (2000) Iron overload and kidney lysosomes. Biochim Biophys Acta 1501: 138-148.

34. Fonseca AM, Preira CF, Porto GA, Arosa FA (2003) Red blood cells upregulate cytoprotective proteins and the labile iron pool in dividing human T cells despite a reduction in oxidative stress free Radical Biology & Medicine. 35: 1404-1416.

35. Pedraza-Chaverrí J, Barrera D, Maldonado PD, Chirino YI, Macías-Ruvalcaba NA, et al. (2004) Sallylmercaptocysteine scavenges hydroxyl radical and singlet oxygen in vitro and attenuates gentamicininduced oxidative and nitrosative stress and renal damage in vivo. BMC Clin Pharmacol 4: 5.

36. Reddy GD, Reddy AG, Rao GS, Haritha C, Jyothi K (2010) Interaction study on garlic and atorvastatin with reference to nephrotoxicity in dyslipidaemic rats. Toxicol Int 17: 90-93.

37. Hassan HA, El-Agmy SM, Gaur RL, Fernando A, Raj MH, et al. (2009) In vivo evidence of hepato- and reno-protective effect of garlic oil against sodium nitrite-induced oxidative stress. Int J Biol Sci 5: 249-255.

38. Chung LY (2006) The antioxidant properties of garlic compounds: allyl cysteine, alliin, allicin, and allyl disulfide. J Med Food 9: 205-213.

39. Weiss G, Houston T, Kastner S, Jöhrer K, Grünewald K (1997) Regulation of cellular iron metabolism by erythropoietin: activation of iron-regulatory protein and upregulation of transferrin receptor expression in erythroid cells. Blood. 89: 680-7.

40. Joseph JA, Shukitt-Hale B, McEwen J, Rabin B (1999) Magnesium activation of GTP hydrolysis or incubation in S-adenosyl-l-methionine reverses iron-56-particle-induced decrements in oxotremorine enhancement of K+-evoked striatal release of dopamine. Radiat Res 152: 637-641.

41. De gobbi M, Pasquero P, Brunello F, Paccotti F, Mazza U, et al. (2000) Juvenile hemochromatosis associated with ß-thalassemia treated by phlebotomy and recombinant human erythropoietin. Haematologica. 85: 865-867.

42. Ricci Z, Picca S, Guzzo I, Ronco C (2011) Kidney diseases beyond nephrology: intensive care. Nephrol Dial Transplant 26: 448-454.

43. Munday R, Munday JS, Munday CM (2003) Comparative effects of mono-, di-, tri-, and tetrasulfides derived from plants of the Allium family: redox cycling in vitro and hemolytic activity and Phase 2 enzyme induction in vivo. Free Radic Biol Med 34: 1200-1211.

44. Oboh G (2004) Prevention of garlic-induced hemolytic anemia using some tropical green leafy vegetables. J Med Food 7: 498-501.

30

Attenuation of CCl$_4$ Induced Oxidative Stress, Immunosuppressive, Hepatorenal Damage by Fucoidan in Rats

Mohamed E. El-Boshy[1,2*], **Fatma Abdelhamidb**[1], **Engy Richab**[1], **Ahmad Ashshia**[1], **Mazen Gaitha**[2] and **Naeem Qustya**[2]

[1]*Laboratory Medicine Department, Faculty of Applied Medical Science, Umm Al-Qura University, Makkah, Saudi Arabia*

[2]*Clinical Pathology Department, Faculty of Veterinary Medicine, Mansoura University Mansoura, Egypt*

*Corresponding author: Mohamed E. El-Boshy, Clinical Pathology Department, Faculty of Veterinary Medicine, Mansoura University Mansoura, Egypt, E-mail: drelboshy@yahoo.com

Abstract

The protective and therapeutic effects of fucoidan extract from Laminaria species against liver damage induced by CCl$_4$ in rats was investigated by monitoring the serum level and hepatic m-RNA expression of TGFβ-1, liver and renal markers, as well as oxidative stress and antioxidant biomarker. Thirty six adult male albino rats were divided into 4 equal groups; one was used as a negative control while groups II, III, and IV administrated 0.1 mL/100 g body weight twice a week for 8 weeks with carbon tetrachloride (CCl$_4$), fucoidan (400 mg/kgbw orally/day), and CCl$_4$ plus fucoidan, respectively. Blood samples were collected at the end of experiment and sera were separated to evaluate serum levels and the hepatic m-RNA expression of transforming growth factor beta (TGFβ-1), tumor necrosis factor (TNF α), interferon gamma (IFN-γ.), interleukin (IL), Il-1β, IL-6 and IL-10, antioxidant markers, reduced glutathione (GSH), superoxide dismutase (SOD), catalase (CAT), glutathione peroxidase (GPx) and lipid peroxidation malondialdehyde (MDA) as well as selective biochemical markers of liver and kidney functions were estimated. The results of this investigation revealed that treatment with fucoidan improved elevated expression of liver TGF β-1, Il-1β, IL-6, TNF α and serum level of malnoaldehyde (MDA), total bilirubin (T. Bil), induced by CCl$_4$ at 8th week post treatment. In addition to enhancing the antioxidant enzyme activities, GSH, GPx, CAT and SOD. Also, liver trransaminase (ALT, AST), alkaline phosphatase (ALP), reduced in fucoidan and CCl$_4$ treated group. These results show that crude fucoidan has potential immunomodulatory, antioxidant and hepatoprotective effects against the hepatic damage induced by CCl$_4$.

Keywords: Fucoidan; CCl$_4$; Hepatoprotective; Oxidative stress; Cytokine; Rats

Introduction

Liver diseases are among some of the fatal diseases in the world today, they pose a serious challenge to international public health. Hepatic fibrosis is a wound healing response to chronic liver injury which is characterized by a net accumulation of extracellular matrix (ECM) including collagen, glycoproteins, and protoglycan [1-3]. Hepatic stellate cells (HSCs), previously known as Ito cell that under physiological conditions stores 80% of retinoids (vitamin A), are the cytological base of hepatic fibrosis. The quiescent HSC is transformed with progressive injury into myofibroblast like cells that are characterized by the appearance of cytoskeleton protein α smooth muscle actin (α SMA) and collagen-I considered as a biomarker for HSCs activation. TGFβ-1 is a key molecule and an important fibrogenic cytokine that facilitates the activation of HSCs and converts it from static HSCs to the phenotype of myofibroblast to express α SMA and possess the character of contraction [4-6].

Carbon tetrachloride, CCl$_4$ has been a frequently used chemical to experimentally induced hepatic fibrosis. Depending on the dose and duration, the effect of CCl$_4$ on hepatocytes is manifested histologically as hepatic statues, fibrosis, hepatocellular death and carcinogenici. The hepatotoxic effect of CCl$_4$ is attributed to its immediate cleavage by cytochrome P450 (CYP2E1) in hepatocytes, which generates trichloromethyl radicals leading to lipid peroxidation and subsequently to membrane damage. The activated Kupffer cell produces toxic metabolites (inflammatory cytokines and reactive oxygen intermediates which results in the injury of hepatic parenchymal cells [7-11].

Fucoidans, is a sulfated polysaccharide extracted from the cell wall of brown algae and some marine invertebrates. It contains substantial percentages of L-fucose and sulfate ester groups, thus called Vulcan, fucosan or sulfated fucan. Recently, fucoidan has been extensively studied due to its numerous biological activities including anticoagulant, antithrombotic, antitumor, antiviral, anti-parasitic, anti-complement, antioxidant, and anti-inflammatory activities. In addition, it is used as immunomodulatory and blood lipid reducing agent, and has acted against hepatorenalpathy and possesses gastric protective effect. Moreover, Fucoidan extracted from the brown seaweed Laminaria japonica had a hepatoprotective effect [11-14].

The aim of the present study is to evaluate the hepatoprotective effect of fucoidan on liver fibrosis induced by CCl$_4$ in rats, through detection of gene expression and serum cytokines of TGFβ-1, IL1β, IL-6, TNF α, IFN-γ and IL-10, in addition to oxidative stress reactions and biochemical hepatorenal markers.

Material and methods

Experimental animals

Thirty two, 1-2 month old male albino rats were involved in the present study. The rats were kept in galvanized zinc-plate cages under strict hygienic conditions and were ensured free from any infection.

The rats were maintained for one week on a pelleted diet and water ad Libitam before starting the experiment for acclimatization. The experiment was approved according to the ethical committee of our college.

Chemicals

CCl_4 was purchased from Sigma Aldrich (Co, USA), Primer sequences for PCR amplification The primer of selected pro-inflammatory cytokines were obtained from (Thermo scientific Co. USA) as displayed in Table 1. Fucoidan extract of Laminaria species received as a powder from Sigma Aldrich was used as a freshly prepared solution dissolved in normal saline.

Fibrosis induction and treatment

Rats were divided into 4 groups (with 8 rats in each group) and treated for 8 weeks as follows: Group I served as a normal control received only 0.1 mL/100 g BW of olive oil. Group II, on the other hand, was treated with fucoidan at a dose of 400 mg/kg BW/day and olive oil all over the duration of the experiment according to, while the rats in Group III were intraperitoneal (IP) injected with a mixture of CCl_4 (0.1 mL/100 g body weight) and olive oil [1: 1 (v/v)] every other day for 8 weeks as described by Fue et al., and Group IV was treated with fucoidan and CCl_4. Blood samples were collected individually from heart puncture for serum chemistry, rats were then sacrificed and specimen from liver were cut in pieces and kept in liquid nitrogen for reverse transcriptase polymerase chain reaction (RT-PCR) analyses.

RT-PCR analysis

Expressions of mRNAs for the proinflammatory cytokines, TGF-β1, IL-1β, IL-6, TNF-α, IL-10 and TNF-α, were quantified by real-time RT-PCR. Total RNA was isolated from liver specimens using the RNA Easy kit (QIAamp Blood Kit; Qiagen GmbH, Hilden, Germany), according to the stander technique. The extracted RNA was dissolved in 30 μL nuclease-free distilled water and stored at -30°C until used. The concentration and purity of RNA were determined by Nanodrop Spectrophotometer (Thermo Scientific, USA). Preparation of the RNA / primer mixture was achieved by adding an RNA template. Real-time PCR was performed using 2 μL templates in a 20-μL reaction containing 0.25 μM of each primer and 12.5 μL Sybr Green. The mixture was incubated at 70-75°C for 5-10 min and then placed at room temperature for 5-10 min for denaturation and primer annealing. The RT-PCR mixture was prepared and completed by adding 10 μL of RNA/primer mixture. The thermal profiles that were used consisted of denaturation at 95°C, for 15 s, 60°C for 20 s, and 72°C for 60 s followed by 45 cycles of 95°C for 15s, and a final elongation at 72°C, in a real-time PCR machine (Applied Bio-system Thermo Fisher, USA). The quantitative mRNA expression level of targeted pro-inflammatory cytokines were estimated by determining the cycle threshold (CT), which is the number of PCR cycles required for the fluorescence to exceed a value significantly higher than the background fluorescence. The reference gene, glyceraldehyde-3-phosphate dehydrogenase (GAPDH), was used as a control. The selective cytokine gene expression was calculated using the 2-CT according to Livak and Schmittgen (2001).

Serum cytokine analysis

Elective humoral immunological parameters, such as transforming growth factor-beta (TGF-β), tumor necrosis factor – α (TNF α),

interleukin -6, (IL-6), IL-1 β, IL-10, and gamma interferon (IFN-γ.) were determined by Enzyme Amplified Sensitivity Immunoassay (EASIA, R & D Systems, Minneapolis, MN, USA) using microplates according to enclosed pamphlets (Human Quateo- ELICYS, Germany).

Liver antioxidant analysis

Liver specimens were rapidly detached, rinsed in ice cold saline buffer (20 mM Tris–HCl, 0.14 M NaCl buffer, pH 7.4) and homogenized in the saline buffer (10%, w/v). The homogenate aliquots were kept at -30 °C for MDA and antioxidant markers estimation. The oxidative stress marker, MDA and antioxidant system SOD, CAT, GPx, and GSH were determined enzyme linked immunoassay (ELISA), using ready-made kits (Cayman. Co. USA) according to the enclosed pamphlets.

Serum biochemical analysis

Ready frozen serum samples were analyzed for ALT, AST, gamma glutamyl-transferase (GGT), ALP, total bilirubin, direct blirubin, glucose, total protein, albumin, urea, createnine were determined with a semi-automatic spectrophotometer (BM-Germany 5010) using commercial test kits (Randox Co. UK) according to stander laboratory method.

Statistical analysis

Data were analyzed by means of one way ANOVA using the SPSS software statistical program with post-hoc LSD multiple comparison test using SPSS software (SPSS for Windows ver. 21.00, USA). Data are expressed as the mean ± SE, and P<0.05 was considered statistically significant.

Results

Cytokines parameters

The gene expression and serum cytokines TGF- β1, L-1β, TNF α and IL-6 were significantly higher in the CCl_4-treated group at 8th week post treatment as compared with the control rats (Table 2 and Figure 1). On the other hand, no significant changes were observed in the aforementioned cytokine expression and serum levels in fucoidan treated groups when compared with the control group.

Primer Name	Primer Sequence (5′–3′)	Base pairs
TGF- β1- FW	TAT AGC AAC AAT TCC TGG CG	162
TGF- β1- RW	TGC TGT CAC AGG AGC AGT G	
IL-1β-FW	CAC CTT CTT TTC CTT CAT CTT TG	73
IL-1β-RW	GTC GTT GCT TGT CTC TCC TTG TA	
IL-6-FW	TGA TGG ATG CTT CCA AAC TG	32
IL-6-RW	GAG CAT TGG AAG TTG GGG TA	
TNF-α-FW	ACT GAA CTT CGG GGT GAT TG	84
TNF-α-RW	GCT TGG TGG TTT GCT ACG AC	
IFN-γ	TGG CAT AGA TGT GGA AGA AAA -	75

IFN-γ- RW	TGC AGG ATT TTC ATG TCA CCA -	
IL-10-FW	TGC CTT CAG TCA AGT GAA GAC	74
IL-10-RW	AAA CTC ATT CAT GGC CTT GTA	

Table 1: Primers used for Real- time PCR Amplification.

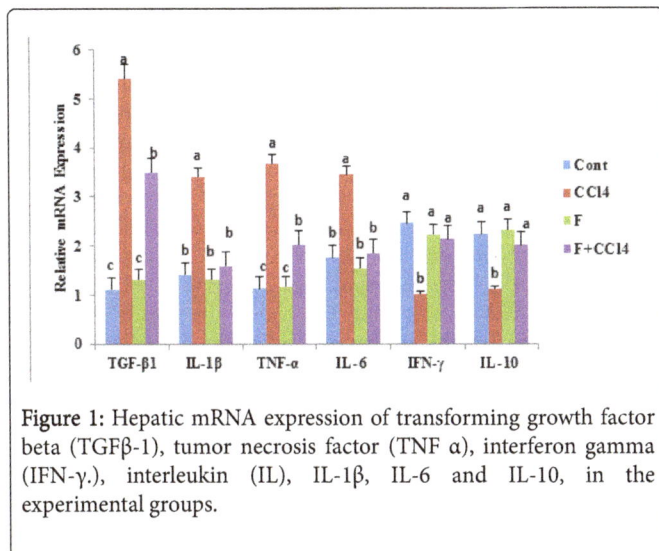

Figure 1: Hepatic mRNA expression of transforming growth factor beta (TGFβ-1), tumor necrosis factor (TNF α), interferon gamma (IFN-γ.), interleukin (IL), IL-1β, IL-6 and IL-10, in the experimental groups.

Additionally, TGF-β1, L-1β, TNF α and IL-6 expression and serum levels were lower in the fucoidan and CCl₄ treated group than CCl₄ treated group. Also, IFN-γ, was reduced in fucoidan and CCl₄ treated group as compared with CCl₄ group, while IL-10 was non-significant differ between all treated groups, as shown in Table 2.

Parameters (Pg/mL)	Experiment Groups			
	Control	CCl₄	F	F+CCl₄
TGF- β1-	14.1 ± 3.42	35.2 ± 2.01	13.2 ± 1.26	19.5 ± 1.18
IL-1β	38.7 ± 2.52	59.5 ± 3.62	38.7 ± 2.52	49.9 ± 3.82
TNF-α	21.5 ± 2.41	65.2 ± 1.71	22.4 ± 0.45	36.6 ± 0.48
IL-6	19.4 ± 1.84	35.3 ± 0.62	18.5 ± 0.78	20.3 ± 0.64
IFN-γ (Pg/mL)	36.8 ± 2.82	22.4 ± 1.86	38.12 ± 3.99	34.9 ± 3.49
IL-10	12.2 ± 0.32	8.1 ± 0.62	13.1 ± 1.58	10.1 ± 0.32

Table 2: Liver Expression and Serum Cytokines Markers (Mean ± S.E) at 8th week Post Treatment with CCl₄, and Fucoidan.

Antioxidant and lipid peroxidation parameters

Results obtained showed a significant decrease (P<0.05) in antioxidant markers, GSH, CAT, SOD and GPx in the CCl₄-treated group when compared with the control rats. In addition, lipid peroxidation MDA was significantly higher in CCl₄-treated group when compared with the other experimental group. On the other hand, treatment with fucoidan alone caused a significant increase in GSH, and CAT as compared with the control group. The antioxidant markers, GSH, CAT, GPx and lipid peroxidation (MDA), did not

significantly differ in fucoidan and CCl₄ treated group from those of the control group as displayed in Table 3.

Parameters	Experiment Groups			
	Control	CCl₄	F	F+CCl₄
MDA	65.1 ± 3.09	87.4 ± 4.01	68.25 ± 4.36	70.5 ± 5.08
GSH	71.5 ± 3.54	38.8 ± 3.51	82.25 ± 3.66	66.6 ± 4.96
GPx	9.5 ± 0.94	6.45 ± 0.82	0.45 ± 0.98	8.15 ± 1.54
CAT	3.5 ± 0.62	1.88 ± 0.08	6.65 ± 0.68	3.01 ± 0.23
SOD	221.9 ± 5.10	195.2 ± 4.06	216.2 ± 3.09	200.8 ± 2.06

Table 3: Hepatic Antioxidant and Oxidative Stress Biomarkers (Mean ± S.E) at 8th week post Treatment with CCl₄, and Fucoidan.

Biochemical Parameters

Results presented in Table 4 show a significant increase in the ALT, AST, ALP and GGT serum activities and total bilirubin, as well as urea and creatinin, while there was a significant decrease in albumin and glucose and a non-significant change in total protein in CCl₄-treated group when compared with the control group. All of the aforementioned biochemical markers, did not significantly change in the fucoidan treated group alone, as compared with the control group. Furthermore, the hepatic markers only were improved in fucoidan and CCl₄ treated group when compared with CCl₄ treated group alone, as displayed in Table 4.

Parameters	Experiment Groups			
	Control	CCl₄	F	F+CCl₄
ALT (U/L)	20.5 ± 1.24	34.1 ± 1.23	19.5 ± 1.81	30.3 ± 2.19
AST (U/L)	28.1 ± 1.42	38.9 ± 1.26	29.2 ± 1.34	35.3 ± 2.14
GGT (U/L)	18.5 ± 1.05	65.2 ± 4.25	17.6 ± 1.95	41.3 ± 3.18
ALP (U/L)	10.9 ± 0.54	18.4 ± 0.50	9.8 ± 0.41	16.2 ± 0.42
T. Bili. (mg/dl)	0.48 ± 0.03	0.71 ± 0.04	0.52 ± 0.05	0.65 ± 0.06
Dir. Bili (mg/dl)	0.22 ± 0.02	0.46 ± 0.09	0.24 ± 0.04	0.42 ± 0.06
Glucose (mg/dl)	112.8 ± 2.20	87.2 ± 4.53	109.6 ± 2.52	86.6 ± 4.54
T Protein (gm/dl)	4.45 ± 0.21	4.59 ± 0.30	5.53 ± 0.34	5.24 ± 0.36
Albumin (mg/dl)	3.25 ± 0.18	2.98 ± 0.22	3.16 ± 0.25	3.25 ± 0.21
Urea (mg/dl)	55.8 ± 1.28	69.5 ± 1.45	54.2 ± 1.02	66.6 ± 3.23
Creatinine (mg/dl)	0.51 ± 0.01	0.69 ± 0.02	0.54 ± 0.04	0.68 ± 0.03

Table 4: Hepatorenal Biomarker Profiles (Mean ± S.E) at 8th week Post Treatment with CCl₄, and Fucoidan.

Discussion

The liver plays a central role in metabolic homeostasis, as it is responsible for the metabolism, synthesis, storage and redistribution of nutrients, carbohydrates, fats and vitamins. Importantly, it is the main detoxifying organ of the body, which removes wastes and xenobiotics by metabolic conversion and biliary excretion [13].

CCl_4 metabolism is an established model of liver necrosis and fibrosis. The liver damage caused by this metabolism is free radical dependent as CCl_4 is oxidized by cytochrome P450 to the highly reactive trichloromethyl (CCl_3) radicals that are generated by the reductive cleavage of CCl_4 bond and generated oxygen radicals and phospholipid peroxides. These generated trichloromethyl free radicals cause liver necrosis, destruction of ECM and lipid peroxidation of membranes. Results from this investigation revealed that TGF-β1 mRNA expression increased as fibrosis developed in CCl_4 induced liver fibrosis in treated rats. As TGF-β1 activity is enhanced by proteolytic release and activation of latent TGF-β1 from HSC. Other cells, such as kupffer cells, invading mononuclear cells, myofibroblast cells, and endothelial cells can also synthesize and release TGF-β1. A several studies have confirmed that the stimulation and proliferation of HSCs are the crucial points in the production of ECM, resulted in the differential of HSCs into yofibroblasts with production of α-SMA lead to stable liver fibrosis. Moreover, the results show that serum TGF-β1, TNF, and IL-6 were significantly increased in CCl_4 treated group as compared with the control. Tan et al. recorded significant elevation of pro-inflammatory cytokines IL-6, TNF-α, and IL-1β with hepatic fibrosis in mice treated with CCl_4. In the same line, Ahn et al. observed elevated pro-inflammatory cytokines, including TNF-α and IL-1β, mRNA expression with hepatic damage in rats treated with CCl_4. At the molecular level, CCl_4 activates TNF-α, TGF-β1, and IL-6 production that appear to direct the cell toward destruction or fibrosis, while IL-10 counteract the liver fibrogensis. In this context, Fue et al. and Tan et al. concluded the elevation the inflammatory cytokines have a key role in pathogenesis of liver fibrosis and activation of HSCs [14-22].

Fucoidan, a family of sulphated polyfucose polysaccharides, exhibit a variety of biological properties, anti-inflammatory, antibacterial, immunostimulant and antitumor. The biological effects of fucoidan relate to their polysaccharide backbones and sulfate content. Recently, the antifibrotic activity of fucoidan was reported in an animal model of hepatic fibrosis. The serum's TGF-β1, TNF α and IL-6, in addition to m RNA liver expression, were reduced in rats treated with fucoidan and CCl_4 at 8th week post treatment when compared with CCl_4 rats. This is in agreement with results obtained by Shinji and colleagues who discovered that fucoidan treatment attenuates HSCs activation by inhibiting TGF-β1. Also, Jingjing et al. concluded the fucoidan down regulation of TGF-β1 and reduce the HSCs activation and the formation of ECM. In addition, researchers reported that elevation of reactive oxygen species, is the key to HSC activation and release of inflammatory cytokines. In the same aspect, Park et al. concluded that fucoidan applies anti-inflammatory effects by inhibiting the expression of pro-inflammatory cytokines *in vitro* and *in vivo*, together with a restricted antibacterial effect *in vivo*. Furthermore, fucoidan enhanced the production of pro-inflammatory cytokines, IL-6, IL-8 and TNF-α in human neutrophil and delay neutrophil apoptosis [17-26].

Malondialdehyde is a reactive aldehyde, used as an indicator of the amount of lipid peroxidation. This can be ascribed to the polyunsaturated fatty acids' damage caused by ROS; this damage results in different products, including MDA. In the present study, there was a significant increase in serum MDA concentration in the CCl_4 treated group; this agrees with the findings reported by other researchers. Lipid peroxidation (LPO), is one of the principal causes of CCl_4 induced liver and renal injury. Attack by free radical oxygen species (ROS) on the polyunsaturated fatty acids generates different products, including aldehydic products, resulting eventually in a loss in the membrane's integrity. Antioxidant enzymes such as SOD, CAT, GPx and GSH constitute a helpful team of defense against ROS, hydroperoxide and environmental toxicity. Likewise, glutathione is a first line of defense and scavenges ROS. Additionally, GSH-dependent enzymes offer an important line of protection as they detoxify noxious byproducts generated by ROS. The depletion concentration of GSH in the liver may be due to enhanced GSH utilization in the elimination of peroxides or NADPH reduction activity. Several studies showed that GSH plays a key role in detoxifying the toxic metabolites of CCl_4 and that liver injury begins when GSH stores are markedly depleted. Tan et al. and Ahn et al. observed a significant reduction of the antioxidant system, GSH, CAT, GPx and GR, while marked elevation of lipidperoxidation, MDA in mice and rats treated with CCl_4 respectively. In the present study, marked reduction in the antioxidant system (SOD, CAT, GPx and GSH) in CCl_4 treated groups was observed when compared with the control group. Depletion of the antioxidant system in CCl_4 treated group could be attributed to CCl_4 generated cellular ROS production and the subsequent depletion of the antioxidant cellular system [27-35].

In fucoidan treated group, GSH and CAT were higher than that of the control group; this is due to the antioxidant activities of fucoidan which have been documented by Wang et al. Moreover, fucoidan reduced the lipid peroxidation, MDA elevation in CCl_4 treated groups. This is in line with results obtained by other researchers who found that I/P administration of fucoidan extract resulted in reduced high MDA level induced by CCl4 treatment in rats. On the other hand, Lie et al. reported that fucoidan from *L. japonica* had no effect on lipid peroxidation induced by $FeSO_4$ *in vitro*, and Nakazato et al. have indicated that the crude fucoidan extract did not reduce the high MDA level in liver injury induced by N-nitroso-diethylamine. Our results, however, found an elevation in GSH, CAT and Gpx in rats treated with fucoidan and CCl_4 as compared with CCl_4 group. The increase in these enzyme activities was probably a response towards the increase in ROS generation since fucoidan has strong scavenging free radical activity, especially against superoxide radicals. This is in agreement with the findings of Jing et al. who reported that fucoidan exhibit radical scavenging activity, *in vitro* and antioxidative activity against oxidative stress in cellular model. Moreover, fucoidan has been reported to have a great potential in preventing free radical synthesis that mediates diseases and can prevent the increase of lipid peroxide in the serum, liver and spleen of rats and mice (Lie; Omar et al.,). Furthermore, Phull et al. demonstrated the fucoidan is a potent antioxidant that can effectively repeal oxidative stress and arthritis-mediated inflammation. In addition to, the fucoidan inhibit expression of nitric oxide (NO), and exhibited antioxidant activity by reducing the reactive oxygen species (ROS) in microglia cells (Nguyen et al.). In the same line, Subash et al. recorded the levels of oxidative stress markers SOD, GPx, GSH, were reduced in inflammatory hepatocytes of rats treated orally with dexamethasone and fucoidan (300 mg/kg) [33-40].

CCl_4 administration causes severe liver damage demonstrated by a significant elevation of serum AST and ALT levels till the end of the experiment. This elevation may be attributed to the cellular leakage and damage of structural integrity of the liver cells. Similarly, CCl_4

treatment induced elevation of serum GGT and ALP with high level of total bilirubin, and direct bilirubin, which are considered indicators of cholestasis and pathological alterations of the biliary flow. The highest concentration of direct bilirubin in the serum is an indication of liver injury caused by CCl_4. Similar to results, other research groups reported elevation of liver marker enzymes and bilirubin in rats intoxicated with CCl_4. Additionally, nephrotoxicity of CCl_4 in the present study was manifested by elevation of urea and creatinine serum levels at 8th week post treatment (Table 3) in CCl_4 treated groups, as compared with the control group. This is similar to results obtained by others. In the present study, administration of CCl_4 to normal rats induced hepatic and renal toxicity, as CCl_4 mediated peroxidation of lipid structures, enhances reactive oxygen species (ROS) and depletion of protein content of tissues; this results in sub cellular damage. Total blood protein level insignificantly changed in CCl_4 treatment, while albumin was lower than the control group (Table 3). CCl_4 intoxication leads to hypomethylation of cellular components; in the case of RNA the outcome is thought to be inhibition of protein synthesis. Hypoproteinemia and hypoalbuminemia in rats intoxicated with CCl_4 for 6 weeks have been reported by Al-Yahya et al. In the present study, serum glucose was reduced in CCl_4 a treated animal as hepatic glycogen content was decreased, reflecting decreased gluconeogenesis by the liver. Similar results were obtained by Rui et al., who reported that gluconeogenesis and Krebs cycle fluxes are altered in rat livers following CCl_4 intoxication. The elevation of hepatic biochemical marker enzymes (ALT, AST, ALP, GGT) was reduced in fucoidan and CCl_4 treated groups reveled improve liver function. The hepatoprotective of the fucoidan against CCl_4 toxicity could be due to down regulation of inflammatory mediators and antioxidant activity of the fucoidan [33-43].

Finally, we concluded that crude fucoidan inhibit TGF-β, suppresses hepatic inflammation and attenuates hepatic oxidative stress in rats intoxicated with CCl_4. Fucoidan could be a promising potential agent as a hepatoprotective and treatment of hepatic fibrosis.

References

1. Shi-Ling S, Zuo-Jiong G, Quan-Rang Z, Tuan-Xin H (2005) Effect of Chinese traditional compound JinSanE on expression of TGF-B1 and TGF-B1 type II receptor mRNA, Smad3 and Smad7 on experimental hepatic fibrosis in vivo. World J Gastroenterol 11: 2269-2276.

2. Jingjing L, Kan C, Sainan L, Jiao F, Tong L, et al. (2016) Protective effect of fucoidan from Fucus vesiculosus on liver fibrosis via the TGF-ß1/Smad pathway-mediated inhibition of extracellular matrix and autophagy. Drug Des Devel Ther; 10: 619-630.

3. Tan H, He Q, Li R, Lei F, Lei X (2016) Trillin reduces liver chronic inflammation and fibrosis in carbon tetrachloride (ccl4) induced liver injury in mice. Immunol Invest. 45: 371-382.

4. Jiao J, Friedman SL, Aloman C (2009) Hepatic fibrosis. Curr Opin Gastroenterol 25: 223-229.

5. Heekyoung C, Doo-Pyo H, Ji-Youn J, Hyun-Jun K, Ki-Seok J, et al. (2005) Comprehensive analysis of differential gene expression profiles on carbon tetrachloride-induced rat liver injury and regeneration. Toxicol Appl Pharm 20: 27– 42.

6. Semiha N, Ilkin C, Zehra MF (2006) The effect of vitamin A on CCl_4-induced hepatic injuries in rats: a histochemical, immunohistochemical and ultrastructural study. Acta Histochem 107: 421-434.

7. Ebaid H, Samir AE, Ibrahim MA, Ahmed R, Sultan E (2013) Folic acid and melatonin ameliorate carbon tetrachloride-induced hepatic injury, oxidative stress and inflammation in rats. Nutr Metab 10: 20-29.

8. Chun-Ping C, Ping W, Yang L, Da-Jin Z, Li-Sheng W, et al. (2009) The protective role of hepatopoietin Cn on liver injury induced by carbon tetrachloride in rats. Hepatol Res 39: 200-206.

9. Li B, Lu F, Wei X, Zhao R (2008) Fucoidan: structure and bioactivity. Molecules 13: 1671-1695.

10. Wang J, Zhang Q, Zhang Z, Song H, Li P (2010) Potential antioxidant and anticoagulant capacity of low molecular weight fucoidan fractions extracted from Laminaria japonica. Int J Biol Macromol 46: 6-12.

11. Sharma G, Susanta K, Writoban BB, Kuntal G, Pijush KD (2014) The curative effect of fucoidan on visceral leishmaniasis is mediated by activation of MAP kinases through specific protein kinase C isoforms. Cell Mol Immunol 11: 263-274.

12. Fu Y, Shizhong Z, Lin J, Ryerse J, Chen A (2008) Curcumin Protects the Rat Liver from CCl_4-Caused Injury and Fibrogenesis by Attenuating Oxidative Stress and Suppressing Inflammation. Mol Pharmacol 73: 399–409.

13. Joan O, Barbara AF, Qing X, Samuel, WF (2010) The identification of stem cells in human liver diseases and hepatocellular carcinoma. Exp Mol Pathol 88: 331-340.

14. Weber LW, Boll M, Stampfl A (2003) Hepatotoxicity and mechanism of action of haloalkanes: carbon tetrachloride as a toxicological model. Crit Rev Toxicol 33: 105-136.

15. Shana RD, Serene ML, Rachel NK, Amin AN, Kusum KK, et al. (2009) Carbon tetrachloride-induced liver damage in asialoglycoprotein receptor-deficient mice. Biochem pharmacol 77: 1283-1290.

16. Ahn M, Kim J, Bang H, Moon J, Kim GO (2016) Hepatoprotective effects of allyl isothiocyanate against carbon tetrachloride-induced hepatotoxicity in rat. Chem Biol Interact 254: 102-108.

17. Park J, Cha JD, Choi KM, Lee KY, Han KM, et al. (2017) Fucoidan inhibits LPS-induced inflammation in vitro and during the acute response in vivo. Int Immunopharmacol 43: 91-98.

18. Nakazato K, Hisashi T, Masahiko I, Takeaki N (2010) Attenuation of N-nitrosodiethylamine-induced liver fibrosis by high molecular weight fucoidan derived from C. okamuranu. J Gastroenterol Hepatol 25: 1692-1701.

19. Jin JO, Yu Q (2015) Fucoidan delays apoptosis and induces pro-inflammatory cytokine production in human neutrophils. Int J Biol Macromol 73: 65-71.

20. Robert D, Hrvoje J, Cedomila M, Biserka R (2009) Dose- and time-dependent effects of luteolin on carbon tetrachloride-induced hepatotoxicity in mice. Exp Toxicol Pathol 61: 581-589.

21. Khan TH, Sultana S (2009) Antioxidant and hepatoprotective potential of Aegle marmelos Correa. against CCl4-induced oxidative stress and early tumor events. J Enzyme Inhib Med Chem 24: 320-327.

22. Gutiérrez R, Alvarado JL, Presno M, Pérez-Veyna O, Serrano CJ, et al. (2010) Oxidative stress modulation by Rosmarinus officinalis in CCl4-induced liver cirrhosis. Phytother Rses 24: 595-601.

23. Ghaffari H, Ghassam BJ, Prakash HS (2012) Hepatoprotective and cytoprotective properties of Hyptis suaveolens against oxidative stress-induced damage by CCl4 and H2O2. Asian Pac J Trop Med. 5: 868-874.

24. Al-Yahya M, Ramzi M, Mansour A, Mohammed A, Nawal A, et al. (2013) Attenuation of CCl4-induced oxidative stress and hepatonephrotoxicity by Saudi Sidr Honey in rats. Evidence-Based Complementary and Alternative Medicine.

25. Khan R, Khan M, Sahreen S (2012) CCl4-induced hepatotoxicity: protective effect of rutin on p53, CYP2E1 and the antioxidative status in rat. Complement Altern Med 12: 178- 184.

26. Kang KS, Kim ID, Kwon RH, Lee JY, Kang JS, et al. (2008) The effects of fucoidan extracts on CCl(4)-induced liver injury. Arch Pharm Res 31: 622-627.

27. Li N, Zhang Q, Song J (2005) Toxicological evaluation of fucoidan extracted from Laminaria japonica in Wistar rats. Food Chem Toxicol 43: 421-426.

28. Gowri S, Manavalan R, Venkappayya D, David R (2008) Hepatoprotective and antioxidant effects of Commiphora berryi (Arn) Engl bark extract

against CCl4 induced oxidative damage in rats. Food Chem Toxicol 46: 3182-3185.

29. Omar HE, Heba MS, Mohammed SB, Bushra YA, Sary KA (2013) The immunomodulating and antioxidant activity of fucoidan on the splenic tissue of rats treated with cyclosporine A. J Basic Appl Zool 66: 243–254.

30. Phull AR, Majid M, Haq IU, Khan MR, Kim SJ (2017) In vitro and *in vivo* evaluation of anti-arthritic, antioxidant efficacy of fucoidan from Undaria pinnatifida (Harvey) Suringar. Int J Biol Macromol 97: 468-480.

31. Nguyen VT, Ko SC, Oh GW, Heo SY, Jeon YJ, et al. (2016) Anti-inflammatory effects of sodium alginate/gelatine porous scaffolds merged with fucoidan in murine microglial BV2 cells. Int J Biol Macromol 93: 1620-1632.

32. Subash A, Veeraraghavan G, Sali VK, Bhardwaj M, Vasanthi HR (2016) Attenuation of inflammation by marine algae Turbinaria ornata in cotton pellet induced granuloma mediated by fucoidan like sulphated polysaccharide. Carbohydr Polym 20: 151: 1261-1268.

33. Lalitsingh R, Jigar B, Jagruti P (2010) Hepatoprotective activity of ethanolic extract of bark of Zanthoxylum armatum DC in CCl$_4$ induced hepatic damage in rats. J Ethnopharmacol 127: 777-780.

34. Sathesh KS, Ravi KB, Krishna MG (2009) Hepatoprotective effect of Trichosanthes cucumerina Var cucumerina L on carbon tetrachloride induced liver damage in rats. J Ethnopharmacol 123: 347–350.

35. Muhammad RK, Wajiha R, Gul NK, Rahmat AK, Saima S (2009) Carbon tetrachloride-induced nephrotoxicity in rats: Protective role of Digera muricata. J Ethnopharmacol 122: 91–99.

36. Rui AC, John GJ, Chris MG, Dean AS, Craig RM (2002) Hepatic gluconeogenesis and krebs cycle fluxes in a CCl$_4$ model of acute liver faliure. NMR Biomed 15: 45–51.

37. Hayashi S, Itoh A, Isoda K, Kondoh M, Kawase M, et al. (2008) Fucoidan partly prevents CCl$_4$-induced liver fibrosis. Eur J Pharmacol 580: 380-384.

38. Jing W, Quanbin Z, Zhongshan Z, Zhien L (2008) Antioxidant activity of sulfated polysaccharide extracted from Laminaria japonica. Int J Biol Macromol 42: 127-132.

39. Kyoko H, Takahisa N, Minoru H, Kenji K, Toshimitsu H (2008) Defensive effects of a fucoidan from brown alga Undaria pinnatifida against herpes simplex virus infection. Int Immunopharmacol 8: 109–116.

40. Livak KJ, Schmittgen TD (2001) Analysis of relative gene expression data using real-time quantitative PCR and the 2(-Delta Delta C(T)) Method. Methods 25: 402-408.

41. Abdel Salam OM, Sleem AA, Omara EA, Hassan NS (2007) Effect of ribavirin alone or combined with silymarin on carbon tetrachloride induced hepatic damage in rats. Drug Target Insights 2: 19-27.

42. Avasarala S, Yang L, Sun Y, Leung AW, Chan WY, et al. (2006) A temporal study on the histopathological, biochemical and molecular responses of CCl($_4$)-induced hepatotoxicity in Cyp2e1-null mice. Toxicology 228: 310-322.

43. Xiao YH, Liu DW, Li Q (2005) Effects of drug serum of anti-fibrosis I herbal compound on calcium in hepatic stellate cell and its molecular mechanism. World J Gastroenterol 11: 1515-1520.

31

Antidotal Effect of Succimer and CaNa$_2$ EDTA on Workers Exposed to Lead, Cadmium and Arsenic

Georgieva VG[*], **Boyadzhieva V, Kuneva T and Pavlova S**

University Multiprofile Hospital for Active Treatment "St. Iv. Rilski" Sofia, Bulgaria

[*]**Corresponding author:** Georgieva VG, University Multiprofile Hospital for Active Treatment "St. Iv. Rilski" Sofia, Bulgaria, E-mail: viktoria_georgieva2@abv.bg

Abstract

A comparative evaluation was made between the antidotal effect of Succimer and CaNa$_2$ EDTA on workers, exposed simultaneously to lead, arsenic and cadmium. The studied patients were divided into two groups: 1st group -15 individuals, treated with peroral administration of Succimer (DMSA) in a dosage of 2.1 grams per day (3 × 0.7 grams) during the first 5 days and in a dosage of 1.4 grams (2 × 0.7 grams) per day from the 6th to the 20th day; and 2nd group -20 individuals who underwent 3-day intravenous therapy, 1 gram of CaNa$_2$ EDTA per day. Blood concentrations of lead, cadmium, arsenic, copper and zinc were measured before and after therapy, observing their urinary excretion as well. The data obtained show that both drugs have a pronounced antidotal effect on lead. The chelating effect of Succimer on arsenic is much better than that of CaNa$_2$ EDTA. The therapy with Succimer does not lead to higher excretion of copper and zinc in urine, in comparison to CaNa$_2$ EDTA. Appropriate for workers with low-level exposure to lead is a 7-day course of treatment with Succimer in a dosage of 2.1 grams per day.

Keywords: Succimer; CaNa$_2$ EDTA; Arsenic and Cadmium

Introduction

The classic antidote used in lead poisoning is CaNa$_2$EDTA [1-7]. In patients with contraindications for its administration (thrombophlebitis, diabetes, ischemic heart disease, etc.) it is especially important to use other drugs with decorporating efficacy [8-15]. In the literature, one finds a series of studies on the effect of various antidotes, such as trisodium salt of diethylenetriaminepentaacetic acid [16-19], 2,3-dimercaptosuccinic acid (DMSA, Succimer, Chemet) [6,8,9,11,19,], d-Penicillamin [1,10]. We found no data about its application as an antidote in workers, exposed simultaneously to metals. Therefore, we aimed at comparing, in a clinical environment, the curative effect of Succimer and CaNa$_2$ EDTA on workers, exposed to lead, cadmium and arsenic, with no visible clinical signs of intoxication.

Materials and Methods

The study covers 35 workers from a metallurgical plant, exposed to the combined effects of lead, arsenic and cadmium. The selected workers are hospitalized in the Clinic of Occupational Diseases, having no evidence of alcohol or drug abuse and no major organ damage. The studied individuals are divided into two groups:

- 1st group- 15 individuals (average age of 39 ± 8 and specialized length of service 14 ± 7.8 years) were treated with Succimer. The drug was taken orally in a dosage of 2.1 grams per day (3 × 0.7 grams) during the first 5 days and in a dosage of 1.4 grams (2 × 0.7 grams) per day from the 6th to the 20th day.

- 2nd group- 20 individuals (average age of 43.5 ± 5 and average specialized length of service 18.5 ± 6 years) passed a 3-day intravenous therapy with CaNa$_2$ EDTA in a dosage of 1 gram per day.

For all workers, blood and urine concentrations of lead, cadmium, arsenic, copper and zinc were studied, before and after therapy.

The heavy metals were determined using flame atomic absorption spectroscopy Analyst 400 Perkin Elmer.

The processing of the results was made by variation analysis-paired sample t-test. All statistical analyses were performed using Origin 9.0. The quantitative variables are presented as mean ± SD, and the categorical variables are presented as number (%). P-values less than 0.05 are considered statistically significant.

Results and Discussion

The average content of lead in the blood (plumbemia) of the exposed individuals before treatment is in the same range in both groups: for the 1st group - 1.03 ± 0.08 and for the 2nd group - 1.17 ± 0.1µmol/l, thus allowing a comparative analysis to evaluate the efficacy of the two antidotes (Figure 1). On the fifth day after the start of administration of the drugs the level of lead reliably decreases (p<0.05) and is 0.71 ± 0.4 and 0.73 ± 0.09 µmol/l, respectively, i.e. in the said peroral dosage Succimer shows equal efficacy to the intravenously applied CaNa$_2$ EDTA. On the 20th day of the treatment with Succimer the lead content in blood reliably decreases (p<0.05) compared to the 5th day, reaching 0.38 ± 0.06 µmol/l.

The results from the daily administration of Succimer and CaNa$_2$ EDTA show a significant increase in lead excretion for both groups of workers. In all studied days of the treatment the plumburia is many times higher than the basal (Figure 2). It is worth noting that with both antidotes the maximum release of lead is to be observed in the first day and then the excretion gradually decreases. It should be emphasized that after the third intravenous application of CaNa$_2$ EDTA the lead content is still much higher than the baseline (p<0.001).

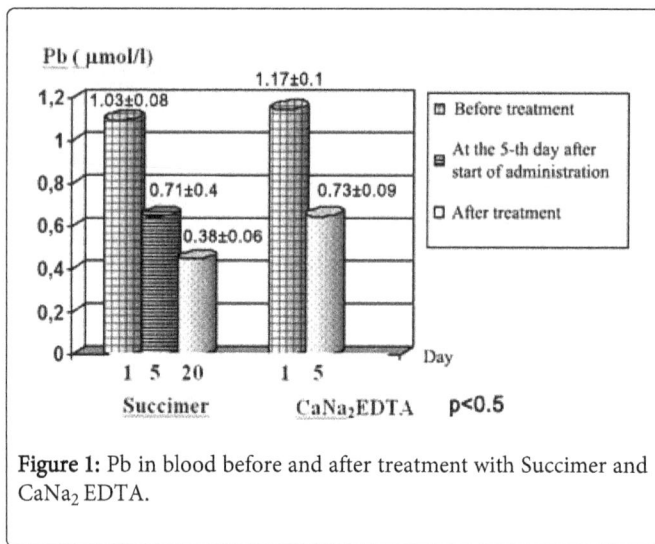

Figure 1: Pb in blood before and after treatment with Succimer and CaNa$_2$ EDTA.

EDTA, which is an evidence of the better chelating effect of Succimer with respect to arsenic.

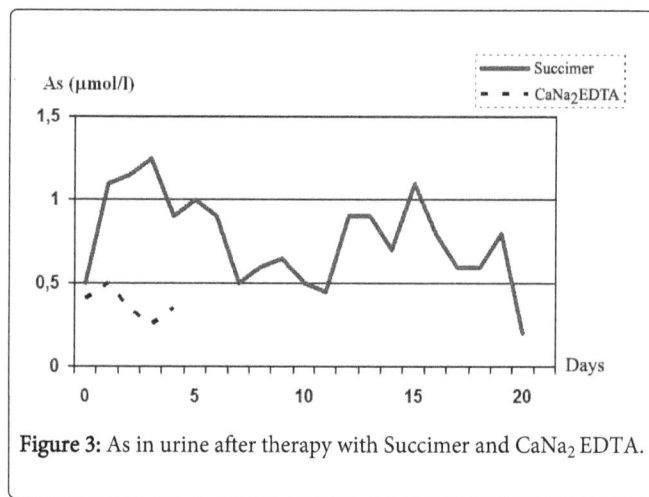

Figure 3: As in urine after therapy with Succimer and CaNa$_2$ EDTA.

In the Succimer treatment after the 5th day is observed a balanced release of lead. After 10 days of drug administration the concentrations of lead in urine reach the reference values, thus indicating the efficacy of the drug at longer administration, very well tolerated and with no danger for the patients. Similar are the results obtained by Restek S et al. in treatment with DMSA - acceleration of urinary lead excretion, mostly during the first five days, followed by a decline in the average plumbemia up to 15% of the levels before the treatment - and they assume that DMSA may effectively reduce chelate lead in occupationally exposed workers.

Observing the urine excretion of zinc of workers, treated with CaNa$_2$ EDTA, striking is the fact of its massive loss (Figure 4). The concentration of zinc on the first day is 155 ± 24 µmol/l, on the second - 114+7 µmol/l and on the third - 125 ± 26 µmol/l, compared to the basal 8 ± 1.5 µmol/l. Zincuria upon the application of CaNa$_2$ EDTA is also reported by other authors, (Graziano JH) [2,3,8]. The zinc content in the urine of the individuals, taking Succimer throughout all 20 consecutive days of treatment, is low–less than 10-15 µmol/l, undergoing no significant changes.

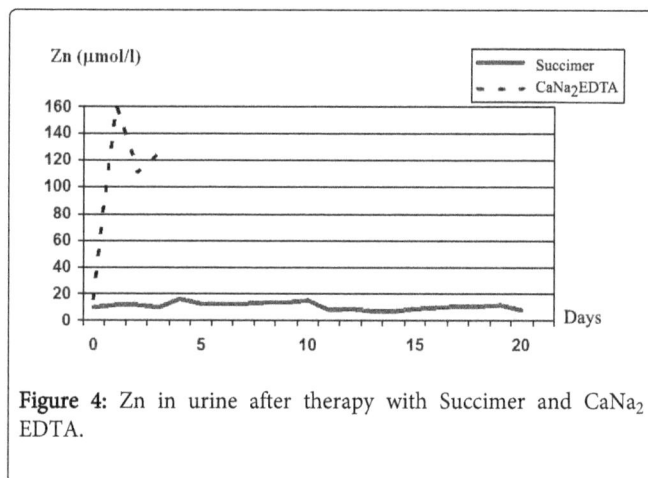

Figure 2: Pb in urine after therapy with Succimer and CaNa$_2$ EDTA.

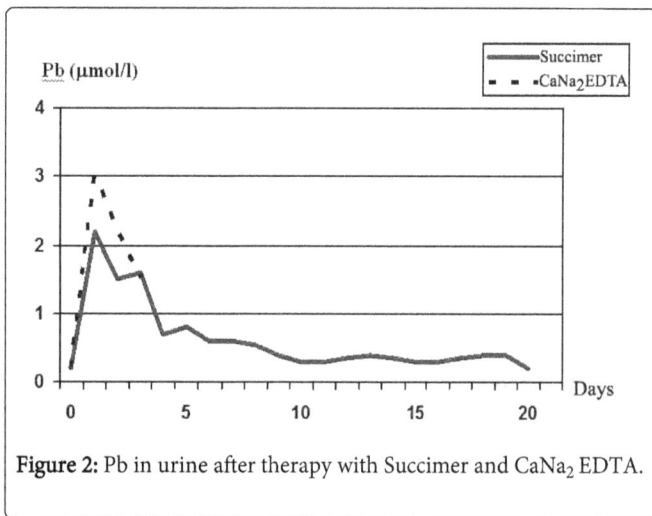

Figure 4: Zn in urine after therapy with Succimer and CaNa$_2$ EDTA.

In the application of both antidotes the average released arsenic content is not above the reference values (1.47 µmol/l), although it is higher than the basal. With one exception, the application of CaNa$_2$ EDTA does not lead to higher excretion above 1.47 µmol/l. Peroral administration of Succimer, however, leads to its increased release compared to the baseline in the first 5 days of the treatment ($p<0.05$) (Figure 3). The individual analysis shows that in 6 out of 15 studied patients the released amount is 2 to 3 times higher than the reference values. It is noteworthy to point out the reliably ($p<0.05$) higher excretion of arsenic at therapy with Succimer in comparison to CaNa$_2$

The release of copper, upon application of both antidotes, is higher than the baseline; however, it is within the range of the reference values. No statistically significant variations were established with respect to the concentrations of cadmium in both groups of individuals, either. The levels of copper and zinc in blood before and after the therapy are within the range of the reference values, which is evidence that they are extracted from the depots of the organism (Figure 5).

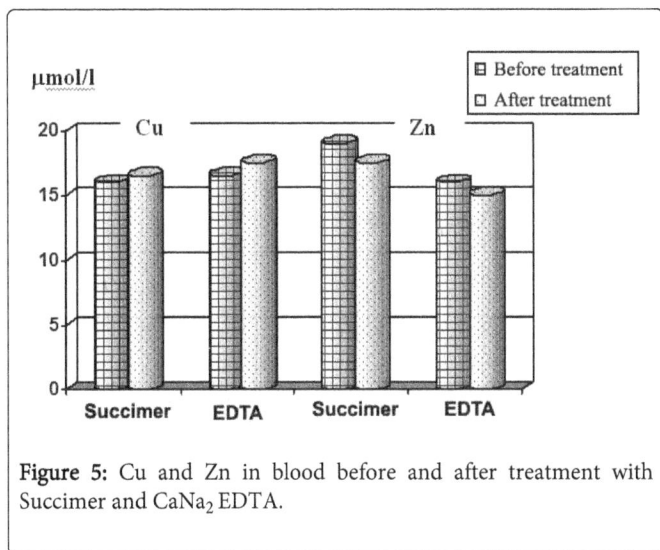

Figure 5: Cu and Zn in blood before and after treatment with Succimer and CaNa$_2$ EDTA.

Conclusion

A comparative evaluation is made between the antidotal effect of Succimer and CaNa$_2$ EDTA on workers, exposed simultaneously to lead, arsenic and cadmium. The studied drugs show a marked antidotal effect on lead. The chelating effect of Succimer on arsenic is much better, compared to CaNa$_2$ EDTA.

The treatment with Succimer results in no change in the excretion of copper and zinc, while CaNa$_2$ EDTA causes daily 10 to 15-times higher release of zinc with the urine than the reference values.

Succimer (DMSA) is an effective chelator, leading to expressed plumburia, suitable for peroral administration, and may be used with patients who are not hospitalized, due to absence of manifested side effects.

In workers with a low-level lead exposure, a 7-day therapy with Succimer is appropriate, in a dosage of 2.1 grams per day.

Patients with symptoms of lead intoxication and high-level lead absorption are recommended a therapy with CaNa$_2$ EDTA for rapid and effective decorporating chelation therapy, with parallel administration of substitution therapy with microelements (copper and zinc).

References

1. Kuneva T (1993) The therapeutic effect evaluation of Cuprenil on chronic saturnism, Hygiene and health, Sofia 23-24.

2. Born T, Kontoghiorghe CN, Spyrou A, Kolnagou A, Kontoghiorghes GJ (2013) EDTA chelation reappraisal following new clinical trials and regular use in millions of patients: review of preliminary findings and risk/benefit assessment. Toxicol Mech Methods 23: 11-17.

3. Bradberry S, Vale A (2009) A comparison of sodium calcium edetate (edetate calcium disodium) and succimer (DMSA) in the treatment of inorganic lead poisoning. Clin Toxicol 47: 841-858.

4. Counter SA, Ortega F, Shannon MW, Buchanan LH (2003) Succimer (meso-2,3-dimercaptosuccinic acid (DMSA)) treatment of Andean children with environmental lead exposure. Int J Occup Environ Health 9: 164-168.

5. Crinnion WJ (2011) EDTA redistribution of lead and cadmium into the soft tissues in a human with a high lead burden - should DMSA always be used to follow EDTA in such cases? Altern Med Rev 16: 109-112.

6. Flora SJ, Flora G, Saxena G, Mishra M (2007) Arsenic and lead induced free radical generation and their reversibility following chelation Cellular and Molecular Biology 53: 26-47.

7. Graziano JH, Lolacono NJ, Moulton T (1992) Controlled study of meso-2,3-dimercaptosuccinic acid for the management of childhood lead intoxication. J Pediatr 120: 133-139.

8. Graziano JH, Lolacono NJ, Meyer P (1988) Dose-response study of oral 2,3-dimercaptosuccinic acid in children with elevated blood lead concentrations. J Pediatr 113: 751-757.

9. Hoet P, Buchet JP, Decerf L, Lavalleye B, Haufroid V, et al. (2006) Clinical evaluation of a lead mobilization test using the chelating agent dimercaptosuccinic acid. Clin Chem 52: 88-96.

10. Kianoush S, Balali-Mood M, Mousavi SR, Moradi V, Sadeghi M, et al. (2012) Comparison of therapeutic effects of garlic and d-Penicillamine in patients with chronic occupational lead poisoning. Basic Clin Pharmacol Toxicol 110: 476-481.

11. Lee BK, Ahn KD, Lee SS, Lee GS, Kim YB, et al. (2000) A comparison of different lead biomarkers in their associations with lead-related symptoms. Int Arch Occup Environ Health 73: 298-304.

12. Mihalache C, Oprea V, Constantin B, Pintilie W, Teslariu E, et al. (2004) Chronic lead poisoning like a group pathology. Clinical report of 12 cases. Rev Med Chir Soc Med Nat Iasi 108: 159-164.

13. Ogawa M, Nakajima Y, Kubota R, Endo Y (2008) Two cases of acute lead poisoning due to occupational exposure to lead. Clin Toxicol 46: 332-335.

14. Petracca M, Scafa F, Boeri R, Flachi D, Candura SM (2013) Imported occupational lead poisoning: report of four cases. Med Lav 104: 428-433.

15. Pollock CA, Ibels LS (1988) Lead intoxication in Sydney Harbour Bridge workers. Aust N Z J Med 18: 46-52.

16. Restek-Samarzija N, Blanusa M, Pizent A, Samarzija M, Turk R, et al. (1988) Meso-2,3-dimercaptosuccinic acid in the treatment of occupationally exposed lead workers. Arh Hig Rada Toksiko 49: 137-145.

17. Roberts DM, Singer RF (2012) Lead mobilization study and the clearance of intravenous CaNa2 EDTA in a patient with end-stage renal failure on hemodialysis. J Clin Pharmacol 52: 110-113.

18. Thomas DL, Chisolm J (1986) Lead, zinc and copper decorporation during calcium disodium ethylenediamine tetraacetate treatment of lead-poisoned children. J Pharmacol Exp Ther 239: 829-835.

19. Torres-Alanis O, Garza-Ocanas L, Pineyro-Lopez A (2002) Effect of meso-2,3-dimercaptosuccinic acid on urinary lead excretion in exposed men. Hum Exp Toxicol 21: 573-577.

Permissions

List of Contributors

Muhammed Majeed
Sami Labs Limited, 19/1 & 19/2, First Main, Second Phase, Peenya Industrial Area, Bangalore-560 058, Karnataka, India
Sabinsa Corporation, 20 Lake Drive, East Windsor, NJ 08520

Kalyanam Nagabhushanam and Anurag Pande
Sabinsa Corporation, 20 Lake Drive, East Windsor, NJ 08520

Sankaran Natarajan, Arumugam Sivakumar and Furqan Ali
Sami Labs Limited, 19/1 & 19/2, First Main, Second Phase, Peenya Industrial Area, Bangalore-560 058, Karnataka, India

Shaheen Majeed
Sabinsa Corporation, 20 Lake Drive, East Windsor, NJ 08520 Sabinsa Corporation, 750 Innovation Circle, Payson, UT 84651, USA

Kuk-Young Moon, Pureun-Haneul Lee, Byeong-Gon Kim and An-Soo Jang
Genome Research Center for Allergy and Respiratory Diseases Soonchunhyang University Bucheon Hospital, Republic of Korea

Moo-Kyun Park
Otolaryngo Rhinology, Seoul National University, Korea

Honghong Li, Lei He, Shuwei Qiu, Yi Li and Ying Peng
Department of Neurology, Sun Yat-Sen Memorial Hospital, Sun Yat-Sen University, Guangzhou 510120, China

Imran Khan, Abd-Ur-Rehman and Samrah Afzal Awan
Department of Botany, PMAS-Arid Agriculture University, Rawalpindi, Pakistan

Abdul Ghani, Attia Noreen and Imran Khalid
Department of Botany, University of Sargodha, Sargodha, Pakistan

Seham Fouad, Nahla Hassan, Nabil Nassief and Rania Hussien
Department of Forensic Medicine and Clinical Toxicology, Faculty of Medicine, Ain Shams University, Egypt

Fathia El- Halawany
Statistics Department, Cairo University, Egypt- King Abdulaziz University, Faculty of Science for Girls, Jeddah

Saritha Suvarna, Sunil K C and Narayana Y
Department of Studies in Physics, Mangalore University, Mangalagangotri, India

Rajesha Nairy
Department of Physics, P.A College of Engineering, Mangalore, India

Cynthia Santos
Emory University School of Medicine, Centers for Disease Control, Atlanta, GA, USA
Icahn School of Medicine at Mount Sinai, New York, NY, USA

Reynolds Kairus
Pontificia Universidad Católica Madre y Maestra, Santiago, Dominican Republic

Ziad Kazzi
Director International Postdoctoral Fellowship in Medical Toxicology, Emory University School of Medicine, Atlanta, GA, USA

Suzanne Bentley
Assistant Professor of Medical Education, Mount Sinai School of Medicine, New York, NY, USA

Ruben Olmedo
Director of the Division of Toxicology, Mount Sinai School of Medicine, New York, NY, USA

Gilles Hanton
GH Toxconsulting, Brussels, Belgium

Roda E, Lonati D, Buscaglia E, Locatelli CA and Coccini T
Laboratory of Clinical & Experimental Toxicology and Poison Control Centre and National Toxicology Information Centre, Toxicology Unit of the Pavia's Hospital, IRCCS Maugeri Foundation, Pavia, Italy

Papa P and Rocchi L
Laboratory of Analytical Toxicology, Clinical Chemistry Service of Pavia's Hospital, IRCCS Policlinico San Matteo Foundation, Pavia, Italy

Bayan Al-Dabbagh
Department of Chemistry, College of Science, United Arab Emirates University, Al Ain, United Arab Emirates

Saeed Tariq
Anatomy, UAE University, Al-Ain, Abu Dhabi, United Arab Emirates

Ying Wang, Bin-yu Chen and Xiang-min Tong
Research Center of Blood Transfusion Medicine, Key Laboratory of Laboratory Medicine (Wenzhou Medical University), Ministry of Education, Zhejiang Provincial People's Hospital, Hangzhou, 310014, China
Clinical Research Institute, Zhejiang Provincial People's Hospital, Hangzhou, 310014, China

Zhi-hui Huang
Clinical Research Institute, Zhejiang Provincial People's Hospital, Hangzhou, 310014, China
School of Basic Medicine, Wenzhou Medical University, Wenzhou, 325035, China

Hilal Ahmad Ganaie
Cytogenetic and Molecular Biology Research Laboratory, Centre of Research for Development (CORD), University of Kashmir, Srinagar-190 006, J & K, India
Phytochemistry Research Laboratory, Centre of Research for Development (CORD), University of Kashmir, Srinagar-190 006, J & K, India

Md. Niamat Ali and Jasbir Kaur
Cytogenetic and Molecular Biology Research Laboratory, Centre of Research for Development (CORD), University of Kashmir, Srinagar-190 006, J & K, India

Bashir A Ganai and Mudasar Ahmad
Phytochemistry Research Laboratory, Centre of Research for Development (CORD), University of Kashmir, Srinagar-190 006, J & K, India

Se Kwang Oh, Hee Jun Shin, Han You Lee and Hye Jin Chung
Department of Emergency Medicine, College of Medicine, Soonchunhyang University, Korea

Neda Amini
Department of Toxicology & Pharmacology, pharmacology & Toxicology Department, Faculty of pharmacy, Pharmaceutical Sciences Branch, Islamic Azad University (IAUPS), Iran

Afshar Etemadi-Aleagha
Department of anesthesiology, Tehran University of Medical Sciences (TUMS), Amir Alam Hospital, Tehran, Iran

Maryam Akhgari
Department Forensic Toxicology, Legal Medicine Research Center, Legal Medicine Organization, Tehran, Iran

Arzu Ulu, Bora Inceoglu, Jun Yang, Stephen Vito and Bruce D Hammock
Department of Entomology and Nematology, and Comprehensive Cancer Center, University of California, Davis, USA

Vikrant Singh and Heike Wulff
Department of Pharmacology, School of Medicine, University of California, Davis, USA

Faheem Jan, Mazhar Ali Khan and Muhammad Taj Akbar
Department of Microbiology, Hazara University, Mansehra, Pakistan

Ifthekhar Hussain
Department of Pharmacy, Hazara University, Havelian Campus, Abbottabad, Pakistan

Naveed Muhammad
Department of Phamacy, Abdul Wali Khan University Mardan, KPK, Pakistan

Muhammad Adnan Khan
Microbiologist BF- Biosciences Ltd Lahore Pakistan

Waqas Ahmad
Faculty of Pharmacy University of Sargodha, Sargodha, Pakistan

Seyit Uyar
Antalya Training and Research Hospital, Antalya, Turkey

Henning Gerlach, Wieland Schrödl and Monika Krüger
Institute of Bacteriology and Mycology, Faculty of Veterinary Medicine, University of Leipzig, An den Tierkliniken 29, D-04103 Leipzig, Germany

Achim Gerlach
Waldstraße 78, D-25712 Burg, Germany

Bernd Schottdorf
Carbon Terra GmbH Gutermannstrasse 25, D-86154 Augsburg, Germany

Svent Haufe
WH Pharmawerk Weinböhla GmbH, Poststr. 58, D-01689 Weinböhla, Germany

Hauke Helm
Südholzring 2, D-25693 Gudendorf, Germany

Awad Shehata
Institute of Bacteriology and Mycology, Faculty of Veterinary Medicine, University of Leipzig, An den Tierkliniken 29, D-04103 Leipzig, Germany
Avian and Rabbit Diseases Department, Faculty of Veterinary Medicine, Sadat City University, Egypt

Masayuki Ohyama
Department of Environmental Health, Osaka Prefectural Institute of Public Health, Japan

Hideki Tachi
Department of Textile & Polymer Section, Technology Research Institute of Osaka Prefecture, Japan

Chika Minejima
Department of Material Science, College of Liberal Arts, International Christian University, Japan

Takayuki Kameda
Department of Socio-Environmental Energy Science, Kyoto University, Japan

Essam Mahmoud Hafez, Milad Gad Paulis and Mostafa Abotaleb Ahmed
Department of Forensic Medicine and Clinical Toxicology, Faculty of Medicine, Minia University, Minia 61519, Egypt

Marian NagyFathy
Department of Pathology, Faculty of Medicine, Minia University, Minia 61519, Egypt

Ahmed Abdel-Lateff
Department of Natural Products and Alternative Medicine, Faculty of Pharmacy, King Abdulaziz University, Jeddah, Saudi Arabia
Department of Pharmacognosy, Faculty of Pharmacy, Minia University, Minia 61519, Egypt

Mardi M. Algandaby
Department of Biological Sciences, Faculty of Science, King Abdulaziz University, Jeddah, Saudi Arabia

Saeeda Almarzooqi, Alia Albawardi and Dhanya Saraswathiamma
Departments of Pathology, UAE University, Al-Ain, Abu Dhabi, United Arab Emirates

Ali S. Alfazari and Hidaya Mohammed Abdul-Kader
Medicine, UAE University, Al-Ain, Abu Dhabi, United Arab Emirates

Sami Shaban
Medical Education, UAE University, Al-Ain, Abu Dhabi, United Arab Emirates

Robert Mallon
RHP Associates, Caldwell NJ

Abdul-Kader Souid
Pediatrics, UAE University, Al-Ain, Abu Dhabi, United Arab Emirates

Santokh Gill and Meghan Kavanagh
Regulatory Toxicology Research Division, Health Canada

Christine Poirier, Dorcas Weber and Terry Koerner
Food Research Division, Bureau of Chemical Safety, Food Directorate, Health, Canada

Frey Francisco Romero-Vargas, Luis Alberto Ponce-Soto and Sergio Marangoni
Department of Biochemistry, Institute of Biology, State University of Campinas (UNICAMP), Campinas, SP, Brazil

Thalita Rocha
Multidisciplinary Research Laboratory, San Francisco University (USF), Bragança Paulista, SP, Brazil
Department of Histology and Embryology, Institute of Biology, State University of Campinas (UNICAMP), Campinas, SP, Brazil

Maria Alice Cruz-Höfling
Department of Histology and Embryology, Institute of Biology, State University of Campinas (UNICAMP), Campinas, SP, Brazil

Lea Rodrigues-Simioni
Department of Pharmacology, Faculty of Medical Sciences, State University of Campinas (UNICAMP), Campinas, SP, Brazil

Yuval Cavari, Shaul Sofer and Isaac Lazar
Pediatric intensive care unit, Soroka Medical Center, the Faculty of Health Sciences Ben-Gurion University of the Negev, Beer Sheva, Israel

Natalya Bilenko
Department of public health, the Faculty of Health Sciences Ben-Gurion University of the Negev, Beer Sheva, Israel

Guy Beck
Division of Pediatrics, Soroka Medical Center, the Faculty of Health Sciences Ben-Gurion University of the Negev, Beer Sheva, Israel

Farrukh Jamal and Quazi S. Haque
Department of Biochemistry, Dr. Ram Manohar Lohia Avadh University, Faizabad-224001, India

Sripriya Sundararajan, Cynthia F Bearer and Dina El Metwally
Department of Pediatrics, University of Maryland, Baltimore, MD 21201, USA

Allison M Blatz
Departments of Pediatrics, Case Western Reserve University, Cleveland, OH 44106, USA

Dorr G Dearborn
Departments of Pediatrics, Case Western Reserve University, Cleveland, OH 44106, USA
Environmental Health Sciences, Case Western Reserve University, Cleveland, OH 44106, USA
Mary Ann Swetland Center for Environmental Health, Case Western Reserve University, Cleveland, OH 44106, USA

Arthur W Varnes
Environmental Health Sciences, Case Western Reserve University, Cleveland, OH 44106, USA

Luana Wlian, Linda Christian Carrijo-Carvalho, Sonia Aparecida Andrade, Durvanei Augusto Maria and Ana Marisa Chudzinski Tavassi
Butantan Institute, São Paulo, Brazil

Silvia Vanessa Lourenço
Dental School, University of São Paulo, São Paulo, Brazil

Consuelo Junqueira Rodrigues
University of São Paulo, São Paulo, Brazil

Hela Ghorbel, Ines FKI and Sami Sayadi
Laboratory of Bioprocess Environnemtaux, Pole regional excellence AUF (PER-LBP), Sfax Biotechnology Centre (CBS), Sfax, Tunisia

Choumous Kalel
Laboratory of Hematology, CHU, Habib Bourguiba, 3029 Sfax, Tunisia

Jamoussi Kamel
Laboratory of Biochemistry, University Hospital, Habib Bourguiba, 3029 Sfax, Tunisia

Mohamed E. El-Boshy
Laboratory Medicine Department, Faculty of Applied Medical Science, Umm Al-Qura University, Makkah, Saudi Arabia
Clinical Pathology Department, Faculty of Veterinary Medicine, Mansoura University Mansoura, Egypt

Fatma Abdelhamidb, Engy Richab and Ahmad Ashshia
Laboratory Medicine Department, Faculty of Applied Medical Science, Umm Al-Qura University, Makkah, Saudi Arabia

Mazen Gaitha and Naeem Qustya
Clinical Pathology Department, Faculty of Veterinary Medicine, Mansoura University Mansoura, Egypt

Georgieva VG, Boyadzhieva V, Kuneva T and Pavlova S
University Multiprofile Hospital for Active Treatment "St. Iv. Rilski" Sofia, Bulgaria

Index